Management of the Voice and Its Disorders
Second Edition

Management of the Voice and Its Disorders
Second Edition

Linda Rammage, Ph.D.
The University of British Columbia
and
Provincial Voice Care Resource Program
Vancouver, Canada

Murray Morrison, M.D.
Professor of Otolaryngology
The University of British Columbia
Vancouver, Canada

Hamish Nichol, M.B.
Psychiatrist
Pacific Voice Clinic
Vancouver, Canada

With

Bruce Pullan, M.A.
Singing Teacher
Vancouver, Canada

Lesley Salkeld, M.D.
Starship Children's Hospital
Auckland, New Zealand

Philip May
Singing teacher
Calgary, Canada

SINGULAR
™
THOMSON LEARNING

Vancouver, Canada · Auckland, New Zealand · Calgary, Canada

SINGULAR
THOMSON LEARNING ™

Management of the Voice and Its Disorders , Second Edition

by Linda Rammage, Ph.D., Murray Morrison, M.D., Hamish Nichol, M.B.

with Bruce Pullan, M.A., Lesley Salkeld, M.D., Philip May

Business Unit Director:
William Brottmiller

Acquisitions Editor:
Candice Janco

Editorial Assistant:
Kristin Banach

Executive Marketing Manager:
Dawn Gerrain

Channel Manager:
Tara Carter

Executive Production Editor:
Karen Leet

Production Editor:
Brad Bielawski

Library of Congress Cataloging-in-Publication Data
Rammage, Linda
Management of the voice and its disorders/ Linda Rammage, Murray Morrison, Hamish Nichol; with Bruce Pullan...[et al.]— 2nd ed
Morrison's name appears first on the earlier edition.
Includes bibliographical references and index.
ISBN 0-7693-0054-5 (pbk. : alk. paper)
1. Voice Disorders. I. Rammage, L.A. (Linda A.) II. Morrison, M.D. (Murray D.) III. Nichol, Hamish IV. Title.
[DNLM: 1. Voice disorders— diagnosis. 2. Voice disorders— therapy. WV 500R174m 2000]
RF510 .R365 2000
616.85'5—dc21

NOTICE TO THE READER

Contents

Foreword

This book provides a wise and useful guide for all professionals involved in the diagnosis and management of voice disorders. Almost twenty years ago, the term Muscular Tension Dysphonia (MTD) was operationally defined by this team, comprised of Linda Rammage, Ph.D., Speech-language pathologist, Murray Morrison, M.D., Otolarynoglogist-Head and Neck Surgeon, and Hamish Nichol, M.D., Psychiatrist. Approaches to management of voice disorders have been greatly influenced by the original concepts of muscle misuse patterns, and have evolved with our understanding of neuromuscular, anatomical, and psychological factors that impact on voice production. The authors refer to "muscle misuse" as the final common path for most dysphonias regardless of the specific components involved in the development of a patient's disorder. The view is that the patient is misusing the laryngeal musculature often as a result of the interaction of a myriad of factors, each of which may need to be considered in the treatment process. A voice disorder usually involves the original pathology, the patient's adaptation to that pathology (although it may no longer be present) and the reaction of others in the patient's environment to their dysphonia. This work presents the science of voice disorders with an excellent review of anatomy and physiology, medical, surgical, diagnosis, assessment and extensive therapeutic methods. However, its major feature is a straightforward presentation on the complexity in dealing with persons and their voice disorders. The case histories make clear that each patient is a complex unison of functional, physical, and emotional factors that contribute to their voice disorder. Clearly, there is no biologic marker for the diagnosis of a voice disorder or its etiology. This is dealt with in a frank and open discussion that addresses the imponderables in finding solutions that usually are unique to the individual when caring for their voice disorder.

Chapters on vocal pedagogy and pediatric voice disorders are provided which further reflect the multidisciplinary focus of this work. Voice pedagogues are now part of the voice care team in large centers where professional voice users are seen. This book enables all members of the team to gain insight into each member's area of expertise. It provides a common ground for discussing the science and art of multidisciplinary voice care.

The hypothesis referred to as "the Irritable Larynx Syndrome" is included in this new edition. The major tenet is that laryngeal irritation due to inflammation or disease may contribute to misuse possibly through plastic changes in central nervous system control. Clinical syndromes such a "paradoxical breathing disorder", which have become apparent in the last decade, may be examples of this hypothesis, and are timely. Although little scientific evidence is yet available to support this hypothesis, it is an interesting and provocative one.

Finally, this book provides all professionals involved with voice care with an illustration of the ideal; a multidisciplinary team of professionals engaged in the best that science, clinical skill and compassion can provide for the care of persons with voice disorders.

Christy L. Ludlow, Ph.D.

Preface

Interest in the human voice and its disorders has spawned the development of voice clinics around the globe, which provide unique interdisciplinary assessment and treatment services, and professional training and research opportunities. Voice clinics that offer interdisciplinary services may include professionals from the fields of speech-language pathology, otolaryngology, psychiatry, vocal pedagogy, neurology, voice science, biomedical engineering, and other peripheral disciplines.

This text has been generated by the professional team members of a single voice clinic, although we acknowledge inspirational contributions from many colleagues around the globe. It is our hope that our presentation will reflect the singleness of direction and purpose that we strive for in our approach to managing patients with voice disorders. As a result of over twenty years of interactive meetings about patients with difficult problems, and cooperative development of classification systems and treatment programs, we feel that we have become a team that is greater than the sum of its individual "parts", and that there is value in sharing our cumulative thoughts with others. This second edition of our text offers expanded ad updated information on assessment, classification, and treatment options that reflect a tremendous growth of knowledge in our specialty areas.

This is not simple laryngology text for otolaryngologists. Neither is it exclusively a speech-language pathology textbook . . . we hope that this text will fill in the gaps between the professions that come together in the interest of individuals with vocal aspirations and problems. It should expand the understanding of scientific and clinical aspects of voice production for the vocal pedagogue; conversely it should help "demystify" the art of vocal pedagogy for the voice clinician. It should help the psychiatrist appreciate ways in which muscle misuse leads to dysphonia, and provide valuable tools to the speech-language pathologist embarking on a therapy program with a psychologically-disordered patient. It should obvious the major advantages to all the team work in this area.

Our voice clinic is the product of who we are, where we live, the politics of our health acre system, where and how we were educated, the expectations of our clientele, and an assortment of personal biases. No other clinical group will share exactly the same philosophies that we have developed, however many may strive for effective interdisciplinary management of individuals with voice disorders. Should you be one of those aspiring teams, we hope that you too will find that learning from each other is fun and rewarding.

Linda Rammage
Murray Morrison
Hamish Nichol

Acknowledgements

The authors would like to thank Christy Ludlow for her helpful insight and introduction. Thanks to Lesley Casson and Michiel Haijtink for their artistic contributions. We acknowledge the inspiration and encouragement that our colleagues and students have offered. Finally, we thank our patients, for providing us with the opportunity to learn from them.

To Our Families

CHAPTER

Evaluation of the Patient with a Voice Disorder[1]

1.1 Principles of Joint Assessment

It is common in medical practice to evaluate a constellation of signs and symptoms and from them to deduce a diagnosis. Once the diagnosis has been secured, treatment is planned. Voice disorders tend to be managed differently because they frequently have a spectrum of causes. A successful treatment program must address all the causative factors. For example, a mild, habitual, technical voice misuse may be exacerbated by psychological factors, whereas smooth operation of the pharyngo-laryngeal esophageal muscular tube is inhibited by gastroesophageal reflux, and the voice disorder is finally triggered by an acute viral infection. The viral trigger will resolve, but the other 3 factors need separate attention. A fully successful result will require coordinated medical treatment, voice therapy, and psychological support that may be most efficiently provided by a multidisciplinary team.

"What one knows, one sees." There is no substitute for an informed and aware clinician in the evaluation of patients with voice disorders. Complete objectivity is a rare achievement for a clinician working alone, and interdisciplinary evaluation offers the best chance of identifying all aspects in the pathogenesis of voice disorders.

A typical story might go as follows. Following the initial interview with a 44–year-old female aphonic patient conducted by the laryngologist, speech-language pathologist, and psychiatrist, the first comment in the ensuing conference was from the psychiatrist: "what an incredible amount of anger is being suppressed by that lady!" She had been whispering for over a year and exhibited symptom inconsistencies that would lead an informed clinician to suspect a psychogenic etiology. Normal cough and laughter were observed, although she was aphonic during speech. Incomplete glottal closure was noted during a sustained /i/ ("ee") on indirect laryngoscopy, whereas complete closure was demonstrated during a spontaneous cough and inhalation phonation. She spent another

[1]The information in this and subsequent chapters assumes familiarity with basic anatomy and current theories of physiology of the speech and voice mechanism. The reader who is not in possession of this knowledge base is encouraged to begin by reading Chapter 8 in this text, supplemented with additional recommended readings.

hour with the psychiatrist, mostly in tears, and normal speech was restored during voice therapy the following day. To the untrained or biased observer, the key etiological factors could have been missed.

In our clinic, we solicit information in advance of the voice evaluation—from patients and from those making referrals. Information from the patient is elicited by means of the intake questionnaire, provided in Figure 1–1. The information received helps determine which members of the voice-care team should be involved in a patient's care from the outset. There may be some disadvantages to use of a preassessment questionnaire, such as a tendency to bias patients toward adopting specific descriptive terms, or, in cases of hypochondriasis or malingering behaviour, inadvertent provision of symptoms that patients may "take on." Nevertheless, we feel the advantages of obtaining preassessment patient profiles to help schedule the most appropriate team members and procedures outweigh any potential complications.

Team evaluation provides a multiple-observer situation. While the otolaryngologist or speech-language pathologist is conducting the interview, other team members are free to make general observations that might be missed by the interviewer. Depending on information known about the patient in advance, additional team members may include a psychiatrist or psychologist; a singing pedagogical specialist, and a neurologist. By joining forces, team members bring different areas of expertise into the evaluation process and dilute each other's reductive biases.

In our experience, it is advantageous to have the otolaryngologist and speech-language pathologist see patients together at the outset, each bringing their own professional skills to the evaluation process. The two professionals can contribute different types of information to a common database while providing a comprehensive assessment service,

and each will learn from the other's skills. In time, the "multidisciplinary" aspects of voice care become "trans-disciplinary," which implies that members of the team develop common skills. An example of this is the speech-language pathologist becoming skillful in laryngeal examination and videostroboscopy, while the otolaryngologist becomes skilled in voice therapy techniques.

The otolaryngologist and speech-language pathologist often call upon the psychiatrist to be part of the voice-care team. Reports from referring consultants and information offered by the patient in the intake questionnaire may give clues about major psychological components so that patients can be scheduled for evaluation at times when the psychiatrist is present. It is obviously not economical or necessary to involve the psychiatrist with every patient, although if he or she is to be participating in a patient's care, it is ideal to make the introduction at the initial interview in a team format. Difficult barriers may be broken down by this interdisciplinary introduction, saving valuable therapy time.

Joint assessment is obviously time consuming and at first may not appear to be cost efficient. Nevertheless, a well-orchestrated interdisciplinary assessment provides for shared observations and may be the most efficient way to reach immediate consensus about treatment priorities and plans.

1.2 History Taking

1.2.1 The First Encounter

In many academic centers, it is a common practice for the patient to be initially "worked up" by students or other persons in training. We feel that there is much useful information to be learned during the first few minutes of the encounter, so at least one senior clinician is present at the outset.

Before coming into the interview room the

$P V C_{RP}$

PROVINCIAL VOICE CARE RESOURCE PROGRAM
Linda A. Rammage, PhD, S-LP(C), Director

PACIFIC VOICE CLINIC, INC.
Murray D. Morrison, MD, FRCSC, Director

www.pvcrp.com

4th floor, Willow Pavilion
Vancouver Hospital
805 West 12th Ave
Vancouver, BC
V5Z 1M9

Phone: (604) 875-4204
Fax: (604) 875-5382

PLEASE PROVIDE THE FOLLOWING INFORMATION AS ACCURATELY AND COMPLETELY AS POSSIBLE:

NAME: _____ TODAY'S DATE: _____

DATE OF BIRTH: _____ AGE: _____   SEX: M   F

TELEPHONE: Res: _____ Work: _____ Fax: _____ email: _____

OCCUPATION: _____ # YEARS : _____ Part-Time OR Full-Time?

REASON FOR VISIT: Describe Symptoms in order of Importance: How Long?

Symptom #1: _____:_____

Symptom #2: _____:_____

Symptom #3: _____:_____

Other Concerns: _____ :_____

work days missed due to throat/voice problems:_____ When? _____

MEDICATIONS AND DOSAGE: _____

_____

_____

ALLERGIES, INCLUDING DRUG ALLERGIES: _____

_____

SURGERIES, SERIOUS ILLNESSES, INJURIES AND HOSPITALIZATIONS (descriptions and dates):

_____

_____

_____

_____ **(Please turn over and complete page 2)**

Figure 1-1. Patient intake questionnaire

3

FAMILY HISTORY OF SERIOUS ILLNESSES, AND SPEECH AND HEARING PROBLEMS: _____

_____

_____

DAILY QUANTITY OF: _____ Coffee, Tea, Coke, Chocolate   _____ Alcoholic Beverages

_____ Cigarettes, Cigars, Other   Quit?: *Yes*   *No*   If *Yes*, When? _____

_____ Water, and other non-caffeinated, non-alcoholic drinks

PLEASE CHECK IF YOU HAVE EVER HAD:

__ AIDS	__ Difficult Nasal Breathing	__ Heart Disease	__ Seizures
__ Allergies	__ Dizziness	__ Hiatal Hernia	__ Sinus Problems
__ Anxiety Disorder	__ Dramatic Weight Gain/Loss	__ Hoarseness	__ Sleep Disorder
__ Arthritis	__ Ear Infections	__ Lump in Throat Sensation	__ Swallowing Problem
__ Asthma	__ Ear Pain	__ Lung Disease	__ Throat-Clearing
__ Bad Bruising	__ Eating/Digestive Disorder	__ Muscle Weakness	__ Throat Pain
__ Breathing Problem	__ Headaches (Chronic)	__ Nasal Discharge	__ Thyroid Problem
__ Chronic Fatigue	__ Head Injury	__ Neck or Back Injury	__ TMJ Disorder
__ Chronic Cough/Choking	__ Head or Ear Noise	__ Neurological Disease	__ Tremor
__ Depression	__ Hearing Loss	__ Post-Nasal Drip	__ Total Voice Loss
__ Diabetes	__ Heartburn	__ Psychiatric Disorder	__ Ulcers

Have you ever had a hearing test? _____ If yes, when? _____ Result? _____

Does your voice change with your emotions? (describe): _____

_____

Do you use your voice in your occupation, or in performance? (describe): _____

_____

Do your symptoms change with the amount and type of voice use? (describe): _____

_____

_____

THANK YOU FOR YOUR COOPERATION! THE INFORMATION YOU PROVIDED WILL HELP US HELP YOU.

Office Use Only: Video Loc: _____   Dx 1: _____   Dx 2: _____   Interview?   *Y*   *N*

Footnote: _____

Figure I–I. (continued)

4

patient is asked to fill out the Voice Handicap Index questionnaire (VHI)[39]. This adds further information about functional, physical, and emotional aspects of an individual's voice function and may also be a useful component of outcome measurement[6,61]. [The VHI is provided in Appendix 1.1.]

When calling patients from the waiting room, we note that a family member, spouse, friend, or vocal trainer or employer may accompany them. It is our usual practice to ask permission to see the patient alone at the outset, promising to bring the accompanying person into the clinic room at a later appropriate stage, with the patient's permission. Persons with voice disorders frequently have others speaking for them, and although this might be useful later on, we really want patients to speak on their own behalf initially. Being alone, patients are also less likely to tell their story in a manner that they think the people close to them want to hear. In several instances, we have recognized early in the interview that a close relationship may be at the centre of an emotional (or physical) conflict that is contributing to the voice disorder. This may not be freely acknowledged if the person accompanying the patient is present and is the source of the conflict. Obvious exceptions to this practice include parents accompanying their young children to provide relevant history and individuals who serve as translators. Even in the case of young children, it is often advantageous to spend some time with them in the absence of caregivers, allowing them to freely represent their perspective on any issues that could affect communication. Many children make their best efforts on assessment tasks when the primary caregiver is not present.

The patient's initial posture and mood are observed; evidence of anxiety, depression, anger, and general psychological demeanor is noted. Because there may be several professionals or students in attendance at the first interview, it is important that each is introduced to the patient and their roles explained. While one clinician takes the history, other team members make observations of behavior that will be helpful in arriving at a diagnosis.

Figure 1–2 illustrates the history portion of the printed form we use in our clinic. It facilitates the orderly movement through the process, regardless of who conducts the interview. The format serves as a quality assurance tool by ensuring that each relevant topic is presented and reported in the history.

Team members need to come to an agreement about the nature of questions asked during the interview. Consistent with principles of objective history taking, each interviewer practices the use of open-ended questions. This strategy guards against simple yes-no responses to specific leading questions that may bias the clinician toward a particular diagnosis before all the facts are available. Ideally, the interviewer's questions guide patients to disclose specific information without leading them to respond in a clinician-biased manner to fit a diagnostic model. Examples of suitable open-ended phrases include:

➤ What can we do for you today?
➤ Tell us all you can about how your speech or throat are troubling you.
➤ Tell us about any patterns that you have noticed in these symptoms.
➤ Tell us about your job, family, childhood, hobbies.
➤ Tell us about your health.
➤ Describe a typical day or week in your life.

1.2.2 Unfolding the Chronology of the Problem

A multiplicity of etiological factors may contribute to symptom formation. Organic disease can trigger a muscle misuse dysphonia, so that what appears initially to be a straightforward viral laryngitis may evolve into a long-lasting voice disorder. Koufman

NAME: _____   AGE: _____   SEX: _____   DATE: _____

Chief Complaint: _____   Duration: _____

History:

Occupation: _____

Type of voice use_____

_____

Voice training_____

_____

Past Medical History:

_____

_____

_____

Allergies _____

Diet/weight: _____

Smoking (1°/2°) _____

Alcohol _____

Coffee/tea_____

Reflux:
- globus _____
- p.n. drip_____
- throat clearing _____
- heart burn _____
- am throat _____
- acid taste _____
- water brash_____
- night chokes_____

Reflux diagnosis? (Y/N)_____

Hearing_____

Audiogram? (Y/N) _____

VOCAL ABUSE HISTORY	Severity/Observations
Throat clearing/coughing	_____
Shouting/cheering/(+ emotive)	_____
Screaming/yelling/crying (–)	_____
Talking over noise (specify)	_____
Talking outdoors/pools etc.	_____
Lecturing, etc. (poor amplif)	_____
Voice use & strenuous exercise	_____
Non verbal vocal sounds	_____
Imitating voices	_____
Stage whisper	_____
Excessive singing, talking, etc	_____
Other: (specify)	_____

FAMILY HISTORY

PSYCHOLOGICAL/STRESS FACTORS

PATIENTS PERCEPTION OF VOICE DISORDER

Severity/Variability _____

_____

Impact/expectation_____

_____

Singer? (Y/N) _____ Status:_____ Range: S A T B

Singers Questionaire filled out? (Y/N) _____

Figure 1–2. Form for history interview.

and Blaylock referred to this as "habituated hoarseness"[43]. In this situation, a subclinical voice misuse may be brought to the surface when coupled with inflammatory edema and then persist when the edema subsides. Muscle misuse or vocal abuse disorders tend to worsen as the day, the week, or the duration of use proceeds, but they may also fluctuate with stresses or other life issues. An open, puzzle-solving frame of mind will help the history taker recognize clues and hypothesize on the significance of symptom patterns.

It is often helpful to begin the history-taking process by asking the patient to describe the current symptomatology in as much detail as possible before going back in time and describing the onset and evolution of the problem. During the initial interview, we capture representative portions of the patient's original history responses on videotape. Our patient interview chair is positioned to allow for easy video recording without disrupting dialogue. Ideally, recordings are made of responses both emotionally charged and emotionally neutral in nature. Speaking of one's close relationships or the voice problem often provides an emotionally charged topic, and describing a typical day may be more emotionally neutral. Incidentally the latter response also provides more insight into the nature and patterns of voice use and vocal demand.

The case history is taken to elicit information about physical, emotional, and behavioral factors in an open-ended way, covering all topics represented in Figure 1–2. We will present a model for this evaluative process in Section 1.3. When the patient is a child, additional information may need to be elicited about events that took place before, during, and after birth and about developmental and behavioral patterns. Relevant issues for evaluation are discussed in greater detail in Chapter 6.

Vocal function testing for acoustic, perceptual-acoustic, and aerodynamic measures are undertaken, including measurement of the patient's initial responses to diagnostic voice therapy techniques. These procedures will be described in detail later in this chapter.

In many instances, a general ear, nose, and throat examination precedes formal evaluation of the larynx. We begin the laryngeal examination by palpation of the muscles around the larynx. Details of laryngeal palpation techniques can be found in Section 1.7.2 below, along with details of other aspects of physical examination.

Videolaryngoscopy with stroboscopy is recorded on tape for each patient seen in our clinic. We usually begin the examination with transoral rigid telescopic laryngoscopy because this gives us the highest quality photographic images and greatest detail about stroboscopy. The telescopic examination is followed by transnasal flexible fiber-optic laryngoscopy in those cases where a full nondistorted view of laryngeal postures is required or when an active gag reflex or other anatomical factors interferes with the examination. Detailed descriptions of the videolaryngostroboscopic evaluation are provided in Section 1.7.3.1.

After the history, observational assessment, vocal function testing, and laryngeal examination and before offering information and management recommendations to the patient, the voice care team holds a brief conference in private to assure that there is general agreement on the problem description and subsequent direction to be followed. This assures that the patient will receive an opinion that all caregivers share. During the conference, formal diagnoses may be generated based on recognizable signs and symptoms of particular organic pathologies. Additionally, 4 patient factors that may contribute to the voice disorder are considered: **(1) technique or level of vocal skill, (2) lifestyle, (3) psychological status, and (4) gastroesophageal reflux.** Because these 4 areas are represented in the discussion so frequently—and generally need to be considered in the treatment protocol—we have developed a model for the management of the patient with dsyphonia based on these etiological platform components.

1.3 A Model for the Evaluation of Dysphonia

1.3.1 Principles

This **model of dysphonia** should help the clinician work through a difficult voice evaluation and come up with a truly helpful treatment plan[51]. Often a number of interrelated factors are involved in the etiology, and all require treatment.

Our model purports that dysphonia in all individuals with voice disorders is built on a **platform** with **4 components**, and each component affects the dysphonia to some degree. The platform components, as listed previously, are **(1) technique** and level of vocal skill; **(2) lifestyle** and matters pertaining to occupation and regular activity; **(3) psychological factors**, including personality and emotional stressors; and **(4) gastroesophageal reflux**. A primary pathology, such as neuromuscular or mucosal disease may lie over the platform created by the 4 interactive components. The impact of the platform components is estimated first, then the presence of a primary pathological process is considered, and the manner in which it interacts with the underlying platform is determined. A treatment program subsequently is planned to take all the relevant factors into account.

Use of this model requires the clinician to follow an orderly analysis of the possible causes for an individual's dysphonia and to adhere to a concept of multiple etiological factors that interact with each other.

The following 6 statements are premises generally accepted as axioms that are helpful

to have in mind when evaluating the patient with a voice disorder.

1. Voice production is an athletic skill requiring coordination of muscle systems throughout the body. A column of air under relatively low pressure must flow upward through the trachea past vocal folds that are held in adduction with a force appropriate to the task. The upper vocal tract resonators are adjusted to provide amplification and the desired tonal focus and articulatory targets.

2. Some individuals are naturally skillful vocal athletes, most are average, and a few are lacking in vocal technical ability. The levels of skill tend to follow a normal distribution curve such as shown in Figure 1–3. Individuals with good voice skills are less likely to become dysphonic in response to psychological distress or to structural changes of the vocal folds than are those at the "poor" end of the spectrum.

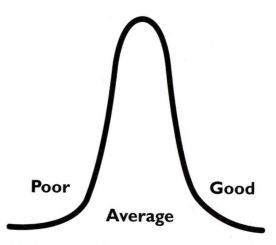

DISTRIBUTION OF VOCAL SKILLS

Figure 1–3. The hypothesized normal distribution curve for individual levels of vocal skill in the community.

3. Speaking or singing with poor technique will lead to more wear and tear on the vocal folds than will the same amount of loud or aggressive voice use produced with skill. Younger adult vocal folds are more resilient than are older ones, therefore older voice users need to be smarter and more skillful to avoid damage.

4. Many people use their voices extensively and exuberantly. They are more susceptible to vocal fold damage and dysphonia if they have poor vocal skills.

5. Psychological distress leads to dysphonia through various mechanisms, but the two most common are (a) increased muscle tension in the larynx, jaw, tongue, neck, and/or respiratory system and (b) suppression or repression of the expression of negative emotion.

6. Gastroesophageal reflux may produce symptoms in 10% of the general population. It increases pharyngolaryngeal muscle tension and is accompanied by chronic laryngeal inflammation. We have demonstrated that there is an increase in thyroarytenoid muscle activity when the lower esophagus is stimulated[26]. The resultant increase in laryngeal muscle tension aggravates any coexistent dysphonia, and treatment of the reflux may be all that is needed for the voice problem to resolve. Reflux amplifies the manifestations of vocal misuse and abuse, therefore a voice therapy program will be more effective when reflux is controlled.

In all individuals with voice disorders, dysphonia is built on a platform made up of the four components. Each component affects the dysphonia to some degree, and although one or two may receive the most attention all four will need to be considered in the treatment plan. Further pathological processes may overlie the platform components and contribute to the voice disorder.

These usually come from one of two broad groups: neurological diseases, and structural changes to the vocal folds. They will be considered later.

1.3.2 Dysphonia Platform Component Assessment

1.3.2.1. Technique and Vocal Skill

Assess and grade the level of vocal technical ability. You will need to

➤ observe general posture; head, neck, and shoulder alignment; and movement
➤ note jaw position and freedom of movement
➤ observe strap muscle activity, especially omohyoid action with speech
➤ watch and feel respiratory action during speech, singing, and other relevant vocal activities
➤ listen for signs of vocal tension and note resonance focus
➤ palpate suprahyoid, thyrohyoid, cricothyroid, and inferior constrictor muscles
➤ observe voice improvement with appropriate diagnostic therapy techniques

1.3.2.2. Lifestyle and Occupation

Consider how general behavioral patterns may affect the voice. Specifically, one would want to know about

➤ excessive talking or singing in poor acoustical environments, such as night clubs, swimming pools, gymnasiums, and so forth.
➤ general talkativeness
➤ smoking
➤ occupational voice demands

1.3.2.3. *Psychological Factors: Personality and Emotion*

Explore possible psychological factors in the production of the dysphonia by seeking in the history for evidence of

➤ a traumatic event around the onset of the dysphonia
➤ difficulties in communicating with significant others
➤ suppression of the expression of negative emotions, such as sadness or anger
➤ abusive relationships in childhood or later
➤ narcissistic preoccupation with voice
➤ overt anxiety or depression[60]

Most people will agree that their voice difficulty gets worse at times of added stress. It is helpful to ask about which stressors seem to affect the voice most noticeably, because this may direct the interview to the source of psychologically based muscle misuse.

1.3.2.4. *Gastro-esophageal Reflux and Associated Medical Conditions*

Determine the relative importance of gastroesophageal reflux in the dysphonia by evaluating symptoms such as

➤ throat sensations in the morning
➤ waking at night coughing or choking
➤ habitual throat clearing
➤ the sense of a lump in the throat (globus pharyngeus)
➤ heartburn
➤ asthma or other chronic breathing difficulties

Look for evidence of reflux laryngitis, usually manifest by excess redness or granularity in the posterior larynx. Consider using special tests for reflux, such as esophageal manometry and 24-hour pH monitoring.

1.3.3 Putting the Platform Components Together

As the clinician works through the voice assessment and considers the relative importance of each of the platform components, a pattern will arise that gives direction to treatment options. To illustrate this, each component can be given a relative size in graphic representation as shown in Figure 1–4.

As an example case, consider the 25-year-old female fitness teacher who is a single parent struggling to access her court-ordered child support. She loses her voice each time she has to talk to her ex-husband. She has moderate-sized vocal nodules. Her nodules would be considered an overlay in the model, but her platform may look like that seen in Figure 1–5.

In another case, a schoolteacher complains of a low-pitched effortful voice by the end of a school day and suffers from throat pain with speech. She complains of a sore throat first thing in the morning and often wakes with a cough. She is overweight. Her platform may look like that seen in Figure 1–6.

1.3.4 The Overlying Pathological Process

The primary pathology that may be identified as the main cause of dysphonia always lies, in this model, over the platform created by the 4 interactive components. Overlying pathologies usually fall into 1 of 2 main groups consisting of the following:

1. disorders of neuromuscular function, such as vocal fold paralysis, dystonia and tremor, Parkinson's disease, ALS and related degenerative disorders, brain injury, and stroke
2. mucosal diseases such as acute or chronic inflammation, vocal nodules, polyps, contact ulcer and granuloma, cysts, sulci, or neoplasia

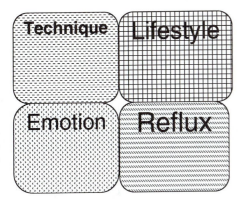

Figure 1–4. The 4 components of the platform on which a dysphonia rests.

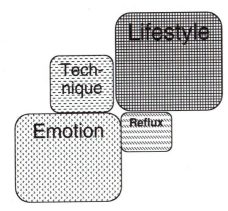

Figure 1–5. Platform components in the case of a 25-year-old fitness instructor.

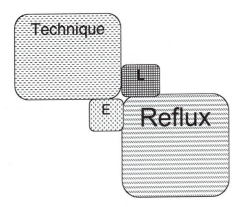

Figure 1–6. Platform components in the case example of a school teacher with reflux.

In some cases, the overlying pathology may have been caused to some extent by action of the platform components. For example, vocal nodules may be caused by postural and muscle misuses, together with vocal abuse. Contact granuloma is caused by reflux plus muscle misuse.

1.3.5 Using the Model

Use of this assessment model involves the following chronology of events and thought processes:

1. During the history taking and physical examination, a primary pathology may be apparent. Set this information aside.
2. Assess the impact of each of the platform components.
3. Consider the manner in which the primary pathological process interacts with the underlying platform.
4. Plan a treatment program that takes all the relevant factors into account.

For example, if technical misuse voice patterns are corrected in voice therapy and any reflux is treated, then an overlying neurological condition may no longer cause a voice concern. Perhaps individuals with a mild laryngeal dystonia who would otherwise be treated with botulinum toxin could be successfully treated at the underlying platform component levels, thus eliminating the need to subject them to repeated injections (Figure 1–7).

Another example is the patient with vocal nodules. It is inappropriate to plan surgical removal unless the platform components have been thoroughly explored and treated. An individual with vocal nodules will typically engage in loud and aggressive vocal behavior, will have developed excessive laryngeal muscle misuse, may have evidence of reflux, and may exhibit personality or psychological characteristics that contribute to vocal abuse, overuse, and muscle misuse.

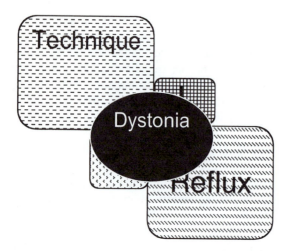

Figure 1–7. In this case example, the component platform underlies a problem with focal dystonia, leading to spasmodic dysphonia.

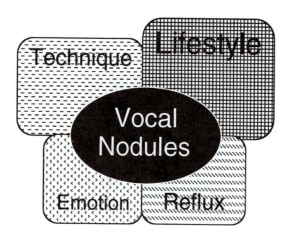

Figure 1–8. Vocal nodules can overlie significant problems with vocal technique, emotions, lifestyle, and reflux.

Management of the platform components is generally what is required in this situation. Graphically the model may look like that seen in Figure 1–8.

Needless to say, there will be as many variations in the model as there are patients

with voice disorders, and the interactions between platform components and the primary pathology will be different for each of the disease processes. When no overlying pathological process is evident, the treatment regimen should focus on resolution of the contributing platform components in proportions representing the degree to which each of them is responsible for the voice disorder. Adherence to this model of patient management should assure that the majority of people that come seeking help with a difficult voice problem will become satisfied customers.

The following sections of this chapter provide details about procedures for assessment of the patient with a voice disorder. These include perceptual and physical assessment methods, the necessary instrumentation, appropriate therapy trials, and psychological evaluation.

1.4 Acoustic and Perceptual Acoustic Assessment

1.4.1 Rationale, Environment, and Basic Recording Hardware

Perceptual assessment methods, both visual and auditory, provide valuable information during assessment of patients with voice disorders. Techniques for visual perceptual assessment of structural and vibratory features of the phonatory mechanism will be discussed in a subsequent section.

Perceptual-acoustic evaluation provides the critical information link between physiological voice function and a listener's perception of the resulting acoustic speech signal. Because the listener's auditory system filters and processes the radiated acoustic speech signal before it is interpreted by the brain, perceptual-acoustic evaluation provides a uniquely "human" set of information regarding voice function or dysfunction; for example, how appropriate is the speaking pitch, loudness, and voice quality to a particular situation?

High-quality acoustic recordings are essential for reliable perceptual and digital acoustic evaluation. Ideally, simultaneous video recordings are made so that acoustic-perceptual evaluation can be assisted by visual cues. This allows for concurrent observation of posture, movement, facial expression, and acoustic aspects of voice productions. A sound-treated recording studio is recommended in cases where the evaluation room is not acoustically appropriate for recording or if it contains noise-generating equipment that must be kept running during the acoustic recording.

High-quality recordings of vocal status before and after clinical intervention are necessary to document treatment effectiveness. Both clinician and patient benefit from documentation, and the medical-legal value of these recordings has been shown on many occasions.

Cassette recorders are used for easy and efficient storage and retrieval of data. Digital recording devices are ideal for acoustic recordings that will be subjected to further acoustic analysis, because they are of superior quality and eliminate the need for analog-to-digital conversion. A unidirectional microphone is generally better than an omnidirectional microphone for recordings that are free of background noise. The microphone needs to have good feedback suppression, a low distortion factor, and a wide frequency range representing the typical spectrum for speech sounds and any atypical speech and voice noise that may characterize dysphoias. An ideal frequency response ranges from near 0 Hz to 20 kHz. It is important to be aware of any special noise-reduction or filtering devices that may be built into recording equipment. In cases where voice disorders are being document-

ed, it may not be wise to engage noise reduction systems or other filtering devices that are considered desirable when recordings are made for entertainment or other purposes.

1.4.2 Acoustic and Perceptual Acoustic Assessment: Instrumentation, Application, Protocols and Interpretation

1.4.2.1. Recording Instrumentation and Protocols

High-quality acoustic recordings, either analog or digital, should be made as a standard assessment procedure for each voice patient, regardless of the etiological factors or treatment plan. Dedicated equipment and software may be used to make physical measures of f_0, vocal intensity, spectral, and timing parameters on a real-time analyzer or from recordings. The comprehensive acoustic evaluation also includes assessment of the perceptual correlates of f_0, intensity, timing, and spectral measures, including pitch, loudness, prosody and rate, and quality. The form in Figure 1–9 is used to guide the clinician through assessment tasks and to record findings. Assessment tasks are designed to elicit "typical" and maximal voice range data and include speech and nonspeech contexts. Ideally, candid recordings of speech or performance in typical voice-use situations are used to assess the range of phonatory behaviors and difficulties experienced by a patient. For the purposes of pretreatment and posttreatment comparisons, it is ideal to obtain some speech samples that have reproducible phonetic, contextual, and emotional features, such as story retelling. When children are assessed, the tasks and protocols need to be modified to reflect appropriate developmental levels.

PERCEPTUAL-ACOUSTIC FEATURES

PITCH PARAMETERS

Singing Range: High:_____ (asc.); _____ (desc.)Register:_____

(Hz/Note) Low: _____ (asc.): _____ (desc.)Register:_____

Total range: _____ Flexibility/continuity: _____

Register transisitions:_____ (asc.);_____ (desc.)

Speaking Range: High: _____ Low: _____ Habitual:_____

(Hz) Situational variability:_____ Intonation: _____ (average)

fo of non verbal vocal sounds: um hm/uh huh: _____

hm/huh: _____ laugh: _____ cough/thr. clear: _____

Appropriateness of speaking pitch, range, register: _____

Pitch-matching: _____ Musicality: _____

Scale markings (right): —2048, —1024 (Hz), —512, —256, —128 (Hz), —64, —32

LOUDNESS PARAMETERS

SPL Range: High: a < _____ ; serials < _____ ; "Hey" _____

Low: a > _____ ; serials > _____ ; "Hey" _____

Habitual (average) SPL Level-Speech: _____ Situational Variability: _____

Cough strength: _____ Pitch/Loudness Interdependence _____

RATE/DURATION PARAMETERS:

Sustained Phonemes: a _____ , _____ , _____ m _____ , _____ , _____

(duration/sec.) max.: _____ Cued? (Y/N) _____

s/z ratio: _____

Connected Speech: Serials max. duration: _____ (rate+3 digits/sec.)

Habitual (average) Rate of Speech: _____ Average Phrase Length:_____

Fluency: _____ Fluency/Rate Variability:_____

QUALITY PARAMETERS:

	0	1 2	3 4 5	6 7
	N	Mild	Moderate	Severe

Voice-Onset Features: Sev. Freq. Consistency/Stimulability

Glottal Attack

Hyperadd-Delayed Onset

Hypoadd-Delayed Onset

Hyperadducted Release

Breath-Intake Features:

Inspiratory Stridor-laryngeal

Audible Inspiration-unvoiced

Inhalation phonation/speech

Stability Features:

Tremolo

Tremor

Pitch Breaks (specify♪♩)

Hyperadd Phonation Breaks

Hypoadd Phonation Breaks

Valving Features: Sev. Freq. Consistency/Stimulability

Breathy

Whisper phonation-unforced

Stage Whisper forced

Hypervalved (squeezed)

Timbre/Dissonance Features:

Strident/Harsh (♪pitch)

Rough/Glottal Fry (♩pitch)

Diplophonic/Glottal Fry

Resonance Features:

Hypernasality/consonant emission

Assimilative nasality-vowels

Hyponasality (m, n, ng)

Fronted Resonance/Artic

Backed Resonance

STIMULABILITY FOR CHANGE IN PITCH, LOUDNESS, RATE, QUALITY PARAMETERS: _____

_____

_____

_____

_____

_____

_____

Figure I-9. Form for acoustic and perceptual-acoustic assessment.

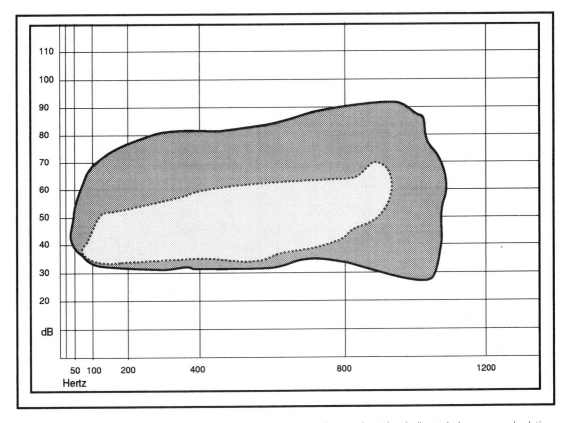

Figure 1–10. Prototype phonetogram: Vocal frequency and intensity are plotted to indicate their ranges and relationships. The X axis represents f_0; the Y axis represents intensity. The phonetogram profiles for a patient pretreatment and posttreatment are demonstrated. The pretreatment plot is in light shading; the posttreatment is in dark shading.

1.4.2.2. Measures of Fundamental Frequency and Pitch; and Intensity and Loudness

In the voice clinic, instrumental measures can be used to define speech averages and dynamic ranges for fundamental frequency (f_0) and intensity of phonation.

Average **speaking f_0 and range** are extracted from contextual speech. A physiologically "natural" range for speaking may be produced during spontaneous vocalizations such as: "uh huh," "m hm," "hm!", "OK", or laughter. F_0 values for these productions can be compared with the typical speaking f_0 range for a determination of the appropriate-

ness of an individual's habitual speaking range. Physiological range for f_0 is measured from singing scales and glissando productions. Because muscle misuses can impose restrictions on f_0 ranges, it is advisable to elicit physiological ranges not only with sustained vowels, but also while using technical "tricks" to minimize the effects of muscle misuses. This is easily accomplished by asking the patient to produce a glissando simultaneous with lip or tongue trilling, during voiced fricative production, or while "blowing" air onto the index finger during an /u/ ("oo") glissando.

Normative data of physiological f_0 ranges

generally cite 2 octaves or greater as "normal." A patient may have a greatly restricted physiological range (for example, less than 1 octave) and yet maintain a fully functional speaking voice with normal intonation patterns. On the other hand, a vocal performer with even subtle changes or restrictions in the dynamic range may suffer great occupational and emotional repercussions. Many vocal performers must produce aesthetically appropriate vocal tones that cover a range of 3 octaves.

The same contextual speech sample may be used to measure **average vocal intensity and range**, whereas "quietest" and "loudest" productions are elicited on a simple word or phrase, such as: "Hey!" or "Hey you!" Many dedicated instruments and software programs are now available to allow for such measures to be made accurately and efficiently in the voice clinic. Tried-and-true basic sound measurement devices such as the oscilloscope (for f_0 measures) and the sound-level meter (for intensity measures) are still valuable instruments. Electroglottography (EGG) can be used for accurate estimates of f_0 provided the voice signal is not too irregular and sufficient vocal fold closure is achieved.

Normative studies of maximum and minimum intensities for different age and gender groups suggest that a minimum dynamic (physiological) intensity range of approximately 30 dB indicates normal voice function for adults[7,31]. It is clear that the f_0 of phonation influences maximum and minimum intensity values, as does age to a lesser degree. (See Baken[4] for a thorough review of data.)

The **phonetogram** provides a clinically relevant display of physiological ranges for f_0 and intensity and their interactions[15,27,42,54]. Several software programs have been developed to measure and plot intensity range against f_0 range on a simple x-y scale (Figure 1–10). This allows the patient and clinician to measure and compare changes in vocal dy-

namics over time. The phonetogram has enjoyed particular popularity within the arena of vocal pedagogy and has been used to document differences between trained and untrained singers[1,2,28].

Although the physical parameters of f_0 and acoustic intensity correspond closely to perceptual judgements of **pitch and loudness** respectively, the unique and complex nature of perceptual processing justifies clinical assessment of psychoacoustic parameters separately. Trained listeners have the unique ability to translate the physical signal to judgements regarding the "appropriateness" of vocal pitch or loudness within a given communication context. The clinician can also determine the extent to which a speaker uses pitch and loudness changes effectively to produce natural suprasegmental characteristics of intonation and stress.

The **pitch** range of an individual's speaking voice may be a problem if it draws undue attention to itself because of its difference from the socially accepted normal range for the age, gender, race, psychosocial, or linguistic code of the person. A speaking pitch range that is too high, too low, or too limited in its dynamics may result in psychosocial difficulties. On the other hand, for some individuals, it may serve to "resolve" psychosocial conflicts (such as inability to accept the responsibilities of adulthood or a gender dysphoria). Speaking pitch ranges that are not representative of natural pitches produced on spontaneous phonation (eg, *um hum; uh huh*; laughing) or during special vocal effects such as lip or tongue trilling or voiced fricative productions (/z/; /v/; /ʤ/) usually are related to muscle misuse. Inappropriate speaking pitch may be associated with monotone speech, glottal fry, falsetto, or a high-pitched, tense voice. If an individual's inappropriate speaking pitch reflects the same range as that produced during spontaneous vocalizations, it usually is related primarily to structural features. Mass-altering lesions, endocrine disorders, neurological disease, or congenital malformations may all lead to abnormally high, low, or restricted speaking pitch ranges.

Vocal tract length and shape and articulatory style can also affect speaking pitch. Longer or larger vocal tracts tend to be associated with lower formant frequencies in men and give the perception of lower pitch; the converse is true for women and children. In the case of a mismatch between resonance tract size and vocal f_0, as with adolescents with transitional voice problems or individuals undergoing gender reassignment, pitch perception may be confounded. If a male-to-female transsexual consciously shortens her vocal tract by raising the larynx, she may overcome the f_0 to resonance mismatch by raising formant frequencies. (Of course if this is done in a way that creates general tension in the vocal tract, some undesirable perceptual features may be created, and speaking may be perceived as more effortful). The feminine voice perception may be further enhanced by a fronted and exaggerated articulatory style and adoption of feminine intonation characteristics, all of which appear to influence listeners' impressions of a higher vocal pitch. If these characteristics are combined with a mean f_0 in the gender-ambiguous range or above (around 160 Hz), the speaker may bias the listener's perception toward a feminine identification[71]. The issue of pitch and vocal identity may pose a problem for some individuals during senescence, because f_0 tends to rise in men, and drop in women as a normal aging characteristic. More details on these natural aging trends are presented in Chapter 8.

A **monotone** speaking style may reflect personality or psychological features. Schizophrenia and affective disorders such as depression have been associated with restricted intonation patterns[17]. Muscle misuse in the larynx and supraglottal musculature may also lead to compromised vocal flexibility and monotone speech patterns. Neurogenic diseases affecting the upper or lower motor neurons may also affect f_0 and pitch control. Lesions of the recurrent or superior laryngeal nerve may result in a restricted pitch range, attributable to impaired vocal fold adduction, cricothyroid muscle dysfunction, or both. Whereas a restricted speaking pitch range may be a consequence of a variety of psychological, muscle misuse, and organic etiologies, abnormally wide speaking pitch ranges are seen only rarely but might be expected in association with certain psychological states, personality disorders, or organic brain syndromes such as Gilles de la Tourette's syndrome.

The appropriateness of an individual's vocal **loudness** typically is determined informally by observation, history, and reports from the patient and others regarding his or her audibility. Restrictions on the upper or lower end of the intensity-loudness range may pose situation-specific problems for an individual. A reduced dynamic intensity range or inappropriate habitual loudness may be indicative of organic or muscle misuse disorders. Various peripheral and central neurological diseases may contribute to problems of vocal fold adduction (too much or too little), which affect one's ability to achieve the appropriate subglottal pressure for intensity increases or decreases. Respiratory diseases or incoordination may also contribute to intensity problems if they impair one's ability to maintain sufficient airflow to create appropriate subglottal pressure. Vocal intensity-loudness ranges may also be affected by resonance characteristics. Structural or neurological disorders and muscle misuse may result in acoustic damping attributable to poor oral opening, losses through the velopharyngeal port, or articulatory postures that affect the vocal tract transfer function. Inappropriate speaking intensity may be related to disease processes alluded to above, such as habitual misuse, hearing deficits, ambient noise levels, psychological conflict, or personality traits.

When a patient's communication partner is complaining of poor audibility, it is important to take into consideration his or her hearing acuity and situations in which conversation is taking place. Often, we arrange audiometric evaluations for both patient and spouse as part of the voice clinic evaluation so that any "listener" components to the communication problem can be addressed.

1.4.2.3. Measures of Duration, Rate, and Prosody

Speaking rate may affect coordination of respiration and phonation, muscle tension in the vocal tract, and intelligibility. Speaking rate may be influenced by situational, physiological, and personality factors. A well-trained speech clinician can generally make a perceptual judgement regarding the appropriateness of an individual's speaking rate. Syllable or word counts for a series of typical speech utterances provide a more objective measure. A review of normative data suggests that the critical range for normal speaking rates may vary from 140 words per minute to 180 words per minute. Of course, the communication context, articulatory proficiency, and other production variables must be considered when one is judging the appropriateness of speaking rate.

Measures of **phonation duration** include the traditional maximum phonation time (MPT) measure for sustained vowels at natural pitch and loudness levels (within the speaking range), as well as measures of speech phrase length. When interpreted in light of other phonatory function measures, MPT values can provide information regarding glottal integrity and respiratory support. The role of MPT in making phonation quotient calculations is discussed in Section 1.5. Normative studies of MPT provide a wide variety of suggested guidelines. Age and gender are clearly both influential in deter-

mining this variability. For children up to age 8, the average normative values range from 13.1 to 16.2 seconds. For adults, average reported values for women vary from 16.7 to 25.7 seconds and for men, from 22 to 34.6 seconds. (See review by Hirano[31].)

Phrase lengths vary normally under the influence of syntax and pragmatics. A syllable or word count per phrase (expiratory breath group) can give the clinician objective data to supplement perceptual judgements of appropriateness of average phrase length, and comparative data for outcome measures. Phrase length may be influenced by rate of speech; longer average breath groups are associated with more rapid speech.

Perceptual, mathematical, or acoustic measures of phonatory **fluency and rhythm** may be included in the rate and duration evaluation. If syllable lengths are grossly variant owing to phonatory or articulatory dysfluencies (for example, laryngeal or oral articulator blocks), then speech may be dysrhythmic or bizarre. Voice-onset delays caused by hyperadduction or hypoadduction of the vocal folds may also disturb speech fluency and rhythm. A frequency and duration count of intensity/f_0 variations, phonation breaks, or delayed onsets can be useful to describe vocal dysfluencies associated with vocal tremors, spasmodic dysphonias, and other motor speech disorders. Figure 1–11 demonstrates a 5 Hz benign essential tremor, as measured from the acoustic signal and a wide-band spectrogram. **Phonation break factor** is a simple episode count for a specified unit of time. This measure may be particularly important to indicate pretreatment and posttreatment values.

An excellent screening tool for identification of prosody and voice disorders has been developed by Shriberg et al[67]. The test battery provides a detailed training program and scoring protocol for delineating phrasing, rate, and stress abnormalities or voice aberrations related to loudness, pitch, and quality that warrant more in-depth evaluation.

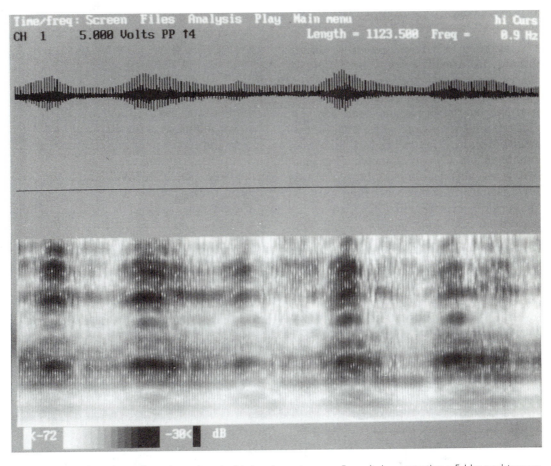

Figure 1–11. Sound waveform (upper) and wide-band spectrogram (lower) demonstrating a 5 Hz vocal tremor. Reprinted with permission from *Voice Care in the Medical Setting*, Copyright 1997, Singular Publishing Group, Inc.

1.4.2.4. Measures of Voice Quality

Perceptual-acoustic terms employed to describe dysphonia features should reflect mechanical or aerodynamic events that account for them. The terms for voice quality measurement listed in our protocol for acoustic and perceptual-acoustic evaluation are based on this philosophy (Figure 1–9). The **Vocal Profile Analysis** protocol employs similar principles for voice quality assessment. It includes perceptual parameters corresponding to long-term postural settings within the phonatory, articulatory, and resonance systems[45,46] (See Figure 1–12). These assessment protocols have been used together in our clinic for comprehensive description of voice quality features. Simultaneous acoustic, laryngoscopic, or EGG measures may be used to confirm the nature of phonatory events that correspond to perceptual judgements of pitch, loudness, rate, duration and quality, as well as to train listeners to use perceptual terms reliably. Team members are trained to apply common operational definitions, and high interlistener reliability scores are needed for judging severity.

It is valuable to include perceptual meas-

Vocal Profile Analysis Protocol

Speaker: .... Sex: .... Age: .... Date of Analysis: .... Tape: .... Judge: ....

VOCAL TRACT FEATURES	FIRST PASS			SECOND PASS							
	Neutral	Non-neutral		SETTING	Scalar Degree						
		Moderate	Extreme		Moderate		Extreme				
					1	2	3	4	5	6	
1. Labial Features				Lip Rounding/Protrusion							
				Lip Spreading							
				Labiodentalization							
				Extensive Range							
				Minimized Range							
2. Mandibular Features				Close Jaw							
				Open Jaw							
				Protruded Jaw							
				Extensive Range							
				Minimized Range							
3. Lingual Tip/Blade Features				Advanced Tip/Blade							
				Retracted Tip/Blade							
4. Lingual Body Features				Fronted Tongue Body							
				Backed Tongue Body							
				Raised Tongue Body							
				Lowered Tongue Body							
				Extensive Range							
				Minimized Range							
5. Velopharyngeal Features				Nasal							
				Audible Nasal Escape							

LARYNGEAL FEATURES	FIRST PASS			SECOND PASS							
	Neutral	Non-neutral		SETTING	Scalar Degree						
		Moderate	Extreme		Moderate		Extreme				
					1	2	3	4	5	6	
6. Phonation Type Features				Modal voice							
				Falsetto							
				Creak(y)							
				Whisper(y)							
				Harsh							
7. Larynx Position Features				Raised Larynx							
				Lowered Larynx							

OVERALL MUSCULAR TENSION FEATURES	FIRST PASS			SECOND PASS							
	Neutral	Non-neutral		SETTING	Scalar Degree						
		Moderate	Extreme		Moderate		Extreme				
					1	2	3	4	5	6	
8. Vocal Tract Tension Features				Tense Vocal Tract							
				Lax Vocal Tract							
9. Laryngeal Tension Features				Tense Larynx							
				Lax Larynx							

Profiles of Speech Disorders' Project, Medical Research Council Grant G978/1192

© University of Edinburgh 1991

Speaker: .... Sex: .... Age: .... Date of Analysis: .... Tape: .... Judge: ....

PROSODIC FEATURES	SETTING	Scalar Degrees		
		Neutral	Moderate	Extreme
1. Pitch Features	High Mean			
	Low Mean			
	Wide Range			
	Narrow Range			
	High Variability			
	Low Variability			
2. Loudness Features	High Mean			
	Low Mean			
	Wide Range			
	Narrow Range			
	High Variability			
	Low Variability			
3. Consistency	Tremor			
TEMPORAL FEATURES				
4. Continuity	Interrupted			
5. Tempo	Fast			
	Slow			
OTHER FEATURES				
6. Denasality				
7. Pharyngeal	Constriction			

OTHER COMMENTS :

Respiratory support :   Adequate   Inadequate

Diplophonia :   Present   Absent

Profiles of Speech Disorders' Project, Medical Research Council Grant G978/1192

© University of Edinburgh 1991

Figure 1–12. Vocal Profile Analysis Protocol form. Reprinted with permission from Vocal Profile Analysis[46]. Copyright 1991, Queen Margaret College and University of Edinburgh Centre for Speech Technology Research.

TABLE 3–5. Bipolar acoustic-perceptual scales for clinical evaluation.

HIGH PITCH __ 1 __ 2 __ 3 __ 4 __ 5 __ 6 __ 7 __ 8 __9 __ LOW PITCH

LOUD __ 1 __ 2 __ 3 __ 4 __ 5 __ 6 __ 7 __ 8 __9 __ SOFT

STRONG __ 1 __ 2 __ 3 __ 4 __ 5 __ 6 __ 7 __ 8 __9 __ WEAK

SMOOTH __ 1 __ 2 __ 3 __ 4 __ 5 __ 6 __ 7 __ 8 __9 __ ROUGH

UNFORCED __ 1 __ 2 __ 3 __ 4 __ 5 __ 6 __ 7 __ 8 __9 __ STRAINED

BREATHY VOICE __ 1 __ 2 __ 3 __ 4 __ 5 __ 6 __ 7 __ 8 __9 __ FULL VOICE

HYPERNASAL __ 1 __ 2 __ 3 __ 4 __ 5 __ 6 __ 7 __ 8 __9 __ DENASAL

ANIMATED __ 1 __ 2 __ 3 __ 4 __ 5 __ 6 __ 7 __ 8 __9 __ MONOTONOUS

STEADY __ 1 __ 2 __ 3 __ 4 __ 5 __ 6 __ 7 __ 8 __9 __ SHAKY

SLOW RATE __ 1 __ 2 __ 3 __ 4 __ 5 __ 6 __ 7 __ 8 __9 __ RAPID RATE

Source: Pausewang Gelfer, Mary Lou, personal communication, June 27, 1996.

Figure 1–13. Bipolar acoustic-perceptual scales for clinical evaluation. *Source*: Mary Lou Pausewang Gelfer, personal communication, June 27, 1996.

ures of social validation in the voice-assessment protocol. This may include use of bipolar, semantic differential scales (eg, "young-old", "steady-shaky") for non-professional evaluation[25] (See Figure 1–13.) By soliciting perceptual ratings from the public, the clinician and patient may gain a more realistic idea of the psychosocial impact a voice disorder has with respect to the "average" listener during day-to-day discourse.

The **voice quality assessment** includes evaluation of upper vocal tract resonance characteristics. The primary evaluation technique used clinically is perceptual-acoustic. The Vocal Profile Analysis Protocol is used to provide a comprehensive assessment of voice quality that includes upper vocal tract settings[46]. Acoustic analysis techniques may provide additional information regarding formant frequencies, which reflect articulatory postures or aspects of nasal resonance. Real-time acoustic software programs can be useful to document and compare resonance features of a voice disorder and those of professional voice users who wish to achieve specific acoustic effects for performance purposes, for example, an enhanced "singer's formant."

Evaluation of upper vocal tract resonance characteristics includes judgement and acoustic measurement of the oral-nasal resonance balance to detect hypernasality or hyponasality. Whereas hyponasality is typically associated with nasopharyngeal obstructions in normally hearing individuals, hypernasality may have organic or muscle-use etiologies (or both). The most obvious causes of hypernasality and nasal air emission on consonants include structural deviations such as cleft palate or iatrogenically induced shortened palate, and these are readily identified during the oral mechanism exam. The common origin of the velar and laryngeal nerve supply (10th cranial nerve) explains why concurrent organic abnormalities in phonation and oral-nasal resonance balance should be documented. In addition, muscle misuses within the vocal tract often result in concurrent voice and resonance quality aberrations; for example, hypertonicity in the tongue base may result not only in phonation limitations but also a degree of hypernasality because of a downward pull on the soft palate via hypertonic palatoglossus muscles.

Concurrent disorders of phonation and resonance may relate to aerodynamic regulation and control mechanisms described by Warren[78,79]. In instances of excessive or insufficient valving forces in the larynx or velopharyngeal port, one valve may compensate for another with greater or lesser closing forces in an attempt to regulate aerodynamic pressures so that they meet requirements for speech. For example, in cases of velopharyngeal valving incompetence and subsequent hypernasality in children with cleft palate, it is common to see hypervalving in the larynx. This laryngeal hypervalving may result in more appropriate intraoral pressure levels for articulation but may lead to dysphonia caused by strain on the phonatory mechanism associated with long-term misuse.

The "human" perceiver has an advantage over software programs when appropriateness of oral-nasal resonance balance needs to be determined. Nasality may be identified as a regional dialectal characteristic; in fact, a frequent finding by Europeans rating North American speech is a level of perceptual nasality that would be considered abnormal in the United Kingdom but is accepted as the norm to North American speakers and listeners. Nasality also may be used for linguistic or psycholinguistic purposes as a critical semantic marker or to indicate social status.

1.4.3 Acoustic Analysis of Speech

The technology for acoustic analysis has developed to the point that an "acoustic blueprint" of the activities in the vocal tract can be generated for almost any speaker. From the voice-source spectrum, measures of frequency and amplitude perturbation (jitter and shimmer, respectively) and signal-to-noise ratios in the acoustic spectrum may be used to supplement the voice quality assessment. To obtain these measures of glottal source features, the acoustic transfer function of the vocal tract is ideally eliminated first by a mathematical process called "inverse-filtering." Jitter and shimmer are measures of stability of the acoustic signal from one period to the next and thus should reflect short-term stability of the phonatory mechanism. (See Figure 8–17, Chapter 8.) Ratio measures of harmonic-to-noise energy indicate the degree to which the signal energy is periodic versus aperiodic and noisy.

Both sustained vowel samples and connected speech may be analyzed acoustically. A minimum protocol would include 3 trials of 2 different sustained vowels—one open and low, the other high and closed—and repetition or oral reading of a standard sentence that samples several different vowels and voiced segments such as; "I will be ready to go soon." By making digital acoustic recordings of phonation simultaneous with laryngostroboscopy, EGG and other measures of vocal fold vibratory characteristics, the team can interpret more accurately the physical correlates of acoustic aberrations from inverse-filtered signals of sustained vowels. Figure 1–11 provides an example of the utility of spectral measures for sustained vowels. In the voice with benign essential tremor, the wide-band spectrogram demonstrates deviations in both intensity and frequency. The frequency deviation is not evident from the acoustic signal alone.

When acoustic measures are being used for pretreatment and posttreatment comparisons, it is critical that vocal production factors of intensity and frequency be controlled because they influence perturbation and noise measures. Ideally, natural discourse samples are analyzed in addition to sustained phonation because articulatory contexts influence glottal-source acoustic parameters, and subsequent effects on vocal quality during speech should be identified[53].

Although a one-to-one correspondence does not exist between single acoustic measures and voice quality labels, in the case of certain perceptual measures, acoustic analysis of the signal may serve to validate and train listeners' judgements. For example, studies have demonstrated that voices judged to have high "breathy-whispery" ratings have acoustic spectra that include one or more of the following features: high levels of interharmonic noise, or replacement of harmonics by noise; regions of high-intensity noise in the spectra above the primary formants (6 kHz and higher); antiformants in the low-frequency spectra related to tracheal resonance; relatively high intensity in the fundamental harmonic (f_0) compared with that of adjacent harmonics, overall spectral energy, or the first formant[21,41,59,66,70] (See Figure 8–16 in Chapter 8 for review.) Sodersten et al have suggested that a different acoustic profile may exist for breathiness associated with hypofunction compared with "hyperfunctional breathiness"[70]. Careful examination of the acoustic profiles may lead us to be more discriminating listeners and to relate perceptual-acoustic features more precisely to phonatory behaviors.

The spectrum of the vocal tract transfer function may also be used to provide information about voice quality. By employing special algorithms (mathematical equations), some programs allow the examiner to locate the frequency of the vocal tract resonances or formants for a given speech or phonation task. Formant features can provide information regarding changes in vocal tract postures (such as tongue, lip, and jaw movements) or vocal tract lengthening and shortening. In the assessment of the singers' vocal technique, the location and intensity of formants can provide clues to the positioning of articulators and may

be used as a feedback tool in training. Numerous dedicated software programs are now available to analyze and display frequency, intensity, and spectral characteristics of speech, as well as irregularities in the vocal signal. The reader is encouraged to review appropriate sections of Chapter 8 (8.4 and 8.5) and figures 8–19, 8–20, and 8–21 to appreciate the nature of the voice source acoustic signal, and the vocal tract acoustic filter function.

Several caveats to interpretation of digital acoustic measures should be considered. First, recording equipment and environment and A-to-D signal processing can influence the perturbation and noise values. In one study, different jitter and shimmer measures were derived for the same signals recorded with 4 different recording devices[18]. Clearly if one is to make valid and reliable comparisons, the recording equipment and environment must be calibrated carefully. Second, it is important to understand that many different algorithms are represented in different software programs for acoustic analysis. Some are better suited to certain clinical measure than others, and it may not be meaningful to compare one with the other[56]. Furthermore, acoustic measures may be based on either time or frequency domains. Even though time and frequency are inversely related in acoustic signals, they may not be equally meaningful for a given perturbation measure such as jitter. Normative data employed as baseline measures against which to compare clinical data must be based on the same hardware, software, and activities.

1.5 Aerodynamic Evaluation

Clinical measures of phonatory flow rates and volumes and subglottal pressure and resistance allow the clinician to obtain information about voice function in a noninvasive manner.

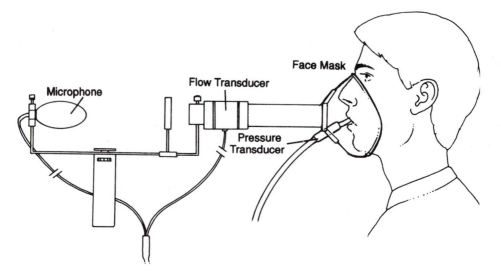

Figure 1–14. Hardware for aerodynamic assessment.

1.5.1 Mean Phonatory Flow Rate

Clinical measurement of flow rates during phonation is typically conducted with a full or partial face mask attached to a flow transducer unit (Figure 1–14). The device that transduces an aerodynamic signal to an electrical signal may be one of several types: pneumotachograph, hot-wire anemometer, plethysmograph, or electro-aerometer. The reader is referred to an excellent text on instrumental assessment by Baken for further details[4].

Mean phonatory flow rates (MFR) measured on steady-state vowel productions provide estimates of glottal impedance, because resistance in the oral cavity is minimal compared with glottal resistance under this condition[4,16]. Measures are usually quantified in milliliters or cc per second. Open vowel productions (for example, /ɑ/) permit the most accurate estimates of laryngeal function to be obtained because they generally offer the least resistance to phonatory flow. Normative data suggests a wide range of variability in this measure: from under 40 to over 300 ml/sec in adults and from 50 to 170 ml/sec in first-grade children[4,13,31]. The clinician is usually interested in the effect that phonetic environment has on vocal function as well, and for this reason, aerodynamic measures should be made during connected speech samples under the most natural conditions possible (considering that the patient is often wearing a face mask). Sentences with a variety of contexts should be elicited to determine the effect on MFR of voiceless versus voiced contexts, loud versus soft speech, different pitch ranges, and other relevant vocal dynamics.

Phonatory flow rates have complex relationships with vocal intensity and fundamental frequency[36,37]. For example, high-intensity phonation at high f_0 levels is generally associated with high MFR; the same relationship may not hold true at lower f_0 levels however. It is critical that production factors of f_0 and intensity be measured simultaneously with MFR to control for reliability and averaging trials and for pretreatment and posttreatment measures. This may be accomplished by time locking separate acoustic measures with the aerodynamic recordings or by using a dedicated device that records the acoustic and aerodynamic signals simultaneously. Because of the complex relationships among production factors, MFR should be determined under a variety of intensity and frequency conditions.

Other production factors held constant, **high phonatory flow rates** (for example, above 300 ml/sec, in men, at normal speaking pitch and loudness levels on /ɑ/) are indicative of poor valving at the glottis, and subsequent DC (direct current) leakage. This could be due to neurological, structural, or muscle misuse factors, for example, vocal fold paralysis, sulcus vocalis, senile atrophy, lesions inhibiting full vocal fold closure, or an habitual glottal posture that does not permit full vocal fold adduction. Phonatory flow rates greater than 900 ml/sec have been reported in individuals with recurrent laryngeal nerve paralysis[31], and in individuals phonating with an intentional posterior glottal chink[59]. Phonatory flow rates also tend to increase with longer open quotients in the vocal fold vibratory cycle. This vibratory feature may be a result of vocal technique or reduced muscle tonus in the vocal folds.

Low phonatory flow rates (below 30 ml/sec for adults at normal speaking pitch and loudness on /ɑ/) most often relate to muscle misuse behaviours that result in excessive vocal fold adductory forces and a high medial compression. Low flow rates have also been reported frequently in singers and are sometimes declared a goal by vocal performers[55]. Neurological conditions, such as laryngeal dystonia, spastic dysarthria, or Parkinson's disease, may also contribute to hypervalving activity and subsequent low MFR. If valving forces in the larynx are hyperkinetic then closed phase increases, amplitude of vibration decreases, and only small amounts of AC (alternating current) flow are released between the vocal folds

during the open phase of the vibratory cycle. Lower intensity phonation is generally associated with lower MFR. One example of a clinical exception to this rule would be loud voice use that is associated with hypervalving laryngeal activity.

The degree of nasal flow can be measured as part of the flow rate protocol if a nasal cone is used rather than a face mask. Some dedicated devices provide a divided mask with 2 transducer channels so that oral and nasal flow can be measured simultaneously.

1.5.2 Flow Volume

Phonatory flow volume indicates the quantity of air that was exhaled during a given phonated segment, as measured with a pneumotachometer, flow transducer, or other standard equipment and quantified in milliliters or cc. As with phonatory flow rates, a wide range has been cited for normal function. Ranges from 1520 to 2723 ml have been reported for women, and 2200 to 4255 ml for men have been reported on maximally sustained open vowels. The ranges for young children reflect their smaller lung capacities, ranging from 700 to 1650 ml[4,31].

When MFR measures are not available, they can be estimated by dividing phonatory volume by maximum phonation time, assuming flow rates are fairly steady. A less accurate, but nevertheless related estimate of flow rate can be obtained from the **phonation quotient** by dividing vital capacity measures by the maximum phonation time[38,82]. This value is generally an overestimate of the MFR because most individuals do not use their entire vital capacity during maximally sustained phonation[81].

1.5.3 Pressure and Resistance

Subglottal pressure and glottal resistance can be measured indirectly using the intraoral method proposed by Smitheran and Hixon[68]. A small tube attached to a pressure transducer is placed between the lips so that its open end rests in the oral cavity and can receive and transmit pressure changes to the transducer (Figure 1–14). This technique is based on the assumption that intraoral pressure equals tracheal pressure when the glottis is open and the lips are sealed for production of the stop consonant. The authors suggested repetition of /pi/ at a rate of 1.5 syllables per second, at habitual pitch and loudness for speech with equal stress allotted to each syllable. Some clinicians feel a more representative speech pressure is obtained with an open vowel, so the syllable /pæ/ is also elicited. Evidence suggests that pressure and resistance values are different for the syllables /pi/ and /pæ/, indicating that the vowel should be controlled for intersubject and pretreatment and posttreatment comparisons[52]. Peak pressure values from /p/ productions can be measured and averaged across several successive productions (a minimum of 10 is recommended) to indicate mean subglottal pressure. Pressure values are traditionally made relative to water pressure, and clinical measures may be cited in centimeters of water pressure (cm H_2O) or in dynes/cm².

Several precautions must be observed to ensure that valid measures are made with the intraoral pressure technique. First, the clinician's description and model of the syllable production must be presented in a manner that does not bias the patient's productions. A clear description of the task, simple modeling, and an instructional "filler" phrase between the clinician's production and patient's response may elicit the most typical production from patients. An example is: "Now I would like you to say the sound /pipipipi . . . / repeatedly in your usual speaking style, until I tell you to stop. Say it at the rate I demonstrated." The goal is to elicit phonatory behavior that is representative of an individual's typical speech patterns, with minimal opportunity to match the clinician's pitch, loudness, or effort level. As with phonatory flow measures, pressure varies with intensity and frequency values in speech. These must be carefully controlled when measures are compared. Most normative data report average subglottal pressure values between 4.5 and 8 cm H_2O as measured either from the indirect method described above or directly from the subglottal space by way of tracheal puncture technique. Lieberman reported subglottal pressures in adults during speech that ranged from 5 to 10 cm H_2O[50].

Phonatory flow measures (MFR) measured on the vowels during the subglottal pressure task can be used in a simple equation to estimate **average glottal resistance** values: average glottal resistance (R_g) = average subglottal pressure (P_s) cm H_2O/MFR (ml/sec): $R_g = P_s/MFR$

Because glottal resistance values are indicative of glottal effort, this formula is particularly helpful in determining how much muscle misuse or compensatory effort is associated with a voice problem at the laryngeal level.

High glottal resistance values are expected in cases where glottal valving forces are exaggerated, and low values are associated with glottal valving incompetence.

Phonation threshold pressure (PTP) measures can be made using the indirect method proposed by Smitheran and Hixon[68]. This measure indicates the minimum subglottal pressure required to initiate vocal fold vibration[75]. This value is expected to be high in the presence of hypervalving activity or structurally based vocal fold stiffness and during high-pitched and loud phonatory activity[76]. Fisher and Swank have indicated that nasal flow measures should be made simultaneously with PTP measures, as changes in the velopharyngeal port may occur when vocal motor control is compromised by attempts to phonate at the low intensity threshold[22,77]. Observations of nasal flow during phonation at threshold levels may account in part for two ongoing problems with the PTP measure:

high variability levels in peak oral pressure values and potential underestimation of subglottal pressures[22]. Clinical application of PTP is still in its infancy but has potential value in defining relationships between vibratory characteristics of the glottal source and aerodynamic features.

1.5.4 Flow Glottograms

If clinical devices are available to obtain inverse-filtered phonatory flow measures, the resultant flow glottogram can provide useful details of vocal fold function[23]. Rothenberg designed a flow mask that performs the inverse filter function while phonation is recorded[63,64]. The resulting signal is relatively free of vocal tract filter functions, and therefore reflects primarily the aerodynamic characteristics related to vocal fold vibratory patterns. Values can be extracted from the signal for peak glottal flow, DC flow offset ("leakiness" factor), open, closed, and closing speed quotients. Simultaneous recordings of flow glottography and electroglottography demonstrate the inverse relationship between the signals as they represent the vocal fold vibratory pattern[29].

A sample protocol of aerodynamic assessment in the voice clinic is offered here. Several trials are recommended for each task so that values representing an individual's average performance can be calculated.

1.5.5 *Protocol for Aerodynamic Assessment*

1. Vital capacity measure: maximum expiratory volume after maximum inhalation.
2. Sustained vowels /ɑ/, /i/ at habitual pitch and loudness, for MFR and flow volume measures. Nasal flow measures can be made if a nasal cone or divided mask is used.
3. Sustained vowels /ɑ/, /i/ at high and low pitch and loudness levels, for MFR, f_0 and intensity measures. Nasal flow measures can be made if a nasal cone or divided mask is used.

4. "Hey!" at loudest level, /ɑ/ at quietest level, for MFR, flow volume and intensity measures.
5. Maximum phonation time on vowels for indications of changes in MFR with vital capacity level and phonation quotient calculations, as necessary.
6. F_0 dynamics: slow glissando up and down throughout entire range for MFR and flow volume measures. Vary intensity with different trials. Nasal flow measures can be made if a nasal cone or divided mask is used.
7. Speech samples for MFR and coarticulatory devoicing effects: "Tell me your name, occupation, and one other thing about yourself." "Count to ten." "Count from 11 to 20." Vary intensity with different trials. Nasal flow measures can be made if a nasal cone or divided mask is used.

    Say these sentences (model verbally, or have patient read from a cue card): "Please seat Shelly, Harriet, and Frederick close to the fireplace." (Look at coarticulatory devoicing effect on MFR of vowels.) "Are you really angrier than you were on Monday?" (Look at MFR in absence of devoicing effect.) Nasal flow measures can be made if a nasal cone or divided mask is used.
8. "Now I would like you to say /pipipi . . . /; /pæpæpæ . . . / repeatedly at the speed I demonstrated until I tell you to stop." "Say it in your usual speaking style." Model 1.5 syllables per second, for estimated subglottal pressure on /p/ and MFR on /æ/, and calculation of laryngeal resistance: P_s/MFR.
9. "Now say /pipipi . . . ./; /pæpæpæ . . . / at the 'softest' or 'quietest' level you can possibly make with your voice." Measure phonation threshold pressure on several trials. Ideally, simultaneous nasal flow measures should be made.
10. Therapy probes (See Section 1.9).

1.6 Musculoskeletal Evaluation

All members of the voice care team are involved in assessing postural and muscle misuses in our patients. Because voluntary muscles are the final common pathway for psychological and physiological function during speech and singing, it is of primary importance to identify specific muscle misuse patterns contributing to voice problems. The musculoskeletal evaluation begins during the history interview, when both the interviewer and observers take note of static postural profiles and changes in posture that may occur with changes in topic. General observations such as "slouching" or "overstraightened" may be used to describe initial clinical observations. Some general postural misuse patterns are depicted in Figure 1–15, along with reference diagrams for ideal body alignment. Because the history interview is the clinical protocol that may elicit the most natural discourse from patients, it is important to document more specific postural misuses as precisely as possible. These observations may be augmented during discussions with the psychiatrist, speech-language pathologist, and singing teacher, with each team member noting specific situations, topics, or voice features that correspond with particular muscle misuse patterns.

It would be an overstatement to suggest that postural abnormalities are always related to muscle misuse or psychogenic factors; a variety of structural disorders and neurological disease processes may result in abnormal muscle tone or misalignment and asymmetry that may contribute to speech and voice dysfunction. Patients with such disorders may show a limited response to the traditional therapy programs for posture retraining. Nevertheless, behavioral or habitual muscle misuse remains the most common cause of postural abnormalities. Postural misuses that may be observed and quantified during the initial interview and subsequent assessment activities are discussed below.

1.6.1 Indicators of Body Misalignment

As part of the postural pattern, the scapulae may be adducted, so that the shoulders are positioned unnaturally posterior, and power in the upper arms is disengaged. If the back and neck muscles are being misused, a "hump" may be observed in the upper back, just below the cervical vertebrae (Figure 1–16).

Misuse of the neck muscles can lead to hyperextension or flexion of the neck (Figure 1–17). Commonly, the head is retracted on the neck so that the jaw extends up and forward, a misuse we refer to as **jaw jut**. The opposite postural misuse is also observed, most commonly in men; in which the head is held forward with neck flexion. It is important to inquire about injuries that may have contributed to postural misuse, in particular, a history of whiplash injuries that may have precipitated splinting of neck muscles. In some, head-neck posture may reflect attempts to compensate for poorly fitting eyewear, bifocal lenses, or some other visual acuity problem.

1.6.2 Specific Muscle Misuses During Phonation

Some commonly observed muscle misuses in patients with voice disorders will be described. For a more detailed and formal assessment of the musculoskeletal system and its use, the expertise of a physical therapist, osteopath, or other professionally trained individual may be sought. Lieberman has described a detailed protocol for assessment of postural patterns associated with hyperfunctional dysphonia[49]. Specialized training in use and interpretation of these assessment techniques provides the voice clinician with a powerful tool to guide the diagnostic and treatment process.

A common misuse of respiratory muscles during phonation, especially for vocal per-

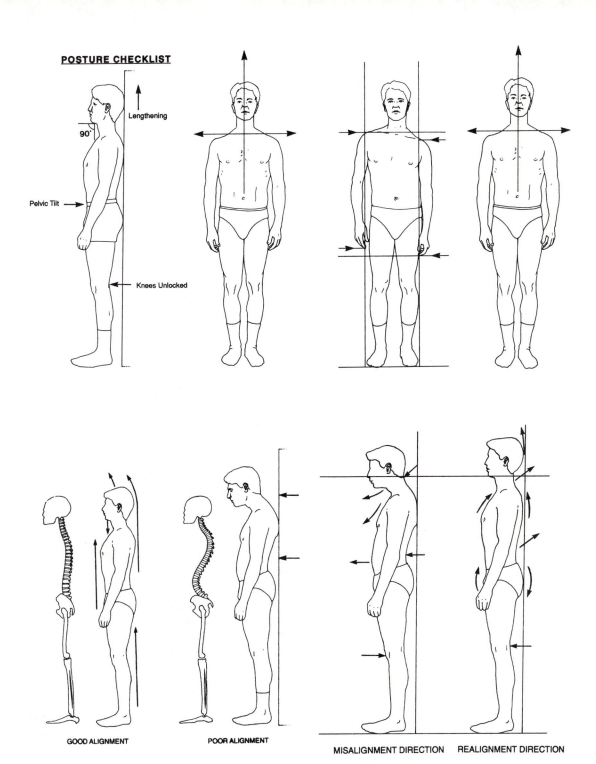

Figure 1–15a. Example of postural misuses, and principles for good alignment: standing.

29

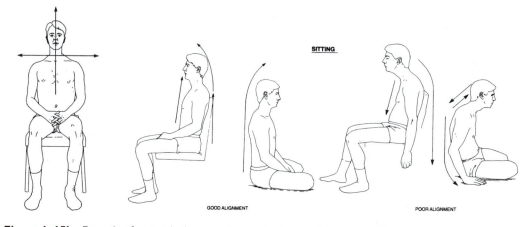

SITTING

GOOD ALIGNMENT   POOR ALIGNMENT

Figure 1–15b. Example of postural misuses, and principles for good alignment: sitting.

formance, is failure to support the lung volume with inspiratory muscle activity once phonation has been initiated (Figure 1–18). This is a function of poor body posture and technical misuse. At high lung volumes, inspiratory muscles (in particular the external intercostals) need to be engaged during phonation so that subglottal pressure does not exceed requirements for the voice task. In instances where subglottal pressure is allowed to exceed the optimal level, the laryngeal muscles may respond by valving to decelerate the airflow at the glottis, which results in excessive glottal compression. Further adjustments in the larynx may be made to allow for continued phonation; for example, contraction of the inspiratory posterior cricoarytenoid muscles may create a posterior glottal chink that acts as a pressure-release valve while medial compression is maintained in the anterior portions of the vocal folds for phonation. This laryngeal isometric laryngeal posture is illustrated and described further in Chapter 2.

Another common misuse of respiratory muscles is tension in abdominal musculature in conjunction with hypertonicity in the pelvic floor muscles. Many patients, particu-larly women, may maintain a tense abdominal "girdle" to satisfy an esthetic goal; others have been told by physical trainers, dance instructors, or their mothers, to "pull your gut in!" In this situation, exaggerated inspiratory movements in the rib cage and auxiliary muscles attached to the clavicles may be observed. These areas may also be held in the inspiratory position to exaggerated degrees during exhalation and phonation. When respiratory movements are restricted, additional auxiliary inspiratory tactics may be observed, including head retraction (jaw jut) and tongue retraction.

A "hands-on" approach to assessment of respiratory function provides useful supplementary information. With the examiner's hands on the abdomen and back and then on lateral portions of the rib cage, we feel for evidence of the appropriate abdominal distension during inspiration at rest and preparatory to various phonatory tasks. Then we feel for lateral expansion of the rib cage during the same activities and maintenance of rib cage expansion through the vocal activity. By palpating the submental region just anterior to the hyoid bone, the examiner can detect inappropriate muscle activity in the suprahyoid muscles during inspiration, which are associated with tongue retraction and sometimes jaw extension. Inappropriate head movements during inspiration may be most easily documented from a lateral view. In instances where a speech-breathing disorder is suspected as a primary contributor to speech and voice dysfunction, a formal examination of the abdominal breathing mechanism should be considered. Hixon and Hoit offer a protocol for this[32].

The diaphragm plays a major role during speech as the primary inspiratory mechanism, and its function should be evaluated. This is typically done informally by observing and feeling movements of the abdominal and rib cage walls during inspiration and inferring the diaphragmatic activity that contributed to these displacements. There is evidence that the diaphragm may also play a role other than inspiratory during some speech-breathing activities[11,34,35]. In instances where diaphragmatic dysfunction is suspected, and to evaluate more specialized functions of the diaphragm during phonation, a formal protocol developed by Hixon and Hoit should be considered[33].

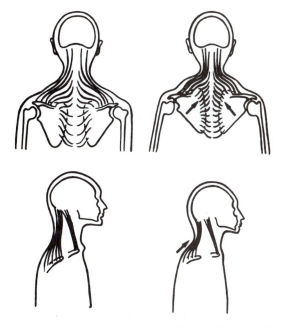

Figure 1–16. Scapulae (shoulder blade) adduction and elevation (right, upper, and lower) compared with normal use (left, upper, and lower).

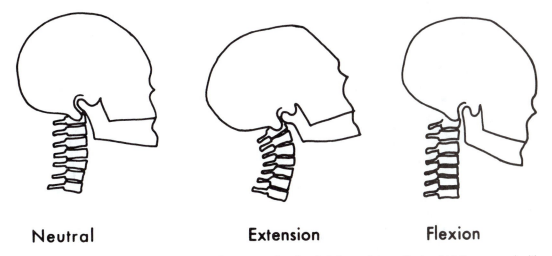

Neutral   Extension   Flexion

Figure 1–17. Inappropriate neck postures: hyperextension (jaw jut) (center); hyperflexion (right), compared with normal use (left).

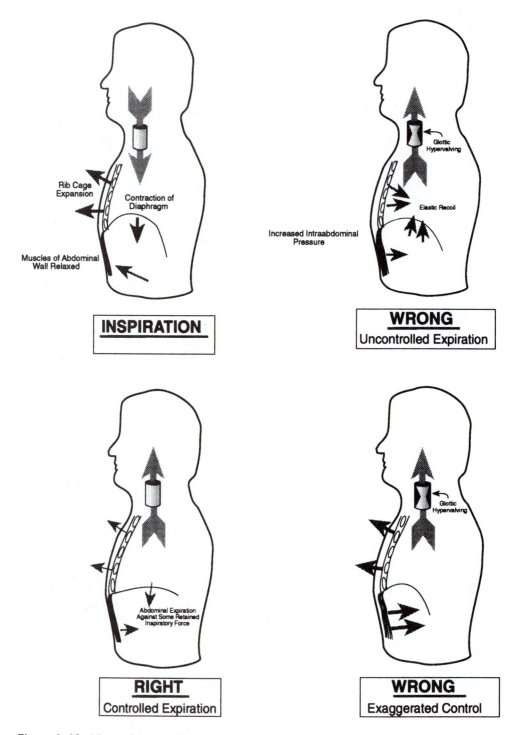

Figure 1–18. Misuse of the breathing system compared with normal use for inspiration and expiration.

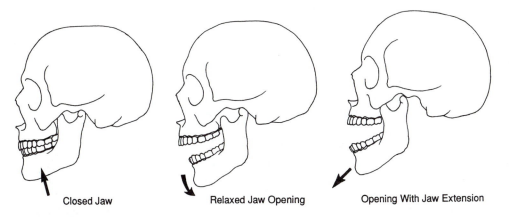

Closed Jaw   Relaxed Jaw Opening   Opening With Jaw Extension

Figure I–19. Misuse of the temporomandibular joint: forward extension during opening (right), compared with normal use for speech (left and center).

Misuse of muscles governing movements at the temporomandibular joint (TMJ) is common. The lower facial muscles may be hypertonic to a degree that minimal or no jaw movement is observed during speech. If the lateral pterygoid muscles are contracted, the mandible may be held forward or pulled forward during opening gestures. (Figure 1–19). With the head of the mandible disengaged from the glenoid fossa and articular capsule, free rotational movements are no longer possible. Thus mandible depression is reduced and any movements observed during speech are effortful. To assess tension in mandible elevators the examiner attempts to rotate the jaw by hand while the patient remains silent. With the examiner's hands placed flat over the TMJ region, "bulging" during speech or jaw opening can be felt if exaggerated or inappropriate forward movements are being made. TMJ dysfunction is common in those with bruxism and grinding. It is helpful to examine dentition for signs of wear and the buccal mucosa for ridges or other hyperplastic tissue.

Further misuse of the tongue-jaw complex may be evidenced by palpation of the suprahyoid muscles during inspiration and phonatory tasks (Figure 1–20). Of particular significance is persistent hypertonicity in the suprahyoid muscles during speech and singing, increased activity during inspiration, and increased activity in association with pitch or loudness dynamics. Often, in untrained or poorly trained singers, the suprahyoid muscles become increasingly tense with rising pitch and around register transitions. The larynx may be pulled upward with this muscle misuse, as confirmed by laryngoscopy or by palpation of the thyroid cartilage during scales and glissando pitch changes. Abnormal tongue posturing and muscle tone may be associated with mild hypernasality, due to involvement of the palatoglossus muscle. When hypertonic, this muscle may effectively pull downward on the soft palate, thus reducing the adequacy of velopharyngeal closure during speech. Further, if the tongue is held posterior to its rest position so it reduces the pharyngeal space, oropharyngeal resonance may be damped, and excessive nasal resonance may be noted because of increased flow through the nasal cavity. Not surprisingly, many individuals with muscle misuse voice disorders also exhibit abnormal resonance features.

If the tongue muscles are hypertonic at rest, the periphery of the tongue may have a "scalloped" appearance, an imprint made by the lower teeth as the tongue is pressed against them for long periods. (Figure 1–21). Conversely, the tongue may be held in a retracted position at rest so that the edges do not rest against the bottom teeth. Observation of the surface of the tongue at rest and on protrusion may reveal excessive narrowing and grooving indicative of intrinsic muscle tension and the tongue surface may tremor inconsistently at rest.

Laryngeal posture at rest and during phonation is of importance to phonatory function and can be assessed informally by palpating the thyroid notch and thyrohyoid muscles. The vertical position of the larynx following a swallow may be used as a reference point for rest while the position of the thyrohyoid notch is determined. Exaggerated excursion of the larynx during speech or singing (more than a few millimeters) is suspect, as is a phonatory posture superior to the rest position. Some singing styles appear to be enhanced by a laryngeal position that is slightly lower than the postswallow rest position. In this case, it is important that the singing posture for the larynx is not maintained after the phonatory activity is completed so that the muscles lowering the larynx are not chronically hypertonic.

Palpation of thyrohyoid, cricothyroid, and pharyngeal constrictor muscles bilaterally provides invaluable information that can be used diagnostically and therapeutically. Procedures for palpating and scoring extrinsic and intrinsic muscle tonicity are offered in Section 1.7.2.

Detailed evaluation of a variety of laryngeal postures is made using the flexible transnasal fiber-optic scope, which permits observation of the larynx during speech and nonspeech activities. This technique is discussed in Section 1.7.2.

The functions of the facial muscles are many

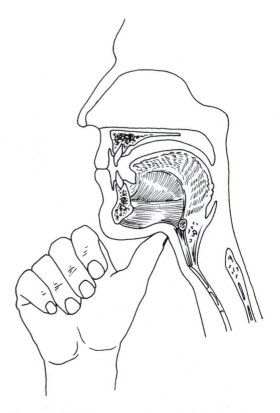

Figure 1–20. Detecting hypertonicity in the suprahyoid muscle complex by palpation.

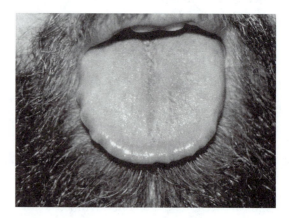

Figure 1–21. Tongue scalloping caused by hypertonicity in tongue muscles at rest; tongue pushes forward into lower teeth, or forward and upward into upper teeth, leaving an imprint of the teeth on the tongue periphery.

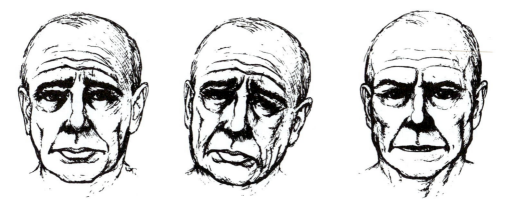

Figure 1–22. Faces showing muscle misuses associated with repressed emotions: chronic anxiety (left); suppression of the impulse to cry (center); and suppressed anger (right).

and varied. Beyond its perceptual, respiratory, and deglutition functions, the face serves as a platform for revealing prevailing conscious or unconscious emotions and the intent behind communicative gestures such as speech. This may explain why facial muscles are so susceptible to misuse. The freedom of speech and voice movements can be jeopardized by tension in muscles in the upper, middle, and lower face areas. Observe signs of anxiety, depression, or denial in the upper face, such as eyebrows elevated or adducted, cheeks elevated, or gaze fixed for long periods. In the lower face, the lips may be pressed together at rest, the upper lip retracted and virtually immobile during speech, the jaw immobile during speech, the mentalis muscles of the chin puckered, all signs of muscle misuse that may be indicative of ongoing emotional distress. If upper and lower facial postures are functioning to inhibit emotional expression, then the specific muscle misuse governing movements of the lips, jaw, and tongue during phonation may be fairly easy to identify but difficult to treat without psychiatric intervention.

1.7 Physical Examination of the Larynx and Vocal Tract

1.7.1 Basic Equipment Needs

Examination with the head mirror and laryngeal mirror remains the clinical standard for laryngeal observation, and coupled with a full head and neck examination, this technique is used for the vast majority of patients with voice disorders being assessed in general clinics. Because invaluable clinical information is obtained with rigid and flexible fiberoptic instruments, particularly when they are attached to a video camera and stroboscope, this section focuses on the most common instrumentation used currently in voice clinics. Hardware equipment systems for a voice clinic evolve rapidly, and as with computers, one always wants to have next year's model.

Flexible Fiber-optic Laryngoscope

Several excellent models are available, and important variables include the diameter of the instrument, the amount of light transmitted, and the magnification offered when connected to the camera. Pediatric models are usually slimmer and easier to pass but may sacrifice brightness and image size. The transnasal flexible fiber-optic scope is depicted in Figure 1–23.

Rigid Glass Rod Laryngoscope

As with the above, the brightness, ease of focusing, size, and clarity of the image are all paramount. The main difference between available models is in the light beam angulation at the tip, with both 70° and 90° scopes offered. To some extent the difference comes down to personal preference and experience. Some of the 90° laryngoscopes have a focusing ring that permits a wider aperture lens and therefore more available light, but it is sometimes difficult to get a sharply focused image. It is probably a good idea to get an instrument that has the fiber-optic cable permanently attached to the telescope because the detachment junction provides a zone for damage and light loss. The transoral rigid glass rod laryngoscope is depicted in Figure 1–24.

Light Source

Both laryngoscopes have fiber-optic cables that are connected to a light source. Reliable halogen lights are available without spending too much money. Expensive xenon arc lamps are not necessary because the quality and light sensitivity of video cameras has improved.

Video Camera

Yanagasawa was a pioneer in the development of video techniques for laryngology[80]. A number of good video cameras are now available at a reasonable price if you do not require one that has a sterilizable endoscope connector for use in the operating room. Most of these have a single chip camera on a C-mount attached to a connector that clips on to most rigid or flexible laryngoscopes. For more money, one can purchase a 3-chip camera or a flexible scope that has the video-recording chip at the tip of the scope.

Stroboscope

The advent of the videostroboscopic technique for laryngeal examination provided voice clinicians with the ability to easily identify structural vocal fold abnormalities such as sulcus vocalis and cysts[10]. By providing information about vibratory characteristics of the vocal folds, video-laryngostrobosopy allows the clinician to document aspects of voice problems related to structure, function, and use. The engineering challenge to marry a strobed light source (which flashes in synchrony with the fundamental frequency of a vocal signal) to a fiber-optic light cable and then provide an image that is easily captured by a video camera attached to a rigid or flexible fiber-optic laryngoscope has been met by a number of companies. Wolff and B&K were two early German companies that pioneered these developments during the late 1970s, followed by Kay in the United States, Atmos in Germany, and Nagashima in Japan. It has been a pleasure to watch these companies compete for the market by constant refinements in light generation and acoustic tracking, as well as in the addition of numerous "bells and whistles." It is now common to see the stroboscope coupled to a recording microphone so that fundamental frequency and loudness are displayed on the video monitor, as well as various forms of digital image capture and manipulation. By the time this book is in print, there will undoubtedly be many more advances. Still, there are a few attributes that a clinician interested in a new stroboscope purchase should be looking for:

1. The light intensity of the strobe source should be such that picture captured by the video camera in strobe mode is similar in brightness to the "regular" light nonstrobed video.
2. The color temperature of the two examinations (strobed and nonstrobed) should be similar. For example the shade and intensity of the reds should be the same.
3. The strobe light should "lock on" to the acoustic signal quickly. If the strobe takes too long to pick up the frequency at which it should flash, important clinical information may be lost.
4. It should be easy for the examiner to switch from regular light to strobed light without using the hands, and the laryngeal video recording of this transition should be smooth.

Audio microphone

A relatively inexpensive, lapel-mounted microphone is used for most situations, but it may be desirable to use a unidirectional headset-mounted microphone to maintain high fidelity and a constant distance if the recordings are also used for a computerized acoustic analysis or perceptual-acoustic ratings. Newer videostroboscopy systems are supplied with the microphone attached to the laryngoscope near the camera coupling.

Video Recorder

Most voice clinic assessments are video recorded, including images of both flexible and rigid laryngeal examination, external recordings of portions of the patient interview, and responses to some probe therapy techniques. It is generally desirable to have quick and easy access to a comparative review of previous recordings of the same patient and be able to edit clips of several tapes together for presentations off site. For a teaching environment, one may also want to have a video monitor located in another room where stu-

dents (or the teacher) can watch the proceedings. To achieve these ends, we have set up our clinic in the following manner, using standard commercial equipment.

We use two S-VHS video recorders with one serving as the master. Four separate inputs for the video signal are available, and it is easy to alternate between them. The "line 1" S-VHS input comes from the laryngoscope camera and "line 2" from the second recorder. The "line 1" non-SVHS "video-in" input is from a home-type video camera mounted across the room to record the interview and general scene, whereas line 2 comes from an old three-quarter inch Sony VCR that was used in previous decades. The master VCR video-out and audio-out signals go to the monitor in the room, whereas the RF cable outlet goes to a video monitor located in another room for outside observation. Patient consent is obtained for any outside observation.

We use half-inch Super VHS videotapes that are 1 hour in length. Unless it has to be removed to allow for presentation editing, the tape stays in the master recorder until it is full. Patient assessments are recorded sequentially, and a card that fits over the tape jacket is filled out with details including the time, name, age, gender, diagnosis codes, and date, along with notations that indicate the inclusion of an interview or whether the picture is a particularly good example of the pathology identified. When the tape is full, this information is transferred to a computer database that can be sorted depending on clinical or academic needs. Because the most recently recorded tapes are easily accessible, it is convenient to slip a tape from a previous visit into the second recorder for comparison with a current image.

Instrument Cart

A cart with drawers for all the bits of paraphernalia is of great help. Tissues, gauze,

Table 1-1. Technique of Palpation

Suprahyoid muscles (S):

Midline upward palpation in submental space with middle finger

Observe: (1) tension at rest

(2) contraction during low-pitched /ɑ/ follow by high-pitched /u/ phonation

Thyrohyoid muscles (T):

Palpate both thyrohyoid spaces with the thumb and forefinger

Observe: (1) tension at rest

(2) contraction during connected speech (count 1 to 5) and with an easy hum

Cricothyroid muscles (C):

Feel the cricothyroid space in midline with tip of the index finger

Observe: (1) position of the cricoid arch relative to the thyroid cartilage

(2) size of the space at rest

(3) closing and opening of the space during high-pitched and low-pitched phonation

Pharyngolaryngeal muscles (inferior constrictor; P):

Rotate the larynx, hook posterior edge of thyroid cartilage with index finger and draw forward, feel the posterior aspect of the cricoid cartilage with middle and ring finger

Observe: (1) tension in pharyngeal muscles

(2) associated aryteniod movement and posterior cricoarytenoid (PCA) muscle contraction during sniffing

---

Important note:

- Laryngeal palpation should be done before any intraoral or larngoscopic examination to avoid changes in muscle tension caused by the manipulation associated with the evaluation.
- Some tenderness may be found in these muscle groups and should be noted.
- Examination is best done from the side with the head, neck, and shoulders in a neutral position.

defoggers, cleaning solutions, biopsy forceps, gloves, anesthetic spray, tongue depressors, and so forth all need a place.

1.7.2 Regional Examination

Tongue and Oral Cavity

The tongue and its movements and the oral cavity mucosa are examined for presence of lesions or evidence of neurological disorders. It is advisable to use a standardized oral mechanism exam, such as **the Dworkin-Culatta Oral Mechanism Examination and Treatment System (D-COME-T)**, which assists the clini-

cian in developing a comprehensive description of structural and neuromotor deficits, differential diagnosis of motor speech disorders, and the relevant treatment programs[20]. Because the D-COME-T provides a screening tool, it can be used in a time-efficient manner with each patient, with more detailed examination procedures used only as indicated by screening test results. During an oral mechanism exam, indicators of certain muscle misuse patterns can also be identified, such as tongue scalloping or jaw and tongue tension. Attention is paid to jaw movement patterns and to the presence of any malocclusion or other dental abnormalities. Any suggestion of

Table 1-2. Criteria for Extra-Laryngeal Muscle Tension Grading System

Suprahoid muscles (S):

0 = soft at rest, may contract slightly on phonation

1 = soft at rest, mild low pitch and moderate high-pitch contraction

2 = some tension at rest, tense with jaw protrusion on phonation

3 = tense all the time, maximally tight on phonation

Thyrohyoid muscles (T):

0 = no muscular contraction at rest, mild on phonation

1 = soft thyrohyoid space at rest, some contraction on phonation

2 = tense, narrow thyrohyoid space at rest, moderate contraction on phonation

3 = very tense with closed thyrohyoid space all the time

Cricothyroid muscles (C):

0 = normal cricothyroid space and phonatory movement

1 = narrowing of cricothyroid space at rest, some movement on phonation

2 = anterior displacement of cricoid cartilage with narrowing of cricothyroid space at rest, closing of the space on phonation

3 = very tense with closed cricothyroid space all the time

Pharyngolaryngeal muscles (inferior constrictor; P):

0 = soft, easy to rotate the larynx 90° and palpate posterior cricoarytenoid (PCA) muscle and arytenoid movement on sniffing

1 = slightly tense, cannot palpate posterior cricoarytenoid muscle movement

2 = moderately tense, difficult to rotate the larynx but still can palpate the posterior edge of thyroid cartilage

3 = very tense, cannot rotate the larynx at all

articulatory or resonance problems will draw attention to associated orolabial, tongue, or velopharyngeal difficulties, and systematic use of the standard oral mechanism will allow for refinement of the clinical description.

Larynx and Pharynx

In the past, physical examination of the larynx was the primary responsibility of the laryngologist, who would report the observations and interpretations to other professionals involved in caring for a patient. The indirect laryngoscopic exam now is conducted regularly by speech-language pathologists as well. With modern equipment, we can document the laryngoscopic examination on videotape, show the patient his or her own larynx, and interpret the findings together as a voice care team. This is the principal reason that voice clinic teams have evolved and that there has been so much interest in voice and in the understanding of voice disorders.

Because the extrinsic laryngeal musculature that suspends the larynx also plays an important role in the process of voice production, palpation of these muscles may provide some information about tension in the intrinsic laryngeal muscles. Palpation of paralaryngeal muscles can yield information about laryngeal posture at rest and during phonation. Integration of this examination technique into routine laryngeal examinations, particularly in patients with voice disorders, can help the clinician make a more accurate diagnosis and plan appropriate management[49].

Details of this technique are outlined in Table 1–1. We rate the tension in each of four

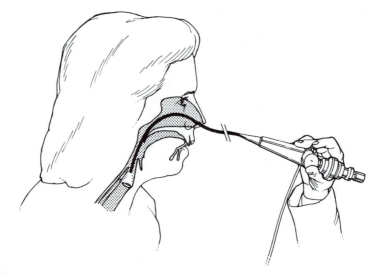

Figure 1–23. Transnasal examination with the flexible fiber-optic scope.

laryngeal muscle groups on a 0-to-3 scale where 0 is normal, 1 is mild, 2 is moderate, and 3 is severely increased muscular tension. Criteria used to make the tension ratings are shown in Table 1–2.

Mirror examination of the larynx is the standard in most otolaryngology offices and shall remain so with good reason. We will not spend time discussing this technique here because it does not offer the multiobserver advantage of video endoscopes. Video imaging of the larynx during endoscopy using transnasal flexible fiber-optic techniques or transoral endoscopy with a rigid telescope does allow multiple observers to view and evaluate laryngeal function.

What are the advantages of flexible fiber-optic endoscopy over use of the rigid telescope? Briefly, the flexible scope is best for "macrolaryngoscopy" and the rigid for "microlaryngoscopy." Transnasal observation using the **flexible fiber-optic scope** of the entire upper vocal tract is essential for full evaluation of connected speech and laryngeal postures, particularly during evaluation of muscle misuse voice disorders (Figure 1–23). Some of the supraglottal postures de-

scribed in Chapter 2 went unrecognized until laryngeal examination could be readily achieved without pulling on the tongue. Because examination with the flexible scope does not need to interfere with articulatory movements in the oral cavity (although it may affect velopharyngeal closure on the side of insertion), it produces a distinct advantage for the documentation of connected speech samples. Examination with the rigid scope generally involves tongue protrusion and is restricted to phonation on a vowel that is associated with anterior tongue displacement, usually /i/, that makes the larynx more visually accessible.

A bonus afforded by the emergence of flexible transnasal fiberoscopy is an excellent view of the nose and nasopharynx. By using this technique routinely with voice disordered patients, we have found unexpected pathology, particularly in the nasopharynx, that may have been related to the problem in question but gone undetected in the standard mirror exam. Inflamed cysts or bursae are examples. The flexible transnasal technique is sometimes employed in place of the rigid transoral approach in severe "gaggers", who generally tolerate a nasopharyngeal approach more easily. There are still those gaggers who cannot be seen by any method other than direct examination under general anesthetic, which one would obviously prefer to avoid and which provides no useful information regarding phonatory patterns and behaviours. Laryngeal examination in children has been facilitated by pediatric flexible scopes. Special techniques and considerations for examining children with voice disorders are presented in Chapter 6.

A tendency for those performing indirect laryngoscopy is to seek a view through the pharynx and supraglottal structures to the vocal folds and then ignore all else. The classification section in Chapter 2 highlights the clinical significance of static and dynamic aspects of glottal and supraglottal postures including false cord adduction and anteroposterior contraction of supraglottal structures. If clinicians are able to video record the examination, they may keep the document and discuss it further after other factors, such as psychological issues, have been considered. In any event, the clinician must make a conscious effort to evaluate the supraglottal structures before passing on to a close view of vocal fold activity.

Although the flexible scope gives the best overview, **the transoral rigid telescope** with its clarity of optics and greater magnification is the best for looking at the details of vocal fold structure. The features we seek to examine with the strobe light such as glottal closure, phase symmetry, mucosal wave, viscosity, discrimination between cysts and nodules, and so forth are all displayed to the best advantage with rigid video laryngoscopy. The effects of altering head and neck posture during the laryngeal examination must be considered in the final interpretation of clinical data obtained. There may be significant differences in laryngeal closure patterns associated with laryngostroboscopy using the flexible verses rigid laryngoscopes,

in particular the perceived magnitude of posterior glottal chinks may be larger in recordings made with the transoral rigid technique[69]. This finding may be related to the typical posture adopted by patients to facilitate an easy view of the larynx. If the laryngoscope is placed centrally in the mouth, the patient's head must generally be retracted, and this may bias laryngeal posture and affect vibratory patterns.

We have found that lateral placement of laryngoscopes allows for an excellent view of the vocal folds without undue neck extension. The scope can be pivoted on the first or second molar for stability and the angle of the image corrected by rotating the camera at its attachment to the laryngoscope. On the other hand, a more central placement with the superior tip of the scope resting against the soft palate eliminates the need to rotate the scope for a symmetrical view and often is well tolerated. Figure 1–24 demonstrates the effects of two different positions of the rigid scope on the laryngeal view and the head and neck postures associated with each examination approach.

Because different types of information can be gleaned from flexible and rigid laryngoscopy, both techniques are essential for a comprehensive clinical examination. Both continuous and flashing stroboscopic light sources may be used to obtain visual perceptual information regarding the anatomical and physiological status of the larynx during phonation.

1.7.3 Instrumental Assessment of Vocal Fold Vibratory Patterns

During direct and indirect examination of the larynx, a continuous light source is generally used to examine gross structural and movement characteristics. This examination technique is supplemented in the modern-day voice clinic by use of a flashing "stroboscopic" light source coupled with fiber-optic or

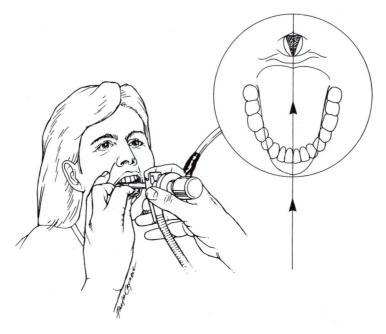

a.

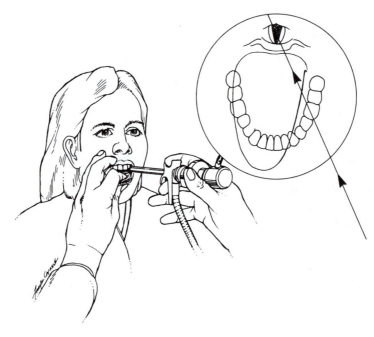

b.

Figure 1–24. Transoral examination with the rigid laryngoscope; (a) Frontal placement of the rigid scope. (b)Lateral placement of the rigid scope.

telescopic hardware and video-audio recording devices described previously.

1.7.3.1. Phonatory Parameters Assessed with Continuous Light

Rate, Range, and Symmetry of Abduction and Adduction Movements. The rate and excursion of lateral vocal fold movements for nonspeech tasks (such as normal and deep inspiration and vegetative adduction during coughing, swallowing, or gagging) provide information about the functional status of the cricoarytenoid joint and the muscles that govern movement from this joint. Slow, incoordinate, asymmetrical, or reduced movements may indicate central or peripheral neurological disease, fixation, or dislocation of the cricoarytenoid joint.

Laryngeal Diadochokinesis. This evaluates the rate of repetition of the vowel /i/ and the syllable /hi/ that requires a devoicing gesture for voiceless articulations in speech. The normal range in adults is 4 to 7 repetitions per second[7]. Rates below the norms may indicate central or peripheral neurological disease, fixation of the cricoarytenoid joint, or laryngeal muscle hypertonicity.

Glottal and Supraglottal Postures and Gestures. This includes the general relationships of laryngeal structures to each other during phonation and at rest. During phonation, we assess the degree of anterior-posterior and lateral compression of the supraglottal structures and the phonatory closure patterns at the glottis elicited with a variety of speech tasks. Posture patterns outlined in Chapter 2 provide a guideline for assessment of glottal and supraglottal postures. Closure patterns are assessed in greater detail for sustained vowels with the stroboscopic light.

Vocal Fold Edges. This implies the straightness and smoothness of the medial edges of each vocal fold. Lesions, scarring, and other organic problems can result in irregular margins.

1.7.3.2. Phonatory Parameters Assessed with Stroboscopic Light (Laryngostroboscopy)

Videostroboscopic techniques have been used in routine voice evaluation for more than a decade. The principles of stroboscopic imaging are based on perceptual features of the optical system. The human visual system is temporally limited in its ability to perceive more than about 5 images per second. Because the vocal folds vibrate at much higher speeds than this during phonation (100–1000 vibrations per second) the examiner is not equipped to distinguish details of movement patterns associated with each vibratory cycle. The stroboscope provides a flashing light source that can solve this perceptual dilemma in the examination of phonatory patterns.

The fundamental frequency of vocal fold vibration (f_0), detected by a microphone placed on the anterior neck, is transmitted to the stroboscope to drive the light generator. By flashing at approximately the same frequency as the f_0, the stroboscopic light illuminates an image of one portion of each vibratory cycle. The visual system then takes over by creating an "averaged" image of the vocal fold vibratory pattern over many cycles (Figure 1–25). If the stroboscopic light is set to flash at exactly the same rate as the f_0, the optical image is of a constant phase of the vibratory cycle, for example the beginning of closing (Figure 1–25). This setting allows the examiner to perceive the averaged degree of irregularity or aperiodicity from one cycle to the next.

A different setting will allow the stroboscopic light to be driven at a frequency several hertz different from the f_0, thus illuminating the vocal folds at a slightly different phase than the f_0, as seen in Figure 1–25. This allows for a slow-motion visual effect that gives the perceiver an impression of the approximate or average movement pattern of successive vibratory cycles. Although the visual perception created by this system is not as accurate as slow-motion photographic images, it is a much easier and faster clinical procedure. Unless the vibratory cycles are extremely irregular, stroboscopic imaging provides a good approximation to the pattern of single, successive vibratory cycles for a given phonatory task[8,40].

Because of their superior quality, we favor telescopic images viewed from the transoral rigid endoscope for our detailed stroboscopic evaluation. This hardware limits the speech task to approximation of a target /i/ vowel and may involve holding the tongue forward to give adequate visual access to the larynx. Wherever possible, the lateral scope placement is used to minimize the need for neck extension, and if the larynx can be visualized without holding the tongue, the patients are requested to position their tongues forward during the exam. Despite the obvious speech limitations, we feel that by recording a wide variety of vocal tasks, the examiner can gain a good understanding of an individual's vocal fold vibratory patterns using the rigid endoscope. A variety of parameters are judged, and these are presented below, followed by a sample protocol used to elicit the phonatory behaviours being observed.

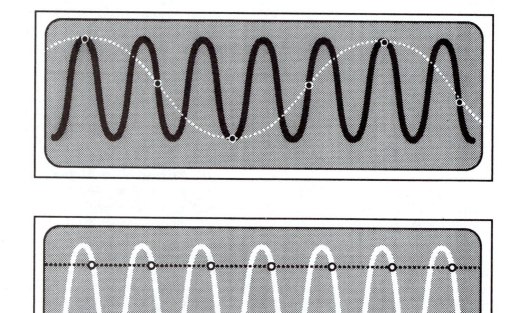

A

B

Figure 1–25. Principles of stroboscopy: (a) If the light is set to flash slightly off the f_0, a slow-motion image will be perceived. (b) If the light is set to flash at the same frequency as f_0 (phase-locked), the image will give the impression of a still frame.

Depending on the parameter being observed and the scoring preferences of the examiners, degrees of abnormality may be rated using an equal-appearing interval scale, a verbal summary scale (eg., "mild-moderate-severe"), a percentage scale, or by indicating on a standard score form the location and degree of impairment. We are employing a new score form for rating stroboscopic features of phonation, developed by Poburka, which is included at the end of this section for reference[57].

Although clinical judgements regarding appropriateness of parameters are generally made during phonation at typical pitch and loudness levels (in modal register), a protocol is used to elicit phonation under a variety of pitch and loudness conditions. This provides the clinician the opportunity to observe variability in vibratory characteristics under a variety of vocal dynamics, which may provide valuable diagnostic and prognostic information. In the case of vocal performers, stroboscopic evaluation may be conducted with a more detailed protocol to examine subtle changes in vibratory features through a wide range of phonatory dynamics and activities. Simultaneous spectral-acoustic, electroglottographic, or photoglottographic measures may be useful to highlight subtle changes.

Amplitude. The extent of vertical-lateral excursion of the vocal folds (Figure 1–26a) is the amplitude. With stroboscopy, amplitude is rated as lateral displacement from the glottal midline. Greatest amplitude is seen during loud phonation in modal register unless this is accompanied by laryngeal constriction. Reduced vibratory amplitude during phonation at typical speaking pitch and effort levels is related to excessive or reduced glottal valving, low subglottal pressure, vocal fold stiffness, poor respiratory support, or a combination of those parameters. Typically, amplitude is rated with reference to modal register phonation at habitual effort and loudness level.

Amplitude Symmetry. This is the degree to which amplitude is the same for each vocal fold, regardless of phase symmetry. Amplitude asymmetry may indicate greater stiffness (due to scarring, tension or both), greater flaccidity (due to denervation), or greater mass (due to lesions) on one vocal fold.

Glottal Closure Pattern. The overall shape of closure during the most closed phase of phonation is known as the glottal closure pattern (Figure 1–26b). Possible descriptors for this characteristic include:

➤ *Complete*
➤ *Posterior chink*: commonly associated with muscle misuse, but also seen to a smaller magnitude in women without voice complaints
➤ *Anterior chink*: usually related to a structural defect

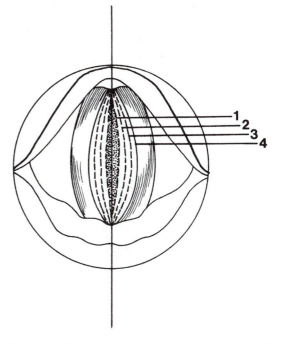

Figure 1–26a. Amplitude of vibrations: from small (most medial position) to large (most lateral position). Symmetry of amplitude should also be noted.

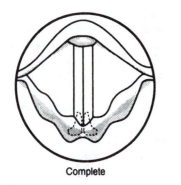

Complete

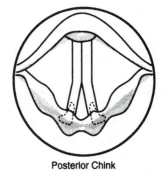

Posterior Chink

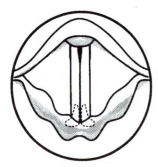

Anterior Chink

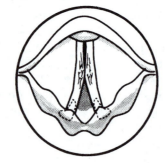

Anterior & Posterior Chink

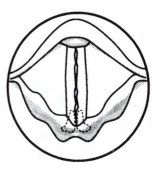

Irregular

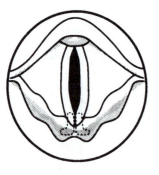

Bowed

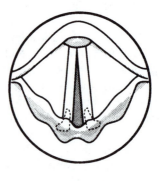

Incomplete

Figure 1–26b. Glottal closure patterns (during most closed phase) of phonation.

➤ *Anterior and posterior chink: hourglass* configuration, commonly associated with bilateral nodules

➤ *Irregular chink*: often associated with irregular vocal fold edges, scarring, and/or lesions

➤ *Bowed: spindle-shaped* configuration associated with neurogenic, psychogenic, muscle misuse, or the aging processes

➤ *Incomplete*: a v-shaped opening along the entire length of the vocal fold margins, commonly associated with paralysis or psychogenic conversion aphonia

➤ *Variable:* any combination of the above, from which any predominant one should be identified.

Mucosal Wave. The mucosal wave is the extent of the traveling wave on the vocal fold mucosal cover (Figure 1–26c). This can be seen as a line or horizontal light travelling from the medial to the lateral surface of the vocal folds. The mucosal wave is dependent on a different tissue viscosity between the mucosal cover and the stiffer muscle, ligament, and collagen layers. (See Chapter 8 for details of the vocal fold layer structure.) It is most evident during loud phonation in modal register unless this is accompanied by laryngeal constriction, but clinical judgements are made under typical pitch and loudness conditions.

It is not always easy to decide whether an immobile vocal fold is paralyzed. Observation of the mucosal wave under stroboscopic examination can be helpful in determining the presence of muscle tone or revealing the gradual return of tone. The atonic flaccid cord tends to flap in the breeze like a flag. Think of it as a "flaccid flap." On the other hand, mass-altering lesions or tissue scarring that results in tethering of the mucosa to deep lamina propria and muscle layers may result in reduced mucosal wave with associated vocal fold immobility.

Phase Closure. The ratio of open-to-closed phase during the averaged vibratory cycle is the phase closure. This can be estimated from the recorded stroboscopic video image by counting the number of video frames occupied by the most closed phase of several successive cycles, the number of frames for the complete cycle, and calculating a separate mean ratio for each condition of phonation examined to yield a *closed quotient*. Phase closure may vary considerably with pitch and loudness conditions. For this reason, it should be estimated separately for each evaluation activity. The clinical judgement for phase closure is based on observation of the phonation pattern during pitch and loudness typical for speech. Closed phase duration may be reduced by conditions limiting medial compression or arytenoid adduction, such as decreased muscle tone, large posterior glottal chinks, or paralysis. Closed phase duration may be increased by hyperkinetic behavior such as excessive laryngeal valving due to muscle misuse and psychopathology.

Phase Symmetry. Phase symmetry is the degree to which the vocal fold excursions represent mirror images of each other regardless of amplitude symmetry (Figure 1–26d). To perceive asymmetrical function, one asks whether one vocal fold leads in the opening-closing phases or if the folds are 180° out of phase. (Is one opening while the other is closing?) Vibratory movements may be out of phase to variable degrees, and we attempt to estimate the degree of consistency for this parameter. Unequal vocal fold mass, muscle tone, or position may result in phase asymmetry.

Regularity and Periodicity. This is the degree to which successive averaged oscillatory cycles resemble each other. It is assessed in phase-locked setting when the strobe is driven at the same frequency as the f_0 so that the same part of the phase is sampled for each perceptual image. In the video image, the

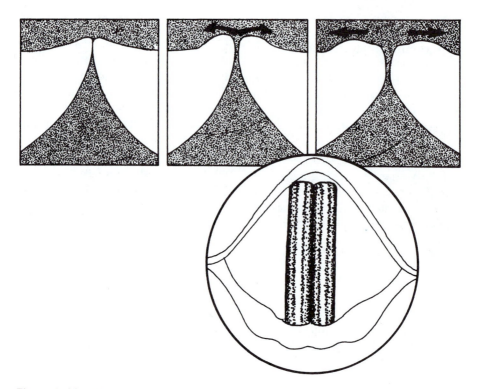

Figure I–26c. Mucosal wave: the perception of a "travelling wave" from medial to lateral on the surface of the vocal folds.

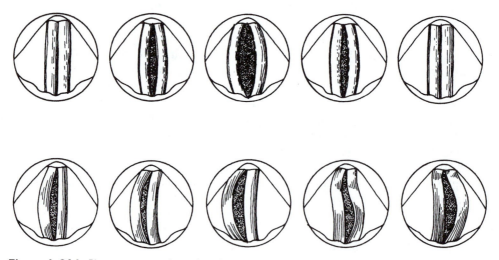

Figure I–26d. Phase symmetry (upper) and asymmetry (lower): the degree to which the vocal folds represent mirror images of each other with respect to rate of opening and closing.

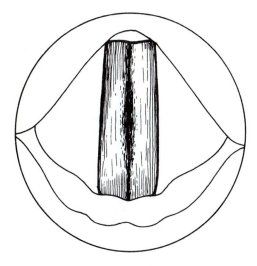

Figure 1–26e. Irregularity (aperiodicity): the degree to which the averaged cycles resemble each other, as measured with phase-locked stroboscope setting. In this case the visual image is blurred because successive cycles are different.

degree to which the image remains still or "jitters" reflects the degree of regularity or irregularity (Figure 1–26e) or percentage of time it is evident. It is important to account for variability in this characteristic based on pitch, loudness, and postural changes. Irregularity or aperiodicity in the vocal fold vibratory patterns should relate closely to measures of perturbation in the glottal source acoustic waveform. Phase asymmetry may confound perceptual judgements of regularity-irregularity, especially if the phase-locked setting is not employed.

Vertical Level of Vocal Fold Approximation. This is the degree to which the vocal folds appear to adduct in the same horizontal plane during phonation. If a discrepancy exists between the vocal fold levels while they are adducted, the closure and vibratory characteristics may be affected to varying degrees. Vocal fold approximation that is off-plane may be related to unilateral paralysis, dystonia, dislocation of the cricoarytenoid joint or laryngeal injury.

Viscosity and Stiffness: Nonvibrating Portions. This is a clinical judgement of the degree to which the vocal folds are not vibrating under normal phonatory conditions and identification of specific vocal fold regions that are not vibrating. The parameter depends on a cumulative perceptual impression based on ratings for amplitude, mucosal wave, and symmetry. Stiffness may be symmetrical or asymmetrical and may be related to muscle hypertonicity, scarring, or lesions, which will have a pervasive influence on stiffness judgements under all pitch, loudness, and posture conditions.

Supraglottal Activity. Signs of muscle misuse in the supraglottal structures should be documented as they relate to specific stroboscopic features. In addition to documenting the supraglottal pattern on anterior-posterior and medio-lateral scales (Figure 1–27), the postural misuse patterns described in Chapter 2 can be used to highlight relationships between these supraglottal activities and other muscle misuses.

1.7.3.3. Protocol for Video Laryngostroboscopic Assessment

The following is a list of tasks to be performed and recorded during laryngoscopic examination for comprehensive evaluation of vocal fold vibratory patterns. Several trials are recommended for each task so that values representing an individual's average performance can be calculated.

A. With continuous light source:

➤ Regular, quiet respiration
➤ Deep inspiration
➤ Cough and swallow
➤ Connected speech and singing
➤ Loud and soft speech and singing
➤ Sustained phonation on vowels
➤ Glissando pitch changes

Stroboscopy Evaluation Rating Form (SERF)

Bruce J. Poburka, Ph.D.

Rater: _____
Client: _____
Date: _____

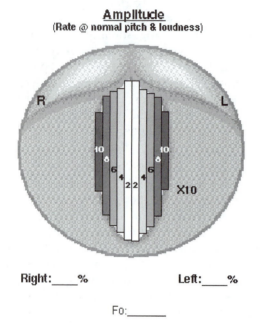

Amplitude
(Rate @ normal pitch & loudness)

Right:____%   Left:____%

Fo:_____

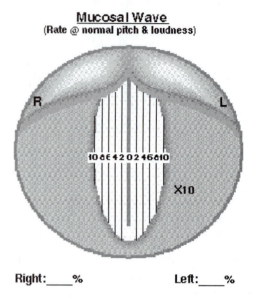

Mucosal Wave
(Rate @ normal pitch & loudness)

Right:____%   Left:____%

Fo:_____

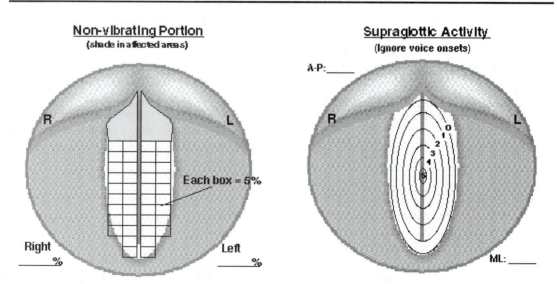

Non-vibrating Portion
(shade in affected areas)

Each box = 5%

Right   Left
____%   ____%

Supraglottic Activity
(Ignore voice onsets)

A-P:_____

ML: _____

Figure 1–27. Stroboscopy Evaluation Rating Form (SERF). Reprinted with permission, from *Journal of Voice*[57]. Copyright 1999, Singular Publishing Group, Inc.

Vocal Fold Edge Smoothness

Right Fold

0   1   2   3   4   5

smooth   rough

O circle on

Left Fold

0   1   2   3   4   5

smooth   rough

Vocal Fold Edge Straightness

Right Fold

0   1   2   3   4   5

straight   irregular

O circle on

Left Fold

0   1   2   3   4   5

straight   irregular

Rate @ normal pitch & loudness

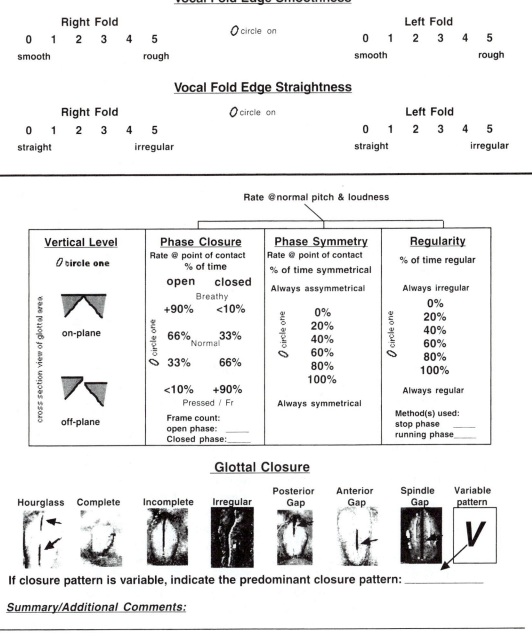

Vertical Level	Phase Closure	Phase Symmetry	Regularity
O circle one	Rate @ point of contact % of time	Rate @ point of contact % of time symmetrical	% of time regular
cross section view of glottal area.	open closed	Always assymetrical	Always irregular
on-plane	Breathy +90% <10%	0% 20% 40% 60% 80% 100%	0% 20% 40% 60% 80% 100%
	66% 33% Normal		
off-plane	33% 66% <10% +90% Pressed / Fr	Always symmetrical	Always regular
	Frame count: open phase: _____ Closed phase: _____		Method(s) used: stop phase _____ running phase _____

Glottal Closure

Hourglass   Complete   Incomplete   Irregular   Posterior Gap   Anterior Gap   Spindle Gap   Variable pattern

If closure pattern is variable, indicate the predominant closure pattern: _____

Summary/Additional Comments:

_____

_____

_____

_____

Figure 1–27. (*continued*)

B. With the stroboscopic light and the target phoneme /i/:

➤ Sustained phonation: within habitual speaking pitch and loudness range; include stroboscopic settings for apparent motion (frequency different from f_0) and phase-locked (frequency = f_0)

➤ Pitch glissandos on sustained phonation: slowly ascending and descending pitch to demonstrate maximum range parameters and all register transitions

➤ High-pitched and low-pitched sustained phonation: target several different pitches above and below habitual speaking pitch range

➤ High-intensity and low-intensity phonation: request loud-loudest and soft-softest voice

➤ Sustained inhalation phonation: used primarily when muscle misuse patterns obstruct view; especially useful if A-P contraction is obstructing view of anterior commissure or if excessive lateral contraction of ventricular folds is obstructing view of true vocal fold vibratory characteristics

➤ Probe therapy to determine potential for change with therapy techniques: coughing, pushing, nasalizing, inhalation phonation, relaxation, low or high lung volume phonation, exaggerated flow phonation (such as the sigh) are all possible during stroboscopic evaluation.

Biasing effects

Although a comprehensive assessment requires that all relevant data on history, physical status and other instrumental measures be obtained, the examiners must appreciate the biasing power that predetermined information may have on their perceptual judgements. It is conceivable that objective measures of voice function and aspects of medical and psychological history will influence the acoustic or visual perceptual judgements of preinformed examiners[58,73]. In light of the evidence for examiner bias, it is advisable to have acoustic and stroboscopy recordings rated by experienced clinicians who are not informed of a patient's history and phonatory function data so that the most reliable perceptual judgements can be obtained.

1.7.3.4. Other methods for evaluating vibratory patterns

Electroglottography. Electroglottography (EGG) is a procedure for measuring changes in electrical impedance of the glottis or the degree to which a high frequency (but low-voltage) electric current passes between the vocal folds. This is accomplished by means of two or more electrodes placed on the surface of the neck external to the larynx, with one over each thyroid lamina. Because human tissue conducts the current well but air does not, the degree of impedance is constantly changing with the degree of contact between the two vocal folds during phonation. Thus, aspects of the vocal fold contact area can be illustrated on a cycle-to-cycle basis. Perhaps the greatest clinical value derived from EGG recordings thus far is the extraction of f_0. Unless a vocal signal is very aperiodic, the rate of repetition of signals recorded with EGG provides an accurate and reliable representation of vocal f_0[5]. On the other hand, the amplitude of the signal during the high-impedance (open) phase is not directly related to acoustic amplitude or intensity. A multichannel EGG system reduces measurement artifacts and thus most accurately represents vocal fold contact area[62].

Because of the difficulties encountered in interpreting EGG, it often is combined with other measures of vocal fold vibratory patterns[3,12,19,29,48]. As a result, guidelines for interpreting EGG signals are evolving, and its usefulness and limitations are becoming better understood[74]. Certain precautions and caveats need to be observed for this measure to be used in clinical decision making[14].

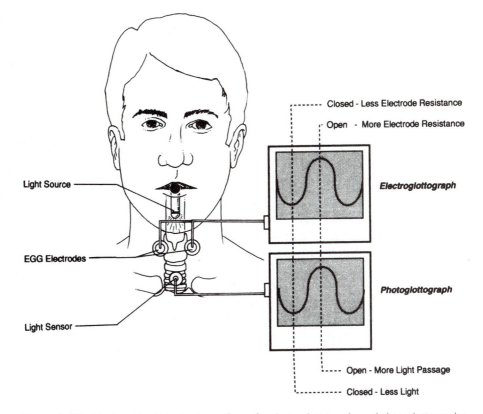

Light Source

EGG Electrodes

Light Sensor

Closed - Less Electrode Resistance

Open - More Electrode Resistance

Electroglottograph

Photoglottograph

Open - More Light Passage

Closed - Less Light

Figure I–28. Hardware and idealized waveforms for electroglottography and photoglottography.

Figure 1–28 demonstrates the placement of EGG electrodes and the nature of the resulting waveform.

Photoglottography. Whereas electroglottography provides information about vocal fold contact area and thus is based on the degree of the closing-closed phases of phonation, photoglottography (PGG) takes advantage of the degree of opening during phonation by continuously measuring the amount of light that is transmitted through the glottis. PGG is a more invasive procedure than EGG because a light and light sensor must be placed in opposition to each other, one above and one below the glottis (Figure 1–28). This probably explains why PGG is used less frequently in clinical settings.

Typically the light source for a transoral or transnasal endoscope may be used, although one study reported success with placement of a high-intensity flashlight placed in the mouth[24]. A surface light sensor may be placed in the region of the cricothyroid membrane to detect the light during glottal opening, or a sensor may be suspended under the glottis through the interarytenoid space. Photoglottography provides the raw material to make temporal estimates of vocal fold vibratory patterns, including time of opening and closing, opening-open quotients, and speed quotients. As with EGG, it provides the most useful details of phonatory function when combined with other simultaneously recorded clinical measures such as stroboscopy, EGG, and inverse filtering of acoustic or flow signals.

Flow Glottography. The inverse-filtered flow signal provides specific information about vocal fold vibratory patterns and is therefore an instrumental measure relevant to this portion of the physical examination. Its use is discussed briefly under Aerodynamic Measures (Section 1.5).

Videokymography. Stroboscopy is based on the assumption that vibration of the vocal folds is stable and regular. Irregular vibrations, which are common in voice pathology, cannot be studied easily nor described in a reliable way. Videokymography overcomes most of these drawbacks. Instead of displaying the video stroboscopic image on the monitor at 60 frames per second, a high-speed mode of nearly 8000 images per second is displayed from one line taken through the glottis and displayed on the X axis of the monitor while the Y axis represents the time dimension. Videokymography visualizes small left-right asymmetries, open quotient differences along the glottis, lateral propagation of mucosal waves, and movements of the upper margin and—sometimes during the closing phase—the lower margin of the vocal folds. Vocal fold vibration can be observed from normal vocal cords and from those affected by various pathologies. At the time of writing, this technique is in the developmental stage, and its usefulness as a standard clinical tool has yet to be established[65]. Sung et al have applied the kymography technique to conventional videostroboscopy, hybridizing the two technologies[72]. Rearrangement of one active horizontal line from successive frames of prerecorded stroboscopic images, displayed from top to bottom along the time axis, provide a static image of vibration at a specific part of the vocal folds over time. Quantitative parameters such as open quotient and asymmetry index can be calculated from the kymogram.

High-speed Link-Intensified Digital Imaging of the Larynx. This technique for investigating vocal fold vibratory movements is also becoming available in research facilities, as the constant expansion of technological possibility progresses[30].

1.8 Neurological Evaluation

Some neurological diseases have a clinical profile that includes dysphonia, but the voice disorder is not a usual first sign. Cerebrovascular diseases (stroke) or degenerative problems such as Parkinson's disease may have phonatory, speech, and language components that require specific attention. Sometimes patients with motor speech disorders present themselves to the otolaryngologist or speech-language pathologist with a voice disorder being the chief complaint. Benign essential tremor and focal laryngeal dystonia are common examples. Descriptions and classification systems for the motor speech disorders that may have voice dysfunction components are presented in Chapter 2. Application of a standarized oral mechanism examination protocol, such as the D-COME-T, described in Section 1.7.2, will help the clinician delineate the nature of and the most-likely anatomical lesion site(s) for motor speech disorders[20].

Patients with other neurological diseases will and do present to a voice clinic for initial evaluation, so the voice care team may be the first to suspect the presence of amyotrophic lateral sclerosis because of the associated early dysarthria or early presenting features of multiple sclerosis. Needless to say, a full neurological examination, particularly of the cranial nerves, is essential. For example, tongue muscle fiber fasciculation may be the earliest sign of amyotrophic lateral sclerosis in the head and neck. Referral to a neurologist of all individuals suspected of having neurological dysfunction should be made promptly.

1.8.1 Laryngeal Electromyography

Laryngeal electromyography is a procedure in which electrical activity of laryngeal muscle is recorded, and measures are made of spontaneously emitted signals and response to volitional movement. In many voice clinics, laryngeal electromyography (LEMG) is performed by the otolaryngologist and neurologist working together. The voice clinician contributes detailed knowledge about laryngeal disease and anatomy, whereas an experienced neurologist-electromyographer identifies subtle waveform changes. Koufman & Walker[44] have itemized 5 main indications for use of LEMG including:

1. *Diagnosis and prognosis of vocal fold paresis*
   Findings may include decreased recruitment and spontaneous activity with polyphasic motor unit potentials. "Recruitment" is defined as the orderly activation of the same and new motor units in response to increasing strength of voluntary muscle contraction. The spontaneous activity indicates ongoing degeneration that, in the presence of markedly reduced recruitment, means full recovery is unlikely. EMG testing can aid in establishing evidence of reinnervation activity and assist in predicting future return of function. Because many of the treatments for laryngeal paralysis are not reversible, the EMG results may influence treatment choice and timing.

2. *Site of lesion testing for vocal fold paralysis*
   If the cricothyroid muscle EMG activity is affected in addition to that of the vocal fold, the implication is that the lesion is in the vagus nerve, higher than the takeoff of the recurrent laryngeal nerve in the neck. This usually means skull-base disease.

3. *Differentiation of fixation from paralysis*
   In this situation, the vocal fold does not move but laryngeal EMG findings are normal. There is normal recruitment, normal waveform morphology, and no spontaneous activity.

4. *Diagnosis of neurological disease and laryngeal movement disorders*
   Abnormal EMG findings may be strongly suggestive of some neurological diseases, such as amyotrophic lateral sclerosis, that can produce dysarthrias. Laryngeal EMG may be supportive of a diagnosis of dystonia evidenced by high amplitude and prolonged phonatory burst, but the findings are not generally pathognomonic. It is typical to see a burst of EMG activity that precedes the onset of voice production in adductor spasmodic dysphonia. In those patients with laryngeal dystonia, the results can assist in identifying early manifestations of the disorder and help in determining the optimal injection site for botulinum toxin.

5. *Needle localization for Botox® injection*
   Although some clinicians inject botulinum toxin into the vocal fold transorally, the most commonly used technique is transcutaneous injection using the EMG as a signal for proper needle-tip location. EMG activities of the thyroarytenoid muscles, innervated by recurrent laryngeal nerves, and of the cricothyroid muscles, innervated by superior laryngeal nerves, are studied bilaterally using either monopolar or bipolar electrodes. The needle electrodes are inserted through the skin of the neck with the patient lying down comfortably. Correct placement is judged by the muscle signal observed and changes in the EMG as a result of various voluntary movements and phonation. For example, the thyroarytenoid produces a steady output during phonation whereas the lateral cricoarytenoid shows an early burst of activity at the onset of phonation followed by an easing off of the signal. Cricothyroid

muscle activity increases with pitch, and an increase in motor activity is observed when the subject ascends from low to high pitches. The posterior cricoarytenoid muscles are maximally stimulated by a "sniff."

1.9 Diagnostic Voice Therapy

Diagnostic or probe therapy seeks to specify the degree and conditions of variability for a patient's dysphonia and to establish techniques that improve the condition. Results of the probe therapy can be used to estimate prognosis for improvement in a voice therapy program. By demonstrating variability in function under controlled conditions, the diagnostic therapy process can be used to modify or eliminate the apparent significance of some organic disease processes. For example, the patient with bilateral vocal fold nodules and a large posterior glottal chink may be trained to reduce the magnitude of the chink and concurrently demonstrate measurably reduced dysphonia. In such a case, reduction of muscle misuses contributing to exaggerated PGC, rather than surgical reduction of vocal nodules, becomes the primary management goal.

Although the results of diagnostic therapy may lead us to de-emphasize significance of organic components, this is not by itself a means to confirm a psychogenic etiology (by process of elimination); rather, it may be supportive of the comprehensive psychological assessment results upon which all psychiatric diagnoses are based. In cases where persistent muscle hypertonicity seems to correspond with chronic anxiety states or other psychological manifestations, psychiatric intervention may become the primary management approach or may be initiated in conjunction with voice therapy.

In instances of long-standing muscle misuses that are secondary to psychological or organic pathologies, the diagnostic therapy program may consist of several trial treatment sessions to allow for prognosis to be determined with respect to voice therapy. The initial assessment session does not always provide the clinician with adequate time to create an atmosphere of relaxation and trust to facilitate immediate behavioral or technical changes with patients. Further, a patient's motivation and commitment in the therapy program is not always evident until the clinician can observe his or her response to the therapy program, including cooperation in practicing techniques away from the clinic.

1.9.1 Facilitation Techniques for Probe and Symptomatic Therapy

The techniques described below are used in various combinations during diagnostic probe therapy, and the successful ones may be developed further during ongoing voice therapy. Selection of probes depends on the primary clinical features of muscle misuse or vocal impairment demonstrated. When a technique targets correction of a specific sign or symptom, such as vocal fold hypoadduction or inappropriately high pitch, it is considered a symptomatic technique. A more detailed discussion on procedural aspects of voice therapy is provided in Chapter 4.

The following is a list of commonly used facilitation techniques:

➤ Adduction (forced): pushing; pulling; cough *(Do not use if mucosal edema is present.)*
➤ Articulation exaggeration; increased orality *(Beware of jaw and tongue tension.)*
➤ Auditory masking during phonation *(Do not use if mucosal edema is present.)*
➤ Breathy-flow phonation (Increase MFR.)
➤ Chanting (Decrease intonation and stress.)
➤ Chewing with phonation *(Do not use in individuals with TMJ dysfunction.)*

➤ Character voices, impersonation: eg, impersonate an opera singer, puppet voices

➤ Distraction: eg, hum while walking, turning pages, shaking head

➤ Inhalation phonation *(Do not use if paradoxical vocal fold movements are present.)*

➤ Intonation increase

➤ Loudness change *(Do not use exaggerated loudness if mucosal edema is present.)*

➤ Lung volume change: eg, low-volume: "Hm!, UmHm"; high volume: sigh

➤ Manual manipulation: eg, increase thyrohyoid space *(clinician should be appropriately trained in laryngeal manipulation techniques)*

depress larynx *(clinician should be appropriately trained in laryngeal manipulation techniques)*

hold tongue forward

hold jaw open *(Beware of TMJ dysfunction)*

➤ Pitch, register change: eg, falsetto, glottal fry

➤ Posture adjustments: eg, alter head position; supine position; lean forward, neck flexed

➤ Resonance focus adjustment (forward: humming/buzzing; backed: "covering")

➤ Simultaneous movements with speech: - eg, head nodding/shaking; shoulder rolls; rapid loose jaw movements; rapid lip or tongue movements

➤ Siren imitation

➤ Speech rate change

➤ Spontaneous phonation: extend cough, laugh, /mhm/, /hm/! *(Do not use cough extensively if mucosal edema is present.)*

➤ Tongue position change

➤ Trills: extend voiced lip or tongue trills

➤ Voice mode change: singing→speaking; speaking→singing

➤ Yawn-sigh phonation *(Beware of TMJ dysfunction.)*

Additional facilitation techniques for diagnostic therapy are listed and described in a text by Boone & McFarlane[9].

1.10 Psychological Evaluation

When the psychological examination of a patient is conducted jointly with the laryngologist and speech-language pathologist, the role of the psychiatrist is immediately made clear to the patient. The psychiatrist is an individual with particular interests in, and expertise about, psychological factors that may cause dysphonia or those that arise in consequence of having a poor voice. It helps in establishing rapport if the psychiatrist is not viewed as someone looking for signs of "insanity." It is valuable for the psychiatrist to observe the changes in a patient's voice, emotional status, and posture that may occur while the laryngologist or speech-language pathologist is taking the initial history. During the joint interview, the psychiatrist may interject to elicit additional information specific to the patient's psychological status. As a physician trained to ensure that an underlying physical condition has not been overlooked before one plunges in to the psychological realm, it is reassuring to the psychiatrist to have had the opportunity to view a videotaped image of the laryngeal examination.

The laryngologist uses the videotape to explain the significance of the findings to the patient, who then knows that the psychiatrist is aware of any lesions or lack thereof or any muscle misuses contributing to dysphonia. Where the larynx is demonstrated to be free of organic disorders but is being misused, the stage is set for review of other factors: social, psychological, and emotional.

After the other team members have completed the laryngoscopy and phonatory function measures, an individual interview by the psychiatrist is indicated. It has been our finding that patients are more forthcoming in describing personal problems in this situation. It is useful to begin the interview by reassuring patients that the idea their dysphonia is "all in their heads" is nonsense. By producing a dysphonic voice himself, the psychiatrist demonstrates that misuse of the muscles of phonation is responsible for the dysphonic voice. It is explained that although the clinician is deliberately creating this dysphonia, the patient's voice problem arises from some habitual misuse outside his or her awareness, the causes of which now need to be sought. Dependent on a patient's history, examples are offered of dysphonia resulting from the operation of infection, reflux, or overuse, coupled with a stressful social situation that did not permit the overt expression of the emotions raised by the distressing ideas.

Another example of a common psychological mechanism in symptom formation is apprehension and physical tension produced by the anticipation of a dysphonic voice when answering the telephone. With this type of introduction, some increase in rapport has usually been achieved and patients are generally receptive to the idea of looking for the factors that could have produced the dysphonia. This is especially the case when there is the mutual awareness that no structural abnormalities were found on laryngoscopy or that those identified could not account fully for the dysphonia. In those instances where the psychiatrist was not present for the initial evaluation, it is advisable to review the videotape of the laryngoscopy and any diagnostic therapy, to inform the patient that this has been done, and to establish with the patient a mutual understanding of what had been demonstrated.

Review of the history is then undertaken with particular emphasis on the patient's life situation at the start of each episode of dysphonia. In doing so, close observation is made of any changes in the patient's voice related to specific topics, especially those of emotionally charged situations or significant relationships. Depending on the circumstances, it may or may not be desirable to draw a patient's attention to changes in the dysphonia and to relate this to the topics

under discussion. Usually it is wise to wait until there have been two or three significant voice changes before making the patient aware of the connection. At this point, asking how the patient accounts for the changes will often lead to much more declarative statements about significant psychological factors. It is worthwhile pursuing any events that have impinged on the neck area, such as a thyroidectomy, being choked in a fight, or a whiplash injury sustained in a car accident, which may have occurred prior to any report of dysphonia. A patient often will say that his or her neck has long been a vulnerable area. In addition, it is useful to determine how the patient experiences stress. Dysphonic patients commonly report headaches, shoulder tension, or breathing difficulties.

The usual psychiatric history is obtained with emphasis on how the expression of emotionally charged ideas were accepted in the family of origin and in adult life, at work, or in the family of procreation. The determination of a patient's self-percept is important. Does the patient perceive himself or herself to be passive, unsuccessful, and mild mannered; or domineering, declarative and loudly successful, with no idea of how a dysphonia could possibly have arisen? Individuals falling into the latter group are unlikely to accept the operation of psychological factors in their voice disorders. How much is the patient's voice a valued, central part of his or her central identity? As D.H. Lawrence has written in his poem, "The Oxford Voice":

> When you hear it languishing
> and hooing and cooing and sidling through
> the front teeth
> the Oxford voice
> or worse still
> the would-be Oxford voice
> you don't even laugh any more, you can't . . .
> We wouldn't insist on it for a moment
> but we are
> we are
> you admit we are

superior.
Re-printed[47] with permission from Laurence Pollinger Limited and the Estate of Frieda Lawrence Ravagli.

For a professional voice user or an amateur poseur, any dysphonia strikes close to home. Voices that are indicative of significant personality traits and coping styles invariably require a peculiar use of the muscles of phonation to produce them. It is not a patient's "natural voice" if it is whining, sycophantic, bombastic, or shrill. It is, then, particularly important to determine how patients' premorbid personalities enable them to respond to the advent of a psychiatric disorder, such as a depressive illness, posttraumatic stress disorder, adjustment reaction, or anxiety disorder, to mention the most common we encounter, and how the voice becomes embroiled in an individual's response.

In conducting the direct mental status examination, attention should be paid to the attitude and general behavior of the patient, particularly with regard to voice production. To what extent is a patient's preoccupation with dysphonia at variance with the degree of the disability? It is important to note the patient's affective responses, especially those of anxiety, anger, and sadness, whether covert or overt. These emotions, if not expressed freely without conflict, are particularly likely to have an impact on phonation. Nonverbal cues, such as changes in facial expression or alterations in posture when the patient is talking about certain topics are often revealing, particularly when they are accompanied by changes in the quality, pitch, or loudness of the patient's voice. A worsening of dysphonia may be noted when certain subjects are discussed. Engaging the patient in a lively, affectively charged conversation, thus causing a distraction from the dysphonia, may lead to a significant improvement in voice, a fact that has diagnostic significance.

Having completed the full psychiatric examination including a detailed mental status examination, when indicated, it is often useful to request patients' permission to examine them for evidence of physical tension. The laryngologist and speech-language pathologist already will have examined the head and neck, larynx, oral-nasal cavities, and articulators. Palpating the short rotators of the head and evaluating the movement of the head on the neck, the freedom of neck and shoulder movements, as well as how the patient's respiration changes while this is done, provides useful supplementary information. It is uncommon for the intrinsic muscles of phonation to be misused without having a concomitant inappropriate level of tension in the auxiliary muscles of the head, neck, chest, and abdomen. After all, the larynx is suspended between the jaw, neck, and upper chest. If the intrinsic muscles are tense, the auxiliary muscles usually are too, hence the common postural abnormalities observed in dysphonic patients. It is useful to observe patients' respiration, particularly a tendency to increase intra-abdominal pressure in order to force air through constricted vocal folds. Drawing patients' attention to tightness of the abdominal wall, spasm of the pelvic floor, and rigidity of the chest gives them a much better idea of why they produce peculiar vocal sounds, especially when they are emotionally aroused but not willing to express their feelings fully.

Depending on the degree of psychological factors producing the dysphonia and the receptivity of a patient to the idea that these are in operation, comments are made promptly to the patient. In those instances where a multiplicity of factors exists or in which the patient has a distinct desire for an organic explanation for the dysphonia, little is said. Rather, the need for a conference with the laryngologist and speech-language pathologist is emphasized. In such cases, it is important that the laryngologist and speech-language pathologist provide the summary statement and be the ones to direct the treatment plan, whether it involves primary voice therapy or psychological treatment concurrent with medical procedures, voice rehabilitation, or both. It is often useful for all three professionals to be together with the patient when this is done.

1.11 Summary

Evaluation of the patient with a voice disorder is best seen as a multidisciplinary endeavour. The transdisciplinary approach provides the advantage of allowing clinicians from a variety of disciplines to cooperate in the assessment, bringing different areas of expertise and perspective to the task, while they dilute each others' reductive clinical biases. A myriad of clinical tools are available to help describe, document, and measure features of voice dysfunction, not the least of which are the clinicians' ears, eyes, and hands. In the years ahead, we will no doubt have access to increasingly refined clinical instrumentation. Nevertheless, machines can never replace the skills and perceptions of the experienced clinical team evaluating a "living-breathing-emoting-vocalizing" human.

The assessment activities described in this chapter lead to a comprehensive clinical description of an individual's voice disorder. In some cases, classification or formal diagnosis(es) can be made as a result. In the next chapter, we will explore in greater detail the classification paradigms and specific etiological bases for voice disorders that may be considered as the assessment proceeds.

References

1. Akerlund, L., Gramming, P., & Sundberg, J. (1992). Phonetogram and averages of sound pressure levels and fundamental frequencies of speech: Comparison between female singers and nonsingers. *Journal of Voice*, 6(1), 55–63.
2. Awan, N. A. (1991). Phonetographic profiles and f_0-SPL characteristics of untrained versus trained vocal groups. *Journal of Voice*, 5(1), 41–50.
3. Baer, T., Titze, I. & Yoshioka, H. (1983). Multiple simultaneous measures of vocal fold activity. In D. M. Bless, & J. H. Abbs (Eds.), *Vocal Fold Physiology: Contemporary Research and Clinical Issues* (pp. 229–237). San Diego: College-Hill Press.
4. Baken, R. J. (1987*). Clinical Measurement of Speech and Voice,* San Diego: College Hill Press.
5. Baken, R. J. (1992). Electroglottography. *Journal of Voice*, 6(2), 98–110.
6. Benninger, M. S., Ahuja, A. S., Gardner, G., & Grylaski, C. (1998). Assessing outcomes for dysphonic patients. *Journal of Voice*, 12(4), 540–550.
7. Bless, D. M. , Glaze, L. E., Biever-Lowery, D. M., et al. (1993). Stroboscopic, acoustic, aerodynamic and perceptual analysis of voice in normal speaking adults. In I. R. Titze (Ed.) *Progress report 4, 121–134,* Iowa City: National Center for Voice and Speech.
8. Bless, D. M., Hirano, M., & Feder, R. J. (1987). Videostroboscopic evaluation of the larynx. *Ear, Nose and Throat Journal*, 66(7), 48–58.
9. Boone, D. R. & McFarlane, S. C. (2000). *The Voice and Voice Therapy*, 6th Edition. Boston: Allyn & Bacon.
10. Bouchayer, M., Cornut, G., Witzig, E., et al. (1985). Epidermoid cysts, sulci and mucosal bridges of the true vocal fold: a review of 137 cases. *Laryngoscope*, 95, 1087–1094.
11. Bouhuys, A., Proctor, D., & Mead, J. (1966). Kinetic aspects of singing. *Journal of Applied Physiology*, 21, 483–496.
12. Childers, D., Naik, J., Larar, J., et al. (1983). Electroglottography, speech, and ultra-high speed cinematography. In I. R. Titze & R. C. Scherer (Eds.), *Vocal Fold Physiology: Biomechanics, Acoustics and Phonatory Control.* Denver: Denver Center for the Performing Arts.
13. Colton, R.H., & Casper, J. K. (1990). *Understanding Voice Problems,* Baltimore: Williams & Wilkins.
14. Colton, R. H., & Conture, E. G. (1990). Problems and pitfalls of electroglottography. *Journal of Voice*, 4(1), 10–24.
15. Damste, H. (1970). The phonetogram. *Practica-Oto-Rhino-Laryngologica*, 32, 185–187.
16. Daniloff, R. (1981). Airflow measurements: Theory and utility of findings. *Transcripts of the Tenth Symposium on Care of the Professional Voice.* New York: Voice Foundation.

17. Darby, J. K. (1981). Speech and voice studies in psychiatric populations. In J. K. Darby (Ed.), *Speech Evaluation in Psychiatry.* New York: Grune & Stratton, Inc.

18. Doherty, E. T., & Shipp, T. (1988). Tape recorder effects on jitter and shimmer extraction. *Journal of Speech and Hearing Research, 31*, 485–490.

19. Dromey, C., Stathopoulos, E. T. & Sapienza, C. M. (1992). Glottic airflow and electroglottographic measures of vocal function at multiple intensities. *Journal of Voice, 6*(1), 44–54.

20. Dworkin, J. P., & Culatta, R. A. (1996). *Dworkin-Culatta Oral Mechanism and Treatment System.* Nicholasville, KY: Edgewood Press.

21. Fant, G., & Lin, Q. (1988). Frequency domain interpretation and derivation of glottic flow parameters. *Speech Transmissions Laboratory - Quarterly Progress and Status Reports* 2–3, 1–21.

22. Fisher, K. V., & Swank, P. R. (1997). Estimating phonation threshold pressure. *Journal of Speech, Language, and Hearing Research, 40,* 1122–1129.

23. Fritzell, B. (1992). Inverse filtering. *Journal of Voice, 6*(2), 111–114.

24. Garratt, B. R., Hanson, D. G., Berke, G. S., & Precoda, K. (1991). Photoglottography: A clinical synopsis. *Journal of Voice, 5*(2), 98–105.

25. Gelfer, M-L. (1988). Perceptual attributes of voice: Development and use of rating scales. *Journal of Voice, 2*(4), 320–326.

26. Gill, C., & Morrison, M. D. (1997).The esophago-laryngeal reflex in a porcine model of GERD. *Journal of Otolaryngology, 27*(2), 76–80.

27. Gramming, P. (1991). Vocal loudness and frequency capabilities of the voice. *Journal of Voice, 5*(2), 144–157.

28. Gramming, P., Sundberg, J., Ternstrom, S., et al. (1988). Relationship between changes in voice pitch and loudness. *Journal of Voice, 2*, 118–126.

29. Hertegard, S., Gauffin, J., & Karlsson, I. (1992). Physiological correlates of the inverse filtered flow waveform. *Journal of Voice, 6*(3), 224–234.

30. Hess, M. M., Herzel, H., Koster, O., Scheurich, F., & Gross, M. (1996). Endoscopic imaging of vocal cord vibrations. Digital high speed recording with various systems. *HNO, 44*(12), 685–693.

31. Hirano, M. (1981). *Clinical Examination of Voice,* New York: Springer-Verlag.

32. Hixon, T. J. & Hoit, J. D. (1999). Physical examination of the abdominal wall by the speech-language pathologist. *American Journal of Speech-Language Pathology, 8*, 335–346.

33. Hixon, T. J., & Hoit, J. D. (1998). Physical examination of the diaphragm by the speech-language pathologist. *American Journal of Speech-Language Pathology, 7*, 37–45.

34. Hixon, T., Mead, J. & Goldman, M. (1976). Dynamics of the chest wall during speech production: Function of the thorax, rib cage, diaphragm, and abdomen. *Journal of Speech and Hearing Research, 19*, 297–356.

35. Hoit, J. (1995). Influence of body position on breathing and its implications for the evaluation and treatment of speech and voice disorders. *Journal of Voice 9*, 341–347.

36. Isshiki, N. (1964). Respiratory mechanism of voice intensity variation. *Journal of Speech and Hearing Research, 7*, 17–29.

37. Isshiki, N. (1965). Vocal intensity and air flow rate. *Folia Phoniatrica, 17*, 92–104.

38. Iwata, S. & von Leden, H. (1970). Phonation quotient in patients with laryngeal diseases. *Folia Phoniatrica, 22*, 117–128.

39. Jacobson, B. H., Johnson, A., Grywalski, C., et al. (1997). The Voice Handicap Index (VHI): Development and Validation. *American Journal of Speech-Language Pathology, 6*, 66–70.

40. Kitzing, P. (1985). Stroboscopy—A pertinent laryngological examination. *Journal of Otolaryngology, 14*(3), 151–157.

41. Klatt, D. K., & Klatt, L. C. (1990). Analysis, synthesis, and perception of voice quality variations among female and male talkers. *Journal of the Acoustic Society of America, 87*, 820–857.

42. Komiyama, S., Watanabe, H. & Ryu, S. (1984). Phonographic relationship between pitch and intensity of the human voice. *Folia Phoniatrica, 36*, 1–7.

43. Koufman, J. A., & Blalock, P. D. (1982). Classification and approach to patients with functional voice disorders. *Annals of Otology, Rhinology and Laryngology, 91*, 372–377.

44. Koufman, J. A., & Walker, F. O. (1998). Laryngeal electromyography in clinical practice: Indications, techniques and interpretation. *Phonoscope, 1*(1), 37–70.

45. Laver, J. (2000). Phonetic Evaluation of Voice Quality. In R. D. Kent & M. J. Ball (Eds.), *The Handbook of Voice Quality Measurement* (pp. 37–48). San Diego: Singular Publishing Group, Inc.

46. Laver, J., & Mackenzie Beck, J. (1991). *Vocal Profiles Analysis*. Queen Margaret College (Edinburgh) and University of Edinburgh Centre for Speech Technology Research, Edinburgh.

47. Lawrence, D. H. (1957). *Collected Poems, Volume 2* (p. 162). London: William Heinemann.

48. Lee, C-K., & Childers, D. G. (1991). Some acoustical, perceptual, and physiological aspects of vocal quality. In J. Gauffin, & B. Hammarberg (Eds.), *Vocal Fold Physiology: Acoustic, Perceptual, and Physiological Aspects of Voice Mechanism* (pp. 233–242). San Diego: Singular Publishing Group, Inc.

49. Lieberman, J. (1998). Principles and techniques of manual therapy: Applications in the management of dysphonia. In T. Harris, S. Harris, J. S. Rubin, & D. M. Howard (Eds.), *The Voice Clinic Handbook* (pp. 91–138). London: Whurr Publishers Ltd.

50. Lieberman, P. (1968). Direct comparison of subglottic and esophageal pressure during speech. *Journal of the Acoustical Society of America, 43*, 1157.

51. Morrison, M. (1997). A pathophysiological model for dysphonia. Proceedings from the XVI World Congress of Otolaryngology Head and Neck Surgery. Sydney, Australia, March, 1997.

52. Netsell, R., Lotz, W. K., DuChane, A. S. & Barlow, S. M. (1991). Vocal tract aerodynamics during syllable productions: Normative data and theoretical implications. *Journal of Voice, 5*(1), 1–9.

53. Nittrouer, S., McGowan, R., Milenkovic, P., & Beehler, D. (1990). Acoustic measurements of men's and women's voices: a study of context effects and covariation. *Journal of Speech and Hearing Research, 33*, 761–775.

54. Pederson, M., Munk, E., Moller, S., et al (1984). The change of voice during puberty in girls measured with electroglottographic fundamental frequency analysis and phonetograms compared with changes of androgens and secondary sex characteristics. *Acta Otolaryngologica* (Stockholm), Suppl. 412, 46–49.

55. Peppard, R. C. (1990). Comparison of young adult singers and nonsingers with vocal nodules. *Journal of Voice, 2*(3), 250–260.

56. Pinto, N. B., & Titze, I. R. (1990). Unification of perturbation measures in speech signals. *Journal of the Acoustical Society of America, 87*(3), 1278–1289.

57. Poburka, B. J. (1999). A new stroboscopy rating form. *Journal of Voice, 13*(3), 403–413.

58. Ramig, L. (1975). Examiner bias in perceptual ratings of nasality in cleft palate speakers. Master's thesis, University of Wisconsin-Madison.

59. Rammage, L. A. (1992). *Acoustic, aerodynamic and vibratory characteristics of phonation with variable posterior glottis postures*. Doctoral dissertation, University of Wisconsin-Madison.

60. Rammage, L. A., Nichol, H., & Morrison, M. D. (1987). The psychopathology of voice disorders. *Human Communication Canada, 11*, 21–25.

61. Rosen, C., Murry, T., Zinn, A., Zullo, T. & Sonbolian, M. (1999). Voice Handicap Index change following treatment of voice disorders. Paper Presented at the 28th Annual Symposium of Care of the Professional Voice; June 6, 1999, Philadelphia, PA.

62. Rothenberg, M. (1992). A multichannel electroglottograph. *Journal of Voice, 6*(1), 36–43.

63. Rothenberg, M. (1973). A new inverse-filtering technique for deriving the glottic air flow waveform during voicing. *Journal of the Acoustical Society of America, 53*, 1632–1645.

64. Rothenberg, M. (1977). Measurement of airflow in speech. *Journal of Speech and Hearing Research, 20*, 155–176.

65. Schutte, H. K., Svec, J. G., & Sram, F. (1998). First results of clinical application of videokymography. *Laryngoscope, 108*(8 Pt 1),1206–1210.

66. Shoji, K., Regenbogen, E., Yu, J. D., & Blaugrund, S. M. (1992). High-frequency power ratio of breathy voice. *Laryngoscope, 102*, 267–271.

67. Shriberg, L.D., Kwiatkowski, J. & Rasmussen, C. (1990). *Prosody-Voice Screening Profile*, University of Wisconsin-Madison. Available at: http://www.waisman.wisc.edu/phonology/, Accessed March, 2000.

68. Smitheran, J. R., Hixon, T.J. (1981). A clinical method for estimating laryngeal airway resistance during vowel production. *Journal of Speech and Hearing Disorders, 46*, 138–146.

69. Sodersten, M., & Lindestad, P-A. (1992). A comparison of vocal fold closure in rigid telescopic and flexible fiberoptic laryngostroboscopy. *Acta Otolaryngologica, 112*, 144–150.

70. Sodersten, M., Lindestad, P-A., & Hammarberg, B. (1991). Vocal fold closure, perceived

breathiness, and acoustic characteristics in normal adult speakers. In J. Gauffin, & B. Hammarberg (Eds.). *Vocal Fold Physiology: Acoustic, Perceptual and Physiological Aspects of Voice* (pp. 217–224). San Diego: Singular Publishing Group, Inc.

71. Spencer, L. E. (1988). Speech characteristics of male-to-female transsexuals: A perceptual and acoustic study. *Folia Phoniatrica, 40*, 31–42.

72. Sung, M. W., Kim, K. H., Koh, T. Y., et al. (1999). Videostrobokymography: A new method for the quantitative analysis of vocal fold vibration. *Laryngoscope, 109*, 1859–1863.

73. Teitler, N. (1992). *Examiner bias: Influence of patient history on perceptual ratings of videostroboscopy.* Master's thesis, University of Wisconsin-Madison.

74. Titze, I. R. (1990). Interpretation of the electroglottographic signal. *Journal of Voice, 4*(1), 1–9.

75. Titze, I. R. (1992). Phonation threshold pressure: A missing link in glottal aerodynamics. *Journal of the Acoustical Society of America, 91*(5), 2926–2935.

76. Titze, I. R. (1994). Principles of voice production. Englewood Cliffs: Prentice-Hall.

77. Verdolini-Marston, K., Titze, I. R., & Druker, D. (1990). Changes in phonation threshold pressure with induced conditions of hydration. *Journal of Voice, 4*(2) 142–151.

78. Warren, D. W. (1986). Compensatory speech behaviors in cleft palate: A regulation/control phenomenon. *Cleft Palate Journal, 231*, 251–260.

79. Warren, D. W. (1986). Regulation/control of speech aerodynamics. *Folia Phoniatrica, 38*, 368.

80. Yanagasawa, E., & Yanagasawa, R. (1991). Laryngeal photography. *Otolaryngology Clinics of North America, 24*(5), 999–1022.

81. Yanigihara, N., & von Leden, H. (1966). Phonation and respiration. Function study in normal subjects. *Folia Phoniatrica, 18*, 323–340.

82. Yoshioka, H., Sawashima, M., Hirose, H., et al. (1977). Clinical evaluation of air usage during phonation. *Japanese Journal of Logopedics and Phoniatrics, 18*, 87–93.

Recommended Reading:

Baken, R. J. (1996). *Clinical Measurement of Speech and Voice*. San Diego: Singular Publishing Group, Inc.

Bless, D. M., Hirano, M., & Feder, R. J. (1987). Videostroboscopic evaluation of the larynx. *Ear, Nose and Throat Journal, 66*(7), 48–58.

Dworkin, J. P., & Culatta, R. A. (1996). *Dworkin-Culatta Oral Mechanism and Treatment System.* Nicolasville, KY: Edgewood Press.

Gelfer, M-L. (1988). Perceptual attributes of voice: development and use of rating scales. *Journal of Voice, 2*(4), 320–326.

Hirano, M. (1981). *Clinical Examination of Voice.* New York: Springer-Verlag.

Hixon, T. J., & Hoit, J. D. (1999). Physical examination of the abdominal wall by the speech-language pathologist. *American Journal of Speech-Language Pathology, 8*, 335–346.

Hixon, T. J., & Hoit, J. D. (1998). Physical examination of the diaphragm by the speech-language pathologist. *American Journal of Speech-Language Pathology, 7*, 37–45.

Jacobson, B. H., Johnson, A., Grywalski, C. et al. (1997). The Voice Handicap Index (VHI): Development and Validation. *American Journal of Speech-Language Pathology, 6*, 66–70.

Journal of Voice (1987-). San Diego: Singular Publishing Group, Inc.

Koschkee, D. L., & Rammage, L. A. (1996). *Voice Care in the Medical Setting*. San Diego: Singular Publishing Group, Inc.

Koufman, J. A., & Walker, F. O. (1998). Laryngeal electromyography in clinical practice: Indications, techniques and interpretation. *Phonoscope, 1*(1), 37–70.

Laver, J., & McKenzie Beck, J. (1991). *Vocal Profiles Analysis*. Edinburgh: Queen Margaret College (Edinburgh) and University of Edinburgh Centre for Speech Technology Research.

Lieberman, J. (1998). Principles and techniques of manual therapy: Applications in the management of dysphonia. In T. Harris, S. Harris, J. S. Rubin, & D. M. Howard (Eds.). *The Voice Clinic Handbook* (pp. 91–138*)*. London: Whurr Publishers Ltd.

Poburka, B. J. (1999). A new stroboscopy rating form. *Journal of Voice, 13*(3), 403–413.

Shriberg, L. D., Kwiatkowski, J., & Rasmussen, C. (1990) *Prosody-Voice Screening Profile* (University of Wisconsin-Madison website). Available at: http://www.waisman.wisc.edu/phonology/. Accessed March 2000.

APPENDIX 1.1

Voice Handicap Index (VHI)
(Jacobson, Johnson, Grywalski, et al)[39]
Henry Ford Hospital

Instructions: These are statements that many people have used to describe their voices and the effects of their voices on their lives. Check the response that indicates how frequently you have the same experience.

	Never	Almost Never	Sometimes	Almost Always	Always
F1. My voice makes it difficult for people to hear me.					
P2. I run out of air when I talk.					
F3. People have difficulty understanding me in a noisy room.					
P4. The sound of my voice varies throughout the day.					
F5. My family has difficulty hearing me when I call them throughout the house.					
F6. I use the phone less often than I would like.					
E7. I am tense when talking with others because of my voice.					
F8. I tend to avoid groups of people because of my voice.					
E9. People seem irritated with my voice.					
P10. People ask, "What's wrong with your voice?"					
F11. I speak with friends, neighbors, or relatives less often because of my voice.					
F12. People ask me to repeat myself when speaking face to face.					
P13. My voice sounds creaky and dry.					
P14. I feel as though I have to strain to produce voice.					
E15. I find other people don't understand my voice problem.					

	Never	Almost Never	Sometimes	Almost Always	Always
F16. My voice difficulties restrict my personal and social life.					
P17. The clarity of my voice is unpredictable.					
P18. I try to change my voice to sound different.					
F19. I feel left out of conversations because of my voice.					
P20. I use a great deal of effort to speak.					
P21. My voice is worse in the evening.					
F22. My voice problem causes me to lose income.					
E23. My voice problem upsets me.					
E24. I am less outgoing because of my voice problem.					
E25. My voice makes me feel handicapped.					
P26. My voice "gives out" on me in the middle of speaking.					
E27. I feel annoyed when people ask me to repeat.					
E28. I feel embarrassed when people ask me to repeat.					
E29. My voice makes me feel incompetent.					
E30. I am ashamed of my voice problem					

P Scale _____

F Scale _____

E Scale _____

Total Scale _____

Please circle the number that matches how you feel your voice is today.

Normal		**Mild**		**Moderate**		**Severe**	
1	2	3		4	5	6	7

CHAPTER

Causes and Classifications of Voice Disorders

2.1 Introduction

The voice clinician is lead to conclusions about the cause(s) of an individual's voice disorder after **listening to, observing**, **examining,** and **describing** the patient following standard procedures as described in Chapter 1. After considering all assessment information, the clinician applies knowledge about voice function, and the various mechanisms of dysfunction to reach a conclusion about the cause(s) of an individual's voice problem. A formal diagnosis may be applied if an accepted diagnostic class or label exists (Figure 2–1).

Diagnostic labels and classification systems may serve several purposes:

➤ When based on sound empirical research, they may help us identify specific causes of a disorder.
➤ They may help group problems with similar etiologies or characteristics in a way that enhances our understanding of function and dysfunction.

➤ They may help us develop prescriptive programs of treatment based on the known factors associated with a particular diagnosis or class of disorders.
➤ They may help us determine the prognosis for the course of the disease or disorder process with or without treatment.
➤ They may help us communicate efficiently and effectively with professional colleagues.
➤ They may help access funding for patient management (eg, primary and secondary financial support programs) and for research activities.

Traditionally, voice disorders have been classified as "organic/structural" or "functional/psychogenic" based on the nature of the assumed or confirmed primary etiological factor(s). Clearly, such a simplistic classification system does little to delineate the complex and often multifactorial nature of voice disorders and, taken literally, could lead us to believe that one of two primary treatment pathways should be followed for a given individual.

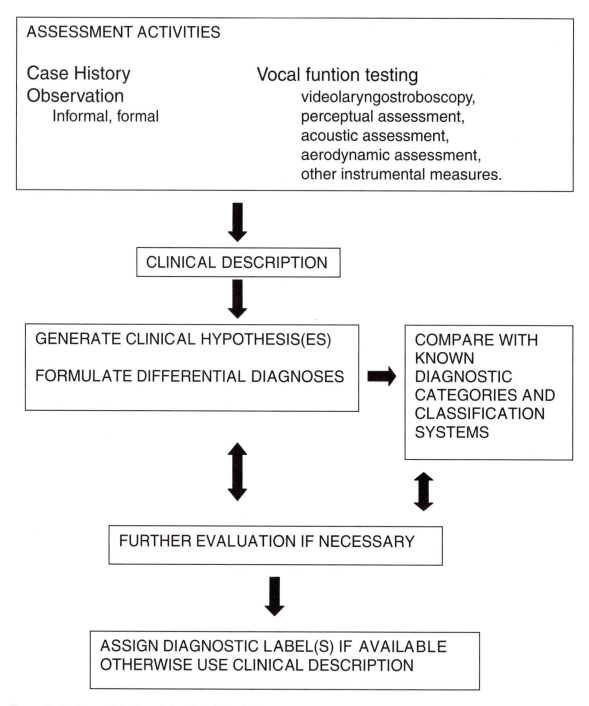

ASSESSMENT ACTIVITIES

Case History   Vocal funtion testing
Observation   videolaryngostroboscopy,
   Informal, formal   perceptual assessment,
                       acoustic assessment,
                       aerodynamic assessment,
                       other instrumental measures.

CLINICAL DESCRIPTION

GENERATE CLINICAL HYPOTHESIS(ES)

FORMULATE DIFFERENTIAL DIAGNOSES

COMPARE WITH KNOWN DIAGNOSTIC CATEGORIES AND CLASSIFICATION SYSTEMS

FURTHER EVALUATION IF NECESSARY

ASSIGN DIAGNOSTIC LABEL(S) IF AVAILABLE OTHERWISE USE CLINICAL DESCRIPTION

Figure 2–1. A model for formulating clinical descriptions, causes, and diagnostic labels for voice disorders.

Many classification systems that are commonly used to label voice disorders are not the product of sound empirical or epidemiological research, and their use is neither standardized nor validated. In some instances, clinicians are too hasty in assigning diagnostic labels to patients' voice disorders and may do a disservice by excluding the possibility of multiple causes. Following the "prescribed" treatment typically associated with an assumed diagnosis and ignoring other relevant interventions may not be efficacious. Despite these important caveats, classification schemes that emerge from many years of clinical observation and experience may help us describe an individual's voice problem, compare it with that of other patients, determine the most likely cause(s), and plan the best course(s) of action.

The process of classifying and labeling voice disorders can be influenced by a number of professional orientations and biases. Classification systems are designed to help organize and explain disorders that are known (or assumed) to originate in a particular physiological system or that generate particular signs or symptoms. Some examples of classification paradigms for disorders of speech and voice are outlined in Figure 2–2.

A comprehensive clinical description of an individual's voice disorder may require application of more than one classification scheme. From the examples in Figure 2–2, a patient might be best described under paradigms 1, 3, and 4, if he or she is found to have bilateral vocal fold nodules, identifiable psychopathology or personality characteristics that contribute to muscle misuse and vocal abuse, and specific muscle misuse patterns that contribute to dysphonia (and to the development of the nodules). This individual might then be described as having a muscle misuse voice disorder Type 1 (laryngeal isometric dysphonia) associated with a bipolar psychiatric disorder and bilateral vocal fold nodules. The order of the contributing factors reflects their relative etiological significance.

In Chapter 1, we presented a model indicating that each person's dysphonia is built over a platform that has 4 components: technique and level of vocal skill, lifestyle, psychological factors (personality and emotion), and gastroesophageal reflux. Our hypothesis is that any of these components could be a primary cause of voice disorders and that all play an etiological role in every patient's dysphonia, if only to a minor degree[51]. Each component may contribute **predisposing, precipitating, or perpetuating** factors. If an additional pathological process appears to be the primary cause the voice problem, it is felt to rest on this platform and interact with the 4 basic components. In this chapter, we will discuss ways that each platform component affects vocal function and present the array of primary pathological processes causing voice disorders. Classification systems that are relevant to voice disorders will also be described.

2.2 The Dysphonia Platform

2.2.1 Platform Component 1: Technique and Level of Vocal Skill

Poor vocal technique may be inborn and habitual. Postural-muscle misuses become densely ingrained through repetition, and central brain processing centers accept them as normal. Physical trauma or disease processes can precipitate or perpetuate muscle misuse. **Whiplash** injuries sometimes result in long-term "splinting" of neck, shoulder, throat, and jaw muscles, which contributes to muscle misuse voice disorders.

Good general posture is necessary to support good voice. Some typical postural misuses include:

➤ head and neck extension with increased cervical lordosis

BY STRUCTURAL/HISTOPATHOLOGICAL CHARACTERISTICS

Location and impact of lesion/defect:
Examples: TNM tumor classification system[2]
vocal fold layer(s) involved
Neoplastic versus Noninvasive
Example: cancer versus vocal nodules
Disease course: acute versus chronic versus progressive
Example: chronic multiple sclerosis versus progressive multiple sclerosis
Congenital versus acquired
Example: cerebral palsy versus dysarthria

BY NEUROPATHOLOGICAL CHARACTERISTICS (site of lesion and associated movement/behavioral/ perceptual features)[17-19,73]

Cerebral palsy classification (see Table 2–1)
Motor speech disorder classification (see Table 2–2)
Examples: UMN: spastic dysarthrias
LMN: flaccid dysarthrias
Extrapyramidal: hyperkinetic/hypokinetic dysarthrias
Cerebellum: ataxias
Multiple sites: mixed dysarthrias
Broca's area: apraxias

BY PSYCHOPATHOLOGICAL/PERSONALITY PROFILE

Classifications based on DSM-IV: Diagnostic and Statistical Manual
of Mental Disorders, 4th ed.[21]
Example: generalized anxiety disorder
Classifications from formal personality inventories
Example: highly extroverted, highly conscientious, low in neuroticism, low in agreeableness, moderate in
openness

BY BEHAVIORAL ETIOLOGY OR SIGNS/SYMPTOMS

Vocal abuse causes:
Example: screamer's nodules
Muscle misuse patterns: laryngeal, extralaryngeal (see Section 2.3)

Figure 2–2. Sample classification paradigms for disorders of speech production.

➤ a tightly held jaw and tongue, producing an upward pull on the larynx (Compensatory contraction of infrahyoid strap muscles may create a muscular "tug-of-war." Common signs include palpable tension and tenderness in the thyrohyoid muscles and visible hyperactivity of the omohyoid muscles with speech.)

Laryngoscopically, the muscular tension can produce various patterns, including:

➤ the laryngeal isometric with an exaggerated posterior chink[29,41,55]

➤ lateral compression of the vocal folds and a long closed phase on stroboscopy
➤ compression of the supraglottal structures with adducted false vocal folds
➤ anteroposterior compression of the supraglottal larynx drawing the epiglottis and the arytenoid cartilages together[39] (This generally accompanies thyrohyoid muscle tension.)

A classification system for muscle misuse voice problems based on the laryngoscopic features is offered in Section 2.3.

2.2.2 Platform Component 2: Lifestyle

Vocal abuses include behaviors that are typically under conscious control or that are manifestations of psychosocial conditions, personality traits, or psychopathologies. The most common vocal abuse behaviors are yelling or screaming, throat clearing, vocalizing to create special effects such as character voices, and imitating animal or engine noises. Creating certain vocal performance effects that require repeated or continuous use of extremes of loudness, pitch, or inappropriate registers can be considered abusive, as can chronic throat clearing and vocalizing in environments that are noisy or otherwise acoustically unfriendly.

Vocal overuse is a lifestyle factor that may have its origins in an individual's personality or occupational demands. Some individuals may have very vocally active lifestyles, in part because of their personality characteristics. The "extrovert" profile typically includes a tendency to seek out environments that provide opportunities to express oneself freely, entertain others, and be surrounded by sensory stimuli. Parties, restaurants, clubs, and bars serve this purpose. Occupational demands or an individual's work style and ethic may also contribute to vocal overuse and abuse. Sometimes occupational environments contribute to vocal abuse. The occupational factors contributing to voice problems are discussed in Section 2.6.

Smoking is another lifestyle factor that is particularly detrimental to vocal health.

2.2.3 Platform Component 3: Psychological Factors

Psychological factors may contribute to voice disorders through mechanisms of the voluntary and involuntary muscle systems and through the sympathetic nervous system. For example, misuse of muscles in the respiratory system and larynx may result in a quiet and monotone voice, which is commonly identified as a sign of depression. Feeling a "lump in the throat" and associated dysphonia is associated with hypertonicity in the pharyngeal constrictor muscles, which may result from gastroesophageal reflux, fear, or both. Voice disorders may be caused by dry mucosa in the vocal tract, which is sometimes caused by an anxiety response of the sympathetic nervous system. Psychological or personality disorders and unresolved emotional conflicts can result in chronic physical conditions that contribute to dysphonia. The American Psychiatric Association has provided a standardized protocol for differential diagnosis of recognized disorders of psychological and personality function: the **Diagnostic and Statistical Manual of Mental Disorders** (DSM). At the time this book was written, the current version was **DSM-IV**[21].

The voluntary muscle system is by far the most common physical mechanism through which psychological factors contribute to voice disorders. We use the words "tense" and "uptight" to refer to the body's reaction to psychological stressors. When these factors are the primary etiology of a voice disorder, a variety of muscle misuse patterns and subsequent dysphonia features may be observed. Common patterns of postural and muscle misuse are presented in Chapter 1, Section 1.6. We discussed the importance of observing signs of muscle misuse in the face that can reveal prevailing emotions, both conscious and subconscious. Psychological mechanisms may result in the use of facial muscles to inhibit emotional expression, particularly in those suppressing the urge to cry in sorrow or shout in anger. Freedom of speech and voice movements can be jeopardized by tension in the muscles of the upper, middle, and lower facial areas. The laryngeal muscle misuse patterns associated with psychogenic factors are presented in Section 2.3.

Emotional distress aggravates most voice disorders by adding muscle misuse to a system that may already be hypertonic. Even in the presence of a primary neuromuscular disorder, such as laryngeal dystonia, the voice may be normal when the individual is relaxed and symptomatic when he or she is experiencing emotional distress.

Vocal abuses may be associated with aggressive or attention-seeking personality characteristics. Certain psychopathologies, such as schizophrenia and obsessive-compulsive disorder, may also lead an individual to abuse the voice. A few researchers have investigated statistical relationships between vocal-abuse-based voice disorders and personality or psychological characteristics[10,22,26,27,30,46,49,58,79,82,84]. This research suggests strong relationships between incidence of vocal fold lesions related to vocal abuses and certain psychobehavioral characteristics including aggression, tension, frustration, argumentative behavior, poor coping skills, and disobedience.

Details on psychological assessment are provided in Chapter 1 (Section 1.10), and treatment of psychological factors is discussed in Chapter 5.

2.2.4 Platform component #4: Gastroesophageal Reflux

Gastroesophageal reflux—retrograde movement of gastric contents into the esophagus—is a transient, usually postprandial event that occurs undetected and without symptoms several times a day in healthy individuals. The disorder has to do primarily with the failure of the lower esophageal sphincter as an antireflux barrier. Gastroesophageal Reflux Disease (GERD) is characterized by a broad spectrum of clinical presentations, from simple heartburn to ulcerative esophagitis. The development and severity of gastroesophageal reflux disease is contingent on the

presence of increased frequency of reflux, increased duration of reflux, and injurious effects of gastric contents on esophageal and laryngeal mucosa.

Although nocturnal reflux has been considered a significant factor in the pathogenesis of GERD, 24-hour pH studies have shown that the majority of patients with either a mild erosive esophagitis or no endoscopic abnormality experience most reflux during the daytime postprandial periods. The progressively greater acid exposure associated with more severe esophagitis is predominantly due to an increase in nocturnal reflux. The longest period of nonbuffered basal gastric output occurs at night. This is because of both impaired clearance of acid from the esophagus and reduced neutralization by salivary bicarbonate. Sleep reduces both salivation and esophageal motility.

GERD is an important cause of both chronic laryngitis and muscle misuse. Its identification and management is essential to effective treatment of patients with voice disorders experiencing reflux, including those with only minor reflux symptoms.

GERD seems to produce increased laryngeal, pharyngeal, and esophageal muscle tone; accompanying symptoms include postnasal drip, a lump in the throat, and the feeling of a need to clear the throat. Habitual throat clearing contributes to vocal abuse and hoarseness. An irritated esophagus reflexly affects the muscles of the pharynx and larynx, causing them to be hypertonic, and the resulting muscle misuse contributes to wear-and-tear injury.

In addition to increasing laryngeal and pharyngeal muscle tone, reflux of gastric contents into the throat produces chronic inflammation. In fact, diffuse chronic laryngitis may be principally due to gastroesophageal reflux.

Typically, the posterior part of the larynx including both the posterior commissure and the interarytenoid area are diffusely reddened, and the mucosa may be hypertrophic.

If the mucous membrane overlying the arytenoid cartilage becomes ulcerated (perhaps associated with hyperfunctional voice use), then the presence of ongoing reflux of gastric acid is felt to prevent normal healing and lead to the development of a contact granuloma. Details about treatment of reflux may be found in Chapter 3.

2.3 Classification of Muscle Misuse Voice Disorders

The term "functional dysphonia" is used by many clinicians to refer to a voice disorder that is unrelated to identifiable organic disease. Unfortunately, the word "functional" is still employed by some clinicians to imply an unspecified primary psychological etiology. This is because comprehensive evaluation of a dysphonic patient with a "normal-looking" larynx that is free of organic disease will often reveal difficulties related both to vocal technique and to psychological distress or conflict. Further, habituated muscle misuse and psychogenic reactions to organic disease frequently interact to produce symptoms that might be broadly categorized under the "functional" label. Finally, habituated muscle misuse that is psychologically based or secondary to organic disease can lead to further organic disease processes (such as vocal nodules), and in such cases the "dysfunctional" aspects of a complex etiological profile may be overlooked by those with a reductive bias toward observable organic pathologies. It is apparent that voice disorders labeled "functional" are associated with laryngeal muscle misuse; because the word is intrinsically ambiguous, we use an alternative term that reflects the final common pathway of dysfunction: **muscle misuse voice disorders.**

The glottal and supraglottal shapes or postures that are noted on indirect laryngoscopy have been used traditionally to classify patterns of muscle misuse. A typical example is the historical term **"dysphonia plica ventricularis,"** in which hyperadduction of the false vocal folds is observed in the dysphonic patient. The full clinical profile typically would include several additional muscle misuses contributing to the voice problem.

Signs of organic change secondary to misuse may complicate the clinician's diagnostic task. Vocal nodules are mucosal changes known to be secondary to vocal abuse and misuse. Nodules often can be identified with a laryngeal mirror and, if assignment of a diagnosis is based solely on this readily identified clinical sign, it seems logical to label the disease process "vocal nodules." Such an approach to classification focuses on organic pathology, often out of context of an individual's habitual voice use patterns and does not allow one to differentiate among the predisposing, precipitating, and perpetuating factors involved in the etiology. The consequences for effective management are considerable. In the example of a vocal nodule diagnosis, this label may bias a clinician to focus on the organic change when planning treatment for his or her patients. If instead, the primary etiology (misuse of muscles) is implied in the diagnostic classification, as in the descriptive term **muscle tension dysphonia with acquired vocal nodules,** then management more likely will be directed appropriately toward reducing chronic dysfunctional muscle use.

In 1983, we coined the term **muscle tension dysphonia** (MTD) to describe the situation where a large posterior glottal chink was related to an overall increase in laryngeal muscle tension, more directly due to inadequate relaxation of the posterior cricoarytenoid muscle during phonation[55]. The term **laryngeal isometric** may better reflect this symptom complex because there are other misuses of the larynx that obviously are manifestations of abnormal muscle tension[29,41]. With this in mind, a currently useful classification is the following [51,54]:

1. The laryngeal isometric pattern
2. Glottal and supraglottal lateral compression
3. Anteroposterior compression
4. Incomplete adduction in conversion reaction dysphonias
5. Psychogenic bowing
6. Falsetto register in adolescent transitional voice disorders

In addition to abnormal laryngeal postures, we see other musculoskeletal misuses that contribute to dysphonia such as:

➤ poor coordination among respiratory, phonatory, resonatory, and articulatory gestures;
➤ excessive or inadequate laryngeal valving;
➤ improper resonance focus; and
➤ improper control of pitch and loudness dynamics.

The final common pathway in symptom formation for many dysphonias is misuse of the voluntary muscle systems that are employed for breathing, phonation, articulation, and resonance. Dysfunctional usage may be the result of a number of interacting factors, including all those represented in the 4 basic etiological platform components. All factors need to be taken into account before making final decisions about classification and therapy.

2.3.1 The Laryngeal Isometric Pattern

The laryngeal isometric pattern is most commonly seen in untrained occupational and professional voice users including singers, teachers, actors, media personnel, and sales representatives. It represents a generalized increase in muscle tension throughout the larynx and in paralaryngeal structures. The etiology usually includes a combination of poor vocal technique, extensive and extraordinary voice use demands, and interacting or secondary psychological factors. Anxiety is most commonly identified, and in some cases, the diagnosis of generalized anxiety disorder is made based on criteria listed in the DSM-IV[21]. Psychological components may be secondary to dysphonia rather than a primary etiological factor, and this implies a perpetuating influence in sign-symptom formation. In instances where psychological factors clearly play a role in muscle misuse symptom formation we, as voice care clinicians, might do our professions and our patients a great service by adopting a psychosomatic approach to diagnostic classification and treatment of the problem. In psychosomatic medicine, the focus is on social and psychobiological factors that precipitate organic disease. In such a situation, a descriptive diagnosis would reflect the etiological significance of these factors, for example *generalized anxiety disorder with associated laryngeal isometric dysphonia and bilateral nodules.*

A key feature of the isometric pattern of laryngeal and paralaryngeal hypertonicity is the role of the posterior cricoarytenoid muscle (PCA) in abducting the glottis. The histological structure of the PCA appears to be well adapted to this role. For example, it has more type 1 muscle fibers than all other intrinsic laryngeal muscles[45]. Type 1 muscle fibers are responsible for by relatively slow-rising but prolonged contractions. Thus, when the larynx is in a general hypertonic state, the sustained contraction of the PCA may deflect the arytenoid cartilages down the cricoarytenoid joint and open the posterior commissure, creating a posterior glottal chink (PGC). This hypothesis was supported by a laryngeal muscle pull experiment that we performed in 1983[6]. Dissected fresh human cadaver larynges were held in a frame with the intrinsic muscles attached to strings pulled in the direction of the muscle contraction. It was easily seen that when the glottis was closed with firm lateral cricoarytenoid and interarytenoid muscle pulls, it took only a light traction on the PCA to open the posterior chink in such a way as to produce the glottal shape seen in this group of patients (Figure 2–3). PGC magnitude also may be associated with hypertonicity in suprahyoid musculature[53].

Studies of clinical populations and normal subjects simulating muscle misuse dysphonias have demonstrated that magnitude of the PGC is directly related to phonatory airflow rate, whispery-breathy perceptions, spectral noise, and distinctive intensity profiles in the acoustic spectra[50,53,62,64]. In clinical populations, other forms of muscle misuse, such as lateral contraction states that can confound aerodynamic and acoustic profiles, may accompany the laryngeal isometric. Disease of the vocal fold mucosa often is identified as a component to the diagnosis and generally assumed to be secondary to the specific pattern of muscle misuses associated with the laryngeal isometric posture.

In cases of tense or very loud phonation, particularly in the presence of hypertonic vocal folds, shearing stresses can injure the delicate tissue of the superficial lamina propria, leading to edema, hemorrhage, or fibrosis. These stresses tend to lead to the development of midmembranous vocal nodules most commonly identified in premenopausal women and prepubertal children. These are also the clinical subgroups that demonstrate the largest PGC magnitudes and widest interarytenoid spaces relative to vocal fold length[55,62]. The posterior margin of the nodules corresponds to the anterior margin of the PGC.

This leads one to hypothesize a specific causal relationship between PGC magnitude and bilateral nodules. Perhaps strong adduction forces employed to overcome exaggerated abduction in the posterior glottis lead to greater shearing stresses on the midmembranous vocal folds at the position where nodules typically develop. Further, lack of adduction posterior to the midmembranous vocal folds would inhibit development of the mucosal disease there. Subepithelial edema or polypoidal degeneration is the usual form of secondary organic disease found in postmenopausal females, particularly in those who smoke. There is evidence that PGC

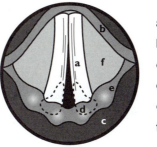

a vocal fold

b epiglottis

c hypopharynx

d arytenoid cartilage

e aryepiglottic fold

f false vocal fold

Figure 2–3. The laryngeal isometric. Generalized tension in all laryngeal muscles often is associated with an exaggerated posterior glottal chink due to persistent posterior cricoarytenoid muscle pull during phonation. This often leads to secondary mucosal lesions, including nodules, chronic laryngitis, or polypoid degeneration.

magnitude and age in women are inversely related[62,64]. This could provide some explanation for the mucosal disease posterior to the typical nodule site in the older female population. Most adult males will develop a diffuse thickening of the cover that is referred to as "chronic laryngitis." Because males have a laryngeal structure that allows for greater closure of the posterior glottis and indeed PGC magnitudes are generally much smaller in the postpubertal male population, it is not surprising that secondary mucosal disease is more diffuse.

The laryngeal isometric frequently is associated with palpable increases in suprahyoid muscle tension on phonation particularly in higher pitch ranges during singing and during high vowels and phoneme transitions in connected speech. Elevation of the larynx in the neck and mandible extension may be observed as the patient ascends a sung scale. "Jaw jut" describes the frequently seen posture that results from simultaneous extension of the neck and mandible.

2.3.2 Lateral Compression

This dysfunctional pattern is a type of tension fatigue syndrome in which the larynx tends to be hyperadducted in a side-to-side direction. It may exist at the glottal level, the supraglottal level, or both. The glottal form usually is related to technical errors, but sometimes acute anxiety states may be identified. By contrast, supraglottal compression (or *plica ventricularis*) is often associated with ongoing psychogenic factors.

2.3.2.1. Subtype A: Glottal Compression

Speech associated with hyperadduction of the vocal folds typically is characterized by a harsh or strident voice quality and aggressive voice onsets (*glottal attacks*; Figure 2–4). Phonation is associated with high laryngeal resistance that explains why patients complain of vocal fatigue and discomfort at the end of a working day. In some situations, an organic illness such as an upper respiratory infection triggers the problem, but persistent hoarseness remains many weeks after the viral illness has resolved. Koufman and Blalock have used the term "habituated hoarseness" to note this relationship[39].

Lateral compression of the vocal folds generally is accompanied by incoordinate breathing, which requires that the larynx function as a valve to control expiratory airflow. As discussed in Chapters 1 and 8, proper speech breathing is associated with a degree of inspiratory muscle activity during exhalation. This

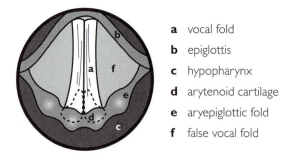

a   vocal fold

b   epiglottis

c   hypopharynx

d   arytenoid cartilage

e   aryepiglottic fold

f   false vocal fold

Figure 2–4. Lateral compression at the glottal level. This frequently is seen with generalized postural misuses and tension. It may be triggered by an infection or chronic gastroesophageal reflux.

normal action creates a push-pull mechanism in the abdominal and thoracic areas to maintain steady flow of air through the trachea. In other words, the larynx is not normally required to function as a flow regulator, as is seen when speech breathing is inappropriate.

Laryngoscopy with stroboscopy will show a prolonged closed phase, reduced vibratory amplitude, and suppression of the mucosal wave in those with lateral glottal compression. Associated ventricular fold adduction may be seen to a limited degree. It may be important to differentiate between primary glottal level compression and primary supraglottal compression because relegation of a patient to the supraglottal contraction category may carry a stronger inference of psychogenic etiology[53].

The glottal form of lateral compression dysphonia can be primarily due to poor vocal habits, posture, and technique. In this instance, the therapy goals are reduction of identified phonatory misuses, because specific psychopathological processes are not usually as evident as in the supraglottal adduction pattern described below.

2.3.2.2. *Subtype B: Supraglottal Adduction*

This pattern is characterized by movement of the ventricular folds toward the midline. It tends to predominate in psychogenic dysphonia[53]. It can exist either with tightly adducted true vocal folds, leading to a high-pitched squeaky voice, or with loose, partially abducted vocal folds, in which case the voice is breathy or a tense whisper (Figure 2–5). In the latter situation, the tips of the arytenoids are brought together, leaving a gap between the loose membranous cords, as well as a triangle between the arytenoid bodies. The anterior gap may not be seen because of adduction of the ventricular folds, which if almost complete may only reveal the small whisper-port posteriorly.

A supraglottal compression pattern is sometimes compensatory to glottal incompetence, such as that created by sulcus vocalis, senile atrophy of the vocal folds, or vocal fold paralysis. In some cases, it may contribute to dysphonia; in other cases, adduction and phonation of the ventricular folds may contribute a desired (if not ideal) sound source. In some rare instances, supraglottal adduction may be intentional, when an individual uses the ventricular folds as a voice source. This might be trained in individuals who have congenital or acquired glottal incompetence that cannot be adequately treated with surgery.

When the voice is strident or squeaky, it may be difficult to identify whether the sound is generated by adducted ventricular

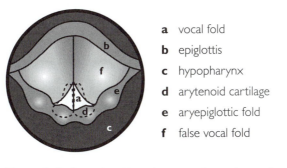

a	vocal fold
b	epiglottis
c	hypopharynx
d	arytenoid cartilage
e	aryepiglottic fold
f	false vocal fold

Figure 2–5. Supraglottal lateral compression or hyperadduction of the false vocal folds. This often is psychologically based.

folds (actual false fold phonation), tightly adducted true folds obscured by supraglottal structures, or true and false folds functioning together as a unit to create the voice. The latter two situations are more likely because in most cases the ventricular folds do not adduct fully to the midline.

In our experience, the lateral supraglottal compression pattern seen on laryngoscopy in patients who do not have glottal incompetence is usually associated with unresolved psychological conflict[53]. Conscious or unconscious repression of anger or sadness is common in depressed patients, and primary or secondary gain may be accrued because of the presence of the voice disorder. Therapy approaches must combine correction of specific misuses with a careful evaluation and management of the psychological factors. It is in this area that the advantages of a joint approach within a multidisciplinary voice clinic—encompassing laryngology, speech-language pathology, and psychiatry or psychology—are most obvious.

2.3.3 Anteroposterior Supraglottal Compression

Koufman and Blalock have presented a voice type labelled "Bogart-Bacall Syndrome," in which patients exhibit a tension-fatigue dysphonia with phonation at the bottom of their vocal dynamic ranges[39]. They describe a contraction pattern that results in reduced space between the epiglottis and the arytenoid prominances in the anteroposterior direction during phonation (Figure 2–6). Individuals using this posture complain of effortful voice and rapid fatigue when speaking at a low pitch, but they are able to talk more clearly and freely at a higher pitch. This kind of voice can be "put on" by those wishing to get a particular effect of authority or sultriness; as a result it is often present in the speech of vocal performers. Singers may exhibit a similar anteriorposterior contraction pattern on phonation in association with tense pharyngolaryngeal postures. This pattern may be used to achieve a particular resonance quality, an example of which is native North American throat singing, but in other singers it may be unintentional and secondary to technical error. Some singing teachers are beginning to use transnasal flexible videolaryngoscopy with their students to provide instant visual feedback that enables them to avoid or create this contraction pattern.

This laryngoscopic pattern is not readily seen with mirror examination or with the rigid telescope because the tongue pull may extend the aryepiglottic length. Transnasal fiber-optic examination during connected speech or singing is the most effective way to demonstrate this misuse. Koufman and

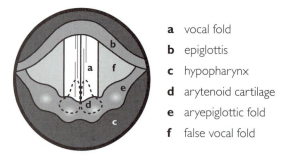

a vocal fold
b epiglottis
c hypopharynx
d arytenoid cartilage
e aryepiglottic fold
f false vocal fold

Figure 2–6. Anteroposterior supraglottal compression. This is a common technical misuse seen in mild, moderate, and severe forms.

2.3.4 Incomplete Adduction in Conversion Aphonia or Dysphonia

The psychological stressor or conflict that leads to a conversion reaction has produced such mental pain that a physical symptom such as aphonia is more bearable to the individual[22,63]. The type of psychological stressors and resulting muscle misuse pattern differ from those associated with other muscle misuse voice problems. In conversion disorder, the misuse may be beyond the patient's awareness, hence the typical *la belle indifference* affect and facial expression. The vocal folds have full movement and can adduct normally for cough or other types of vegetative phonation such as laughter, but they stop short of sufficient adduction for voicing (Figure 2–7). Generalized hypertonicity can be identified in the larynx; when sound does come out, it is usually high pitched and strident or breathy.

2.3.5 Bowed Vocal Folds Associated with Psychogenic Dysphonia

In older patients, presbyphonia is associated with loss of muscle bulk and tone, as well as weakening and fragmentation of elastin and collagen fibers. This often results in a bowed glottal closure configuration. This so-called *senile atrophy* is not necessarily the principal dysphonia factor in patients who have bowed vocal folds (Figure 2–8). Occasionally, patients who appear to have a psychogenic dysphonia will phonate with a bowed glottis but may resume normal phonation and laryngoscopic appearance after voice therapy, psychotherapy, or both. This also may represent one of the forms of dysphonia in "habituated hoarseness" that follows an upper respiratory tract infection or other organic trigger[39].

2.3.6 Falsetto Register in Adolescent Transitional Voice Disorder

Normal adolescent voice change during puberty often is accompanied by pitch breaks, register breaks, and a degree of embarrassment. Psychological factors may lead to inhibition of the transitional event and establishment of perpetual falsetto phonation. Laryngoscopy reveals laryngeal hypertonicity and the cartilaginous glottis may be hyperadducted, restricting phonation to the anterior membranous vocal folds (Figure 2–9). The larynx generally is elevated by suprahyoid muscle contraction so it approximates the hyoid bone or base of tongue. Downward traction on the

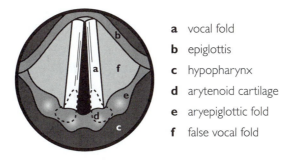

a   vocal fold

b   epiglottis

c   hypopharynx

d   arytenoid cartilage

e   aryepiglottic fold

f   false vocal fold

Figure 2–7. Incomplete vocal fold closure along the entire glottis in the absence of organic or neurological disease, typically is associated with conversion reaction aphonia.

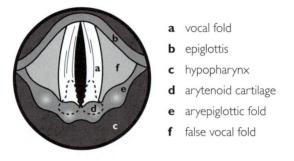

a vocal fold

b epiglottis

c hypopharynx

d arytenoid cartilage

e aryepiglottic fold

f false vocal fold

Figure 2–8. Vocal fold bowing caused by muscle misuse.

thyroid cartilages sometimes results in modal register phonation at a pitch that is more representative of the adult male voice. A detailed case presentation of adult transitional voice disorder is presented in Chapter 4.

2.4 Organic Disorders

2.4.1 Tumors

Tumors tend to produce an indolent, slowly progressive hoarseness, and some patients who are hoarse worry about cancer. In reality, the assurance that there is no cancer present may be all that the patient needs or wants.

Laryngeal tumors may be benign or malignant. A full discussion of this topic is well beyond the scope of this book. The reader wishing more detail should refer to one of the many current references on this topic, but a few general comments are in order.

Laryngeal papilloma is a benign, warty grow that is more common in children than adults and is linked to the human papilloma virus. It is thought that the larynx becomes infected during birth, and treatment generally consists of repeated laryngoscopic laser excision.

The most common malignant tumor in the larynx is squamous cell carcinoma affecting

the glottis. The typical patient with cancer of the vocal fold is a man in his 60s or 70s with a harsh, raspy or breathy voice that came on insidiously. He is almost always a long-time smoker. When laryngeal cancer is suspected, referral to an otolaryngologist is essential. Squamous cell carcinoma can be diffuse or localized, keratotic or erythematous, exophytic or ulcerative; it can appear hard or soft, and may confuse the examiner. A high index of suspicion is necessary to maximize cancer identification.

Airway obstruction and neck nodal metastases usually are not associated with early cancer of the glottis but may develop if the disease is allowed to progress. When neck nodes or airway obstruction accompany the early presenting features, the primary tumor may have started in the supraglottic larynx or hypopharynx, where it can reach a considerable size before symptoms develop.

2.4.2 Infection

Inflammation of the larynx with erythema (redness) and swelling of the mucosal membranes commonly accompanies an upper respiratory tract infection. A typical case is presented in Chapter 3 to illustrate treatment for **viral laryngitis**. There are three main groups of viral infection in the upper aerodigestive tract.

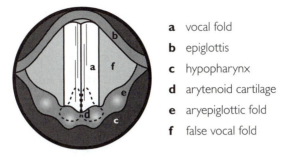

a	vocal fold
b	epiglottis
c	hypopharynx
d	arytenoid cartilage
e	aryepiglottic fold
f	false vocal fold

Figure 2–9. The laryngeal posture for falsetto register phonation typically seen in adolescent transitional voice disorder.

1. The *common cold* viruses principally cause inflammation in the lining of the nose and sinuses. In most cases, the degree of actual laryngitis is slight, but laryngeal edema and consequent hoarseness occasionally accompany the common cold.

2. *Adenoviruses* are the usual culprit in cases of severe sore throat, accompanied by fever, pain on swallowing, tender lymph nodes in the neck, and swollen, red tonsils. As with the common cold, there may be mild hoarseness, but communication is not usually impaired.

3. The organisms that cause *laryngo-tracheo-bronchitis* are often the *influenza* or *parainfluenza viruses*. This is the type of illness that produces the most severe voice change and a sudden curtailment of vocal performance. In children, laryngeal edema leads to narrowing of the airway just below the vocal folds, resulting in inspiratory stridor or croup. Although similar severity of inflammation occurs in adults, the larynx is big enough to avoid obstruction, but the hoarseness, cough, and general misery can be intense. This common illness results in a low pitched, often breathy voice with pitch or phonation breaks or even aphonia. Physical examination shows a thickened, red tra-

cheal and subglottal mucosa. The inflammatory changes may be easier to see in the subglottis than in the vocal folds themselves. This adult variant of the childhood type of laryngotracheitis is probably the most common cause of voice loss due to infection of the larynx.

Bacterial infection may occur primarily, or it may be secondary to a viral illness. The erythema tends to be more severe and accompanied by pain and fever. There may be thick, purulent discharge or ulceration. Bacterial infection with pathogens such as *streptococcus* or *staphylococcus* may produce subglottal thickening and some airway narrowing, as well as severe hoarseness. Supraglottitis caused by *hemophilus influenzae* can lead to major airway emergencies.

In rare cases, **tuberculosis** can affect the larynx, usually secondary to a pulmonary infection. Examination reveals what appear to be fairly smooth subepithelial pale nodules variably located around the supraglottic larynx.

Fungal infection of the larynx is quite common. The usual cause is *Candida Albicans* (Monilia) introduced by regular use of corticosteroid inhalers, particularly in the presence of diabetes or immunological abnormalities. Numerous white flecks of fungal colonies usually scatter themselves around the arytenoid area, aryepiglottic folds, and epiglottis. Thicker, white, keratotic-looking plaques may occur on the vocal folds themselves and be mistaken for dysplastic or malignant lesions. This association with surrounding typical monilial colonies is the giveaway and the vocal fold lesions will disappear with antifungal therapy.

2.4.3 Chronic Noninfective Laryngitis

Chronic inflammatory changes in the glottis can be the result of **smoking**, **allergy**, **gastroesophageal reflux**, or **vocal abuse**. These changes may lead to the development of *nodules* or *polyps* at the middle portion of the vibrating vocal fold or to generalized diffuse thickening of the epithelium and underlying connective tissue.

These diffusely thickened vocal folds may be further affected by **keratosis** or **leukoplakia** (meaning "white plaques"). In this situation, the irritative processes lead to disruption of the normal epithelial maturation and may have malignant potential. This is not to imply that nodules resulting from chronic voice abuse in a singer, or in a child with "screamer's nodules" have any chance of becoming a cancer, but it illustrates the wide range of causes and pathologic processes that may lead to glottal mucosal thickening and the resultant dysphonia.

Although **seasonal allergies** may cause hoarseness similar to that accompanying a cold, it is surprising that this is not a common problem. Even patients with significant nasal allergies or asthma have a low incidence of voice problems. The severity of other allergic signs and symptoms should help identify which patients are suffering dysphonia of allergic cause.

Repeated vomiting associated with **bulimia nervosa** can also produce chronic laryn-

gitis, and this possibility should be considered in dysphonic adolescent females[52].

2.4.4 Mucosal Changes Caused by Misuse and Abuse

Misuse and abuse of the voice can result in wear and tear on the vocal folds with development of epithelial thickening, termed variably "vocal nodules," "polyps," or "chronic laryngitis." The term **misuse** implies that vocal technique is faulty and the true vocal folds, which are made up of voluntary muscle, are forced to vibrate under undue stress and tension. To produce a clear, effortless tone, the vocal folds must be adducted without too much force so that expiratory flow can serve to sustain vibration, rather than force apart a tightly closed valve. A common misuse involves tight glottal adduction and forceful expiration, leading to muscle fatigue, as well as inflammation produced by the shearing stresses on the vocal folds.

Vocal **abuse** refers to exuberant overuse of the voice from such activities as excessive singing, loud talking (especially in noisy places), shouting, cheering, and so forth. People who abuse their voices often tend to have muscle misuse as well, and the cumulative effects can be exponential. Vocal fold changes occur more rapidly with vocal abuse in the presence of misuse, compared with those whose habitual vocal technique is more "correct"[23]. Vocal nodules may be a sign of vocal misuse and abuse, rather than being the primary problem. The presence of nodules does not necessarily mean they should be removed. If the misuse and abuse are controlled, nodules often resolve. Even if the nodules persist, the patient's voice problems may resolve, and the presence of nodules may cease to be an issue. Relevant case studies and figures of vocal fold lesions secondary to muscle misuse and vocal abuse are presented in Chapters 3 and 4.

2.4.5 Laryngeal Trauma

External trauma to the larynx, such as that which may occur in a motor vehicle accident, can result in laryngeal disorganization or scarring, producing voice alterations. Nonetheless, this is relatively uncommon and usually does not present a diagnostic dilemma. Internal trauma to the vocal folds from surgical treatment or intubation is more frequent, however, and often can be overlooked. Although direct injury to vocal folds at the time of intubation for a surgical procedure is unusual, its voice effects can be severe, particularly if the patient is an occupational or professional voice user. Physicians who are planning to pass an endotracheal tube in a patient who relies on voice for income should discuss this possibility with the patient beforehand, use the smallest tube that is sufficient for adequate ventilation, and take available measures to prevent injury. Injury may occur from subluxation of the cricoarytenoid joint or tearing of the vocal cord structure, if the tip of an endotracheal tube catches in the laryngeal ventricle and then is pushed against this resistance. When this occurs, it tends to be in a situation in which the intubation is a life-saving measure, and a subsequent voice problem initially is not high on the list of concerns.

Another major cause of internal laryngeal injury is excessive removal of mucosa or glottal tissue at the time of surgical treatment of disease, whether benign or malignant. It was relatively common in the past to see well-healed, white vocal folds in a woman still complaining bitterly about a harsh, squeaky voice several months after surgical "stripping" of glottal mucosa. Any resultant scar on the vocal fold can inhibit normal vibration and leave the patient with an unpleasant dysphonic voice. Stroboscopic examination now readily shows the damage that was done: tethering of the mucosa to the deeper vocal fold layers and stiffness of the fold through scar formation that accompanies re-epithelialization. Happily, surgical techniques have changed so that, with mucosa sparing procedures, this problem is less common. Of course, it is an expected and accepted side effect of endoscopic removal of neoplastic diseases.

2.4.6 Contact Ulcer and Granuloma

Contact ulcers and granulomas in the larynx are inflammatory lesions that occur over the vocal processes and medial surface of the arytenoids in the posterior larynx. They usually are unilateral, but bilateral lesions do occur. In the typical case, the contact granuloma occurs in someone who is suffering from gastroesophageal reflux disease and has a habitually aggressive style of voice use. A less common variety of this disorder is the true postintubation granuloma, which is usually bilateral. Management of contact granulomas may entail biopsy early in the course of treatment but generally centers on reflux management and close follow-up because the granuloma may resolve spontaneously under this therapy. Chapter 3 includes a relevant case study and figure of contact granuloma.

2.4.7 Cysts, Sulci, and Mucosal Bridges

Mucosal changes not directly related to muscle misuse and vocal abuse, such as intracordal cysts and vocal fold sulci, were not well recognized until video magnification and stroboscopic study of vocal fold vibration enhanced the ability to examine the larynx. Bouchayer et al described these lesions as representing a spectrum of disorders related to abnormal embryological development[7]. Hypothetically, cysts are caused by a failure of development that leaves a remnant of mucosa in Reinke's space below the "normal" mucosal cover. The cyst that develops in Reinke's space often contains a white, mucoid substance and has a delicate mucosal lining. The overlying vocal fold mucosa is usually loosely adherent to the cyst, but the cyst is densely stuck to the underlying lamina propria (Figure 2–10).

The lesion can also be open to the laryngeal lumen as a sinus or "sulcus vocalis." An overlying flap of mucous membrane may be present that makes the sulcus difficult to see even with videostroboscopy. Commonly only the densely stuck deep part of the sulcus exists, and this is observed as a groove along the free edge of the fold. Bouchayer referred to this as "sulcus vergeture"[7] (Figure 2–11). Although in regular light the folds look bowed, stroboscopic exam clearly shows the sulcus is tethered to the underlying vocal ligament. In Western Canada, this lesion seems to be prevalent in the population from the Indian subcontinent.

2.4.8 Congenital and Acquired Webs

Webs at the anterior commissure of the vocal folds are typically congenital but also can occur following surgery or other treatments that ablate tissue at the anterior commissure, particularly if the intervention was bilateral (Figure 2–12). The web illustrated in Figure 2–12 formed following laser ablation of anterior commissure laryngeal papilloma. Although webs may often look simple and thin, the thinness is usually only found at the posterior free margin of the web. Anteriorly they splay superiorly and inferiorly into a thick base that includes a firm fibrous core. This makes what should seem to be an easy endoscopic division likely to fail and necessitates special procedures for successful ablation. By contrast, the mucosal microweb that, until the advent of video stroboscopic examination techniques, was not seen or deemed important, may produce a subtle loss of vocal power and can be dealt with by a simple "snip". Large webs are obvious and produce significant degrees of hoarseness and if extensive can also cause airway obstruction.

2.4.9 Cricoarytenoid Joint Problems

The synovial cricoarytenoid joints may be subject to the same arthritic problems that affect other joints, although involvement is remarkably uncommon in rheumatoid disease. Most joint mobility difficulties are related to intubation trauma, either from prolonged intubation or acute injury producing subluxa-

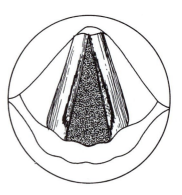

Figure 2–11. Sulcus vocalis vergeture. The mucosa is densely adherent to the fibrous layer of the lamina propria and does not vibrate well.

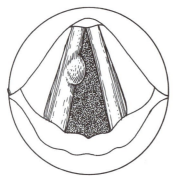

Figure 2–10. Intracordal cyst of the left vocal fold.

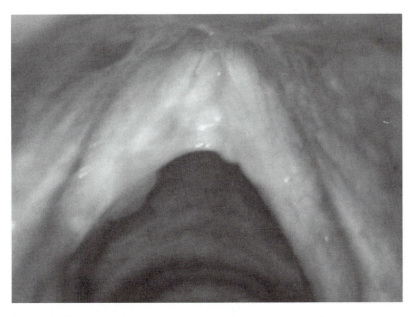

Figure 2–12. An acquired anterior glottic web that developed after repeated laser excision of laryngeal papilloma. A small persistent papilloma can be seen below the free edge of the left vocal fold.

tion. The subluxed arytenoid is asymmetrically positioned, and the vocal process is more anterior and inferior compared with the normal side. The ipsilateral vocal fold appears shorter and thicker and may look bowed.

Chronic gastroesophageal reflux can also promote periarticular inflammation and fibrosis that can stiffen the joint and limit mobility. Laryngological examination will reveal erythema of the posterior glottis and limited excursion, with or without ulceration or granulation tissue medial to the arytenoid cartilage.

2.5 Neurological Factors: Motor Speech Disorders

Speech and voice disorders that are related to neurological disease or dysmorphology are **motor speech disorders** and are broadly classified as **dysarthrias** and **apraxias.** They may be congenital or acquired.

Congenital and early-childhood motor speech disorders are typically associated with **cerebral palsy (CP).** This is a general term encompassing a variety of neuromotor disorders that are caused by nonprogressive lesions in the developing brain or disruption in brain development. CP affects mobility, posture, and balance. These motor-control problems can affect speech and voice development in indirect and direct ways. First, a child's inability to independently explore the environment deprives him or her of essential input and motivation to learn to communicate. Second, motor weakness or incoordination may affect speech and voice muscles directly, making it difficult for a child to develop the fine motor movements associated with vocal communication. Because of the effects of the developing brain on motor skills, the physical manifestations of CP often change with time.

Acquired motor speech disorders are caused by lesions in the brain or peripheral nervous system resulting from traumatic brain injury, cerebrovascular accidents (CVA; strokes), chronic and degenerative neuromuscular diseases (e.g., multiple sclerosis; amyotrophic lateral sclerosis), iatrogenic causes (e.g., surgery that requires sacrificing a peripheral nerve), or viral and infectious illnesses. They are often associated with dysfunction of similar nature in other parts of the body; for example an individual suffering a CVA in the cerebral motor strip may experience spasticity and weakness that affects arm, leg, and facial movements, as well as speech.

Classification systems for motor speech disorders have been developed and used clinically for many years. They are based on well-documented associations between specific neurological lesion sites and their effects on motor activities, including those of speech.

The classification system that has evolved for describing CP and its associated impairments is based on 3 primary parameters: severity, physiological state related to site of lesion, and extent and location of motor impairment. Table 2–1 describes each category briefly and demonstrates the format for deriving a diagnostic label, for example, "moderate spastic hemiplegia"[73].

The most widely used classification system for differential diagnosis of motor speech disorders was developed by Darley, Aronson, and Brown. [17,18,19]. Motor speech disorders are broadly classified as dysarthrias or apraxias of speech. **Dysarthria** is a term used to en-

Table 2-1. Classification Parameters for Cerebral Palsy[73]

Severity (Mild, moderate, severe)	Physiological Features (Site of lesion)	Anatomical Features (Location and extent)
Mild	**Spastic—Pyramidal** ➤ upper motor neuron system pyramidal lesion (motor strip and pyramidal tracts); muscles have high tone ➤ isometric contractions around joints affect voluntary movement ➤ contralateral side of body	**Monoplegia** ➤ one limb affected (rare) **Hemiplegia** ➤ one side affected (arm, leg, and other structures, same side)
Moderate	**Choreoathetoid—Extrapyramidal** ➤ basal ganglia or cerebellar lesion ➤ involuntary extraneous movements ➤ reduced resting muscle tone and force common: poor posture maintenance ➤ 6 possible types of associated involuntary movements: dystonia, athetosis, chorea, ataxia, rigidity, dyskinesia	➤ arm often more involved ➤ loss of sensation common **Quadriplegia** ➤ entire body affected ➤ legs and feet more involved
Severe	**Mixed-Pyramidal + Extrapyramidal** ➤ high muscle tone and involuntary movements	**Diplegia** ➤ primary involvement of lower limbs, with mild involvement of upper limbs

compass a group of motor speech disorders characterized by disturbed neuromuscular control, caused by lesions in the central or peripheral nervous system (or both). It can involve weakness or incoordination of voluntary movements in the respiratory, phonatory, resonance or articulatory systems. **Apraxia** or dyspraxia of speech is a disturbance of phonetic-motor programming characterized by difficulty initiating, sequencing, or accurately targeting movements for speech in the absence of neuromotor weakness of the speech musculature.

Focussing primarily on dysarthrias of speech, the perceptual classification system proposed by Darley, Aronson, and Brown distinguishes among the various motor speech disorders based on clusters of perceptual acoustic features that characterize each type and relates them to the site(s) of lesion that could explain the observed patterns.

Table 2-2 presents a classification system for motor speech disorders, their neuromotor substrates, and their distinguishing perceptual speech characteristics. Some of the most common causes of motor speech disorders will be discussed in greater detail in the next sections.

2.5.1 Vocal Fold Paralysis

Unilateral vocal fold paralysis (UVP) is the most common motor speech disorder affecting voice. It is caused by a lower motor neuron lesion (CN X: Vagus Nerve) and thus is classified as a *flaccid dysarthria*. Unilateral recurrent laryngeal nerve paralysis may cause a spectrum of problems, such as breathy voice, aspiration, and weakened cough. When the lesion is above the pharyngeal branch of CN X, mild hypernasality also may be a consequence. The most common cause of UVP is stretching or sectioning of the recurrent laryngeal nerve during cardiac or thyroid surgery, but viruses may also lead to

UVP, and often this is usually inferred by reviewing the patient's history. Immediately after onset, the paralyzed vocal fold may be too far lateral from the midline to permit approximation by the mobile fold. As a result, the voice may be weak and breathy. Occasionally, a double-pitched vocal tone, referred to as diplophonia, may be heard. In many patients, recovery of the voice occurs either through a mechanism of spontaneous medialization, without the return of vocal fold mobility, or with full recovery. Medialization may be due to random reinnervation of laryngeal muscles with resultant improvement in muscular tone. The voice may return to normal when this occurs.

The main indication for surgical treatment of vocal fold paralysis is ineffective cough and aspiration, but restitution of voice may also be a reason for surgical intervention, as discussed in Chapter 3.

2.5.2 Dystonia and Tremor

Focal laryngeal dystonias and benign essential vocal tremors are slow hyperkinetic dysarthrias thought to be associated with lesions in the basal ganglia. The term **spasmodic dysphonia** (SD) implies that a patient with a normal-looking larynx at rest has a strained voice quality and vocal dysfluency, typically caused by adductor muscle spasms that create phonation or pitch breaks. It is usually insidious in onset and progresses over months or years. This disorder may be related to stress or psychological factors, but many patients are identified as having a focal dystonia akin to blepharospasm or writer's cramp. Effective management of SD patients requires a team approach including the contributions of an otolaryngologist, speech-language pathologist, neurologist, and psychiatrist. A relevant case example is provided in Chapter 4.

Usually, the larynx of a patient suffering from idiopathic adductor spasmodic dys-

Table 2-2. Classification of Motor Speech Disorders (MSD)

MSD Type	Location Of Lesion	Neuromotor Deficits Conditions	Distinctive Speech Features
Apraxia	Broca's area and other motor and relay areas in the left or dominant hemisphere	May be accompanied by hemiplegia or paresis Often associated with nonverbal oral apraxia	Disturbed timing, rate, prosody: pauses prolongations, equal syllabic stress, delayed onsets
			Sound or syllable substitutions, omissions, additions, repetitions; hesitations and articulatory groping
			Minimal speech sound repertoire or muteness if severe
Dysarthria **Flaccid**	Lower motor neurons: CN nuclei, axons, myoneural junction, muscles	Bulbar palsy: muscle weakness, hypotonicity, reduced reflexes Muscle atrophy and fasciculations if long-standing or progressive	CN V (jaw), *unilateral*: minimal speech effect *bilateral*: imprecise consonants
			CN VII (face), *unilateral*: minimal speech effect *bilateral*: imprecise labial consonants, some vowel distortion
			CN X (velopharyngeal valve; larynx), *above pharyngeal branch*: vocal weakness, breathiness, diplophonia; reduced pitch and loudness ranges; monopitch, hypernasality; nasal emission *below pharyngeal branch*: voice symptoms only
			CN XII (tongue): *unilateral*: mild consonant distortion

MSD Type	Location Of Lesion	Neuromotor Deficits Conditions	Distinctive Speech Features
			bilateral: imprecise articulation, reduced intelligibility
			Phrenic nerve (diaphragm): *spinal intercostal nerves*: reduced VC/breath support
Spastic	Upper motor neurons, bilateral: pyramidal system, 1° motor cortex	Hypertonicity, reduced range, force, speed of movements, exaggerated reflexes	Strained, strangled, harsh voice quality; low pitch; reduced pitch and loudness variability; slow rate hypernasality; imprecise articulation
Unilateral UMN	Upper motor neurons, unilateral: internal capsule, corona radiata, motor cortex, brainstem	Unilateral weakness: face and tongue +/- hemiplegia/paresis	Mild symptoms (LT): Imprecise articulation, irregular breakdowns; slow rate; harsh or hoarse voice; may sound spastic in acute stage
Ataxic	Cerebellum	Hypotonicity, reduced rate, inaccurate timing, range and direction of movements	Dysprosody: "scanning" speech: excess, equal stress; prolongations; repetitions; excess loudness variations; slow rate; irregular articulatory distortion and breakdowns
Hypokinetic	Extrapyramidal system, basal ganglia: dopamine deficiency, depigmentation in substantia nigra	Parkinsonism: rigidity, reduced range of movements, variable rate, arrests of movements, tremor	Rapid and variable rate, monopitch, monoloudness, reduced stress, breathy, weak voice, inappropriate pauses, imprecise articulation

(continued)

Table 2-2. Classification of Motor Speech Disorders (MSD) *(continued)*

MSD Type	Location Of Lesion	Neuromotor Deficits Conditions	Distinctive Speech Features
Hyperkinetic	Extrapyramidal system: primarily basal ganglia	Abnormal, rhythmic or irregular and unpredictable involuntary movements: "quick" or "slow"	
Quick		Unsustained, rapid, random movements, may interrupt intended movement or target	Highly variable and imprecise articulation, sudden loudness variations, episodic hypernasality
chorea			
myoclonus		Sudden jerking movements	Episodic hypernasality, phonation breaks
tics (eg, Gilles de la Tourette's syndrome			Sudden, ticlike, vocalizations, e.g., grunts, snorts, barks, cursing (midspeech or from silence)
Slow		Abnormal, slow and/or sustained involuntary movements, postures, or muscle contractions, sometimes called dyskinesias	
Dystonia **Focal dystonias,** *oralmandibular*		Sustained muscle contractions interrupt jaw, lip, tongue movements	Articulatory distortions, dysfluencies, sometimes voice and resonance changes
laryngeal dystonia		"Spasmodic dysphonia" muscle contractions cause full or partial adduction and/or abduction of the vocal folds; sometimes occurs with benign essential vocal tremors and/or spasmodic torticollis; may exist in absence of neuromotor deficits as a psychogenic or muscle misuse type	Vocal dysfluencies: voice breaks, delayed voice onsets; often strained-strangled voice quality

MSD Type	Location Of Lesion	Neuromotor Deficits Conditions	Distinctive Speech Features
Organic voice tremor		Rhythmic variations in pitch, loudness, or both Benign, often familial; may coexist with other tremors in head, neck, or hands	Rhythmic fluctuations in pitch and loudness that are most evident on sustained vowels; rhythmic spasmodic vocal interruptions if severe or associated with a spasmodic dysphonia; may be articulatory and resonance distortions if associated with lingual, mandibular, labial or palatal tremors.
Mixed dysarthrias	More than one site of lesion	Various, depending on systems involved; often associated with chronic or progressive neurological diseases, eg, amyotrophic lateral sclerosis, multiple sclerosis Wilson's, Shy-Drager Syndrome	Various, depending on systems involved

Classification material adapted from Darley, Aronson, and Brown[17-19].

phonia will look normal, at least with regular light. Stroboscopic exam will reveal the increased closed phase that is typical of a laryngeal dystonia. The excursion of the mucosal wave also will be reduced. The voice and glottal appearance on phonation typically will be more normal at high pitches where less bulk of the vocalis muscle has to be involved with the vibratory cycle, and phonation control may be more aerodynamic than for low pitches in modal register (see Chapter 8). Low-pitched phonation will more likely be spasmodic, even on indirect examination when the tongue is being forcefully extended.

Hyperadducted supraglottal structures may be associated with dystonia.

The term **dystonia** refers to a condition in which a muscle or group of muscles becomes involuntarily hypertonic, and the resultant spasm results in its inability to function normally. Typical examples around the head and neck include cervical dystonia (spasmodic torticollis), blepharospasm, Meige's syndrome (blepharospasm plus oromandibular dystonia), as well as spasmodic dysphonia. Not all spasmodic dysphonia symptoms can be definitely attributed to this hyperkinetic motor speech disorder. Psychopathologies accounting for the muscle misuse patterns creating SD have been identified in a few patients, and treatment usually is directed differently for these patients. The ability to render near-miraculous resolution of SD symptoms using botulinum toxin makes life more pleasant for patients and voice care teams. As mentioned above, spasmodic dysphonia is sometimes confused with tremor, discussed below.

Dystonic adductor spasm of the larynx can also produce difficulties with respiration variously labeled **adductor breathing dystonia**, **vocal cord dysfunction**, or **paradoxical vocal fold movement**. Patients afflicted with this difficulty usually will come to the voice clinic with an airway complaint rather than concern about their voices, although voice symptoms may be present. Typically, they complain of difficulty breathing in, because of a restricted airway. Inspiratory voicing may accompany attempts at inspiration. On laryngoscopy, the true vocal folds can be seen to adduct during inspiratory attempts, sometimes with a posterior chink allowing for a limited airway. Other muscle misuses in laryngeal and paralaryngeal muscles are also often identified, commonly anteroposterior compression. Fortunately these patients may respond to botulinum toxin treatments, but some need airway support via a tracheotomy. The psychiatric interactions in this disorder are probably important but confusing, with the "chicken-egg" dilemma being operant.

In rare cases, focal dystonia may affect other muscles in the larynx. Posterior cricoarytenoid involvement may lead to **abductor spasmodic dysphonia** that is characterized by an inconsistently weak breathy voice and vocal dysfluencies caused by abductor muscle spasms. The clinical picture may be confused with a more common psychogenic hypoadducting dysphonia not unlike that seen in many cases of conversion aphonia. True abductor dystonia appears to exist and may respond to injection of botulinum toxin

into the posterior cricoarytenoid muscles, although the results are often less satisfying than those experienced by individuals treated for adductor SD. Even less common is **cricothyroid muscle dystonia.** This we have documented once with laryngeal electromyography, in a patient who experiences cricothyroid muscle spasms only when singing in upper ranges.

2.5.3 Benign Essential Tremor

Benign essential tremor is another slow hyperkinetic dysarthria associated with basal ganglia lesions. It is often familial and usually begins in late middle age. The family history is positive in 50% of patients. It is characterized by rhythmic contractions of alternating muscle groups producing a shake that may affect the voice, hands, or head. Some feel that the tremor tends to start in the dominant hand and then spread to the voice. Benign essential tremor may be relatively spasm free or combine with an element of spasm that renders diagnostic labeling confusing. One may describe a tremor with associated spasm or without; or a spasmodic dysphonia with associated tremor or without. It may be helpful to consider a list of voice profiles associated with dystonia and tremor as follows:

➤ Adductor spasmodic dysphonia
➤ Benign essential tremor
➤ Adductor spasm-tremor combinations
➤ Abductor spasmodic dysphonia (posterior cricoarytenoid muscles)
➤ Adductor breathing dystonia
➤ Dysphonia with other forms of dystonia (eg, Meige's syndrome).

2.6 Occupational Factors

The vocal demands and environmental conditions associated with certain occupations may contribute to the development of vocal abuse, muscle misuse, and organic pathologies in the larynx[15,25,43,47,57,59,61,66-69,74-76,78]. Voice disorders caused by vocal demands or conditions of an occupation are known as **occupational voice problems**. Some workers' compensation agencies may recognize two categories of occupational voice problems: *occupational voice disease* and *occupational voice injury*. The latter term is typically reserved for cases of identifiable lesions resulting from exposure to a noxious agent or injurious vocal event(s) that take place in the workplace, but it may also be applied to voice problems related to ongoing vocal overuse or misuse, comparable to repetitive strain injuries. Occupational voice disease typically is recognized as a more chronic response to the ongoing vocal demands or environmental stimuli that cause dysfunction.

The comprehensive study of occupational risk factors for voice problems is a relatively new focus, although deleterious effects of speaking in noise have been recognized for many years. The acoustic conditions of many working environments have been extensively investigated by those concerned about risks of hearing loss, reductions in speech intelligibility in noise, and the subsequent effects of poor acoustics on learning and attention[3,8,9,13,14,31,32,33,57,60,80]. Public school classrooms have been identified as a working environment of great concern. In particular, noise and reverberation levels that are higher than the recommended standards have been found in several studies world wide [3,8,31,32,60]. The implications for both teachers and students are numerous. Adverse effects of noise on health, attention and learning have been demonstrated, and preliminary research suggests the effects of noise can contribute to the development and maintenance of voice problems through a variety of physiological mechanisms[9,13,14,31,34,37,38,40,65,70,72,80,83]. Speech in poor acoustic environments may be an occupational voice risk for other occupations as well. Anecdotal and research reports reveal a high incidence of voice problems among swimming instructors and lifeguards, aerobics instructors, cheerleaders, and military instructors[10,43,59,61,67,68]. Individuals in each of these occupational groups are required to use their voices loudly for extensive periods of time over noise, outdoors, or in extremely reverberant spaces.

Additional occupational factors that may contribute to the development and maintenance of voice problems include exposure to chemicals or gases that are known to irritate the upper aerodigestive tract (eg, tobacco smoke, ozone, sulfur dioxide), frequent exposure to viral or other infectious illnesses, inappropriate levels of environmental humidity, high work expectations or performance demands, elevated stress levels, long periods of vocalizing without breaks, extensive voice use on telephones or other communications hardware with poor acoustic specifications, and inadequate vocal training for occupational demands. Among teachers, the most extensively studied population, the risk appears to be higher for women than for men by a factor of at least 2:1[66,75]. Several factors may account for this gender-based difference, among them the ability of the larger male vocal system to withstand extended phonation at high intensities and a higher level of hyaluronic acid in the lamina propria of men, thought to increase the impact resilience of the vocal folds[28,75] (see Chapter 8).

Investigators have taken several approaches to identify occupations and occupational risks associated with voice problems. Studies of individuals seeking treatment yield some consensus on occupations most frequently represented in the clinical population. Survey research has provided data on occupational voice users that includes individuals who may have vocal symptoms but do not seek clinical expertise. Occupational groups that have been identified as having a high prevalence or being at high risk for voice problems include singers, teachers, aerobics and swimming instructors, counselors, salespersons and ticket agents, particularly those working primarily on phones, and other occupational voice users who rely heavily on their voices to do their jobs and are subjected to known risk factors.

2.7 Voice Disorders in the Elderly

Although elderly patients may develop voice disorders from those etiological factors that affect all age groups, such as upper respiratory tract infections, they are also susceptible to changes that are related to growing old. Certain voice changes are a normal part of the aging process and should not be considered disordered, but it is important for the voice clinician to recognize and understand these to be in a position to help out when problems develop. Changes in the aging vocal system are described in detail in Chapter 8. In summary, it seems that there are two primary altered states in the larynx that develop with aging. One, which predominates in women, is a thickened, chronically edematous larynx, resulting in altered voice quality and a naturally lower f_0 that may be below the typical "gender-ambiguous" f_0 around 160 Hz[48]. Atrophic changes predominate in the other state. These patients, most of them men, develop a thin and reedy timbre and a higher pitched voice, which may include phonation above the gender-ambiguous f_0. Other age-related changes—such as reduced vital capacity, reduced elasticity in structures of the chest wall, and reduced strength in articulators—can all contribute to altered speech and voice dynamics[36,42,71,77].

2.7.1 Disorders Caused by Attempts to Compensate for Normal Aging Processes

As already described, the aging process in the male larynx involves muscle atrophy and loss of elasticity. The normal voice effect is increased pitch and "thinning" of the vocal tone. Attempts to compensate for these changes usually result in glottal fry phonation, increased laryngeal effort, and subsequent rapid vocal fatigue. Indirect laryngoscopy reveals apparent shortening and bowing of the true vocal folds. The vocal folds may adduct more efficiently if lengthening can be achieved by higher pitched phonation.

A more masculine-sounding voice in women (particularly those who have smoked for many years), caused by Reinke's edema and polypoid degeneration may be socially unacceptable. Those women who attempt to correct the pitch change by compensatory muscle misuse may develop lateral glottal and supraglottal compression and increased vocal effort. Phonation becomes easier and clearer when the patient is encouraged to allow the vocal tone to drop to a more natural range that is consistent with the age-related mucosal changes.

How far do these changes have to go before they cease to be normal? The answer usually rests with the individual patient's physical and psychological reaction to the changes and the ease and effectiveness with which he or she is communicating. A change in vocal image is often at the core of an individual's concern. When the older woman's voice is so low in pitch that she is addressed as "sir" on the phone, she may consciously or subconsciously make muscular adjustments to raise the pitch. This tactic may work to a point, but soon the dysphonic voice resulting from muscle misuses associated with the attempted compensations are more of a problem than the natural changes causing the low pitch. Similarly, the old man with an easily tiring "glottal fry" phonation and bowed vocal folds may be suffering more from his subconscious attempt to drive the vocal pitch down to the male range than from the muscle atrophy, fragmented collagen, and weakened elastin of his larynx.

2.7.2 Psychogenic Voice Disorders in the Elderly

Vocal folds are made up largely of voluntary muscle, and voluntary muscles move them about. This neuromuscular system may become unbalanced by either psychological or neurological disease processes that are prevalent in the elderly. The elderly are subject to the same psychopathological processes that affect all age groups and may develop voice disorders through the mechanism of muscle misuse at the level of the final common functional pathway. In older patients, loneliness or separation from family, loss of independence, and other lifestyle changes may lead to depression and anxiety. There is, logically, considerable overlap between those patients who have dysphonia as a result of attempting to compensate for age-related or neurological changes, and those patients who have purely psychogenic dysphonias.

2.7.3 Voice Disorders and Neurological Disease in the Elderly

Neurological degenerative disorders, such as Parkinson's disease, can cause impaired vocal coordination, flexibility, and strength due to the same neuromuscular mechanisms affecting other voluntary movements, including those of articulation. Medical and surgical procedures used to treat disorders common to the elderly, such as cardiovascular disease, may result in peripheral nerve damage, most commonly to the left recurrent laryngeal nerve disturbed during cardiac surgery or intubation injuries in the larynx during general anaesthetic.

There are a number of neurological diseases in which the voice may be abnormal but is not the presenting symptom. Examples include stroke, amyotrophic lateral sclerosis, and pseudobulbar palsy. In others, dysphonia may be the presenting symptom of a neurological disorder. Essential tremor is generally a disorder of the elderly and is discussed in Section 2.5.

2.7.4 Miscellaneous causes of dysphonia in the Elderly

Older people are most susceptible to cancers and other systemic ailments such as lower respiratory problems and gastroesophageal reflux disease, which can play a part in forming dysphonia symptoms. Other factors important to the speech chain, including hearing, general alertness and mental status need to be considered as well.

2.8 Voice Disorders in Children

Infants and children are particularly susceptible to certain disease states and pathological processes that may interrupt the normal process of communication development. Congenital or early-childhood disorders that can contribute to voice problems include hearing impairments, structural defects such as cleft palate and laryngeal webs, cerebral palsy, and viruses such as human papilloma virus. We have devoted a chapter to management of voice disorders in children; readers are referred to Chapter 6. Additional therapy guidelines and case studies are offered in Chapter 4.

2.9 The Irritable Larynx Syndrome

We define the Irritable Larynx Syndrome (ILS) as "hyperkinetic laryngeal dysfunction resulting from a variety of specific causes in response to a definitive triggering stimulus". Hyperkinetic laryngeal dysfunction presents in numerous forms:

➤ **Muscle misuse voice disorders** of various forms as described above
➤ **Episodic laryngospasm**, vocal cord dysfunction, paradoxical vocal fold motion,

and adductor breathing dystonia, which are all descriptive terms that relate to a situation in which the glottis closes and inhibits airflow

➤ **Chronic cough, throat clearing, and the sense of a lump in the throat** (globus pharyngeus) are also symptoms that may be tied to muscle tension in the larynx. These symptoms have been attributed to respiratory disease, gastroesophageal reflux[16,44], psychological stress[81] and allergies among other things.

Although the larynx usually looks structurally normal, physical findings include abnormal laryngeal posture and palpable muscle tension in and around the larynx, as described by Lieberman and Harris[41].

ILS symptoms are triggered by something definitive, such as odors, airborne particles, or chemicals. Foods, refluxate, esophageal stimuli, or voice use may also trigger symptoms.

Inclusion criteria for ILS diagnosis are as follows:

1. Symptoms attributable to laryngeal tension such as laryngospasm or muscle tension dysphonia, with or without globus sensation or chronic cough
2. Visible and palpable evidence of tension manifest as laryngoscopic lateral or anteroposterior supraglottal compression plus excessive palpable tension in suprahyoid, thyrohyoid, cricothyroid, and pharyngeal muscles
3. A sensory trigger, such as airborne substances, esophageal irritants, or odors

The ILS diagnosis is excluded if there is organic laryngeal or neurological disease.

We feel that the irritable larynx syndrome develops in individuals as a reaction to a central nervous system change that leaves sensory-motor pathways in a hyperexcitable state. Clinical review of a group of 39 patients made it evident that there are a number of possible causative factors and that several can be active in any one person[56]. Emotional distress, habitual muscle misuse, gastroesophageal reflux, and postviral illness seem to be the most prevalent. There are a number of possible neuropathological processes that may lead to chronic laryngeal motor stimulation and heightened sensory irritability.

A process termed "neural plasticity" may alter central neuronal control of the larynx and related structures and the way that laryngeal motor systems react to sensations or thoughts. There are several processes by which central neurons may undergo plastic adaptation. In response to nerve or tissue injury, afferent inputs are withdrawn from the central neuron, which then makes new connections by resprouting dendrites or reactivating "silent" synapses. Through this process, an afferent stimulus that used to result in one response now may elicit a different one. The body of literature on chronic pain is a helpful source of information and understanding about plasticity and its possible role in development of ILS[12]. We also hypothesize that a change in the sensory-motor control of laryngeal muscle systems can be brought on by viral illness affecting the central nervous system (CNS). Figure 2–13 illustrates this concept.

When the first neurotransmitter stimulus arrives at the CNS neuronal cell wall, it sends a message through the cytoplasm by way of a second messenger to the nucleus where immediate early genes such as c-fos or c-jun are induced. C-fos then moves out to the cytoplasm where fos protein is synthesized. The proto-oncogene fos then moves back into the nucleus where it binds with DNA and regulates the transcription of late response genes.

The periaqueductal grey (PAG) area in the brainstem is involved in vocalization. Stimulation of the dorsal and lateral regions of the PAG evokes vocalization in some animals, and lesions produced here will result in mutism [4,20]. Cells in the caudal areas of the

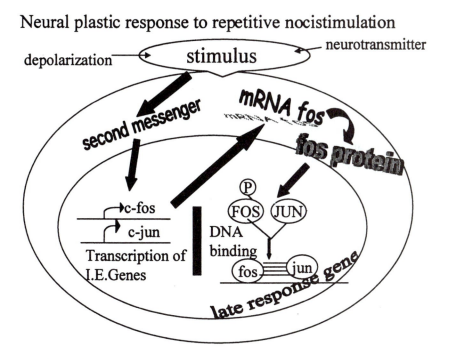

Figure 2–13. Diagram illustrating how a repetitive noxious stimulus may alter the genome of a CNS neuron and lead to neural plastic change in its response to other stimuli.

PAG have been found to have a relationship with laryngeal muscle activity. Supramaximal stimulation of the internal branch of the superior laryngeal nerve in the cat has been shown to increase fos labeling in dorsomedial and dorsolateral regions of the PAG[1]. This evidence suggests that neurons in this area are stimulated by laryngeal sensory fibers coming to the PAG, possibly via the nucleus of the tractus solitarius.

On the basis of these factors, it is hypothesized that central nervous system viral infections, such as Herpes Zoster and others, can and may result in genome changes that alter laryngeal motor control.

Emotional connections affecting the larynx may work through the periaqueductal grey; it is well known that emotional states and defense reactions relate to PAG activity[5,11].

Jurgens has proposed that the PAG serves as a link between sensory and motivation-controlling structures and the periambigual reticular formation, coordinating the activity of the different phonatory muscles[35]. These studies support the obvious association between increased voice tension and psychological stress or repressed emotion.

Asthmalike reactions in parasympathetic parts of laryngeal muscle systems can be expected to respond to irritation in the same way that bronchial muscles respond in lower airway disease. The laryngeal effect may produce muscle misuse voice problems, chronic cough, or laryngeal airway spasm rather than an "asthmalike" expiratory wheeze. As for reflux, we know that there is a direct reflex relationship between stimulation of the lower esophagus and thyroarytenoid muscle activity[24]. It also seems possible that chronic laryngeal reflux irritation affects the PAG, where neural plastic change results in long-term changes to laryngeal function.

Figure 2–14 graphically demonstrates how the laryngeal central nervous system control network may be impacted by all the factors described (habitual muscle misuse, emotional distress, viral illness, and chronic reflux stimulation) to produce a hyperirritable "spasm-ready" state.

Figure 2–15 represents passage from the "spasm-ready" to ILS symptom manifest state. Muscular tone modulators may be present that make the spasm more easily triggered by a sensory irritant. These tone modulators may include general psychological stressors or postural factors. The trigger is usually an episodic sensory irritant, such as acid refluxate, airborne particles, or odors.

Although ILS is only a clinical theory, it may help the voice care team manage what can be a complex set of problems. We believe that an "irritable larynx syndrome" exists in which hyperkinetic laryngeal dysfunction, as manifest by laryngospasm, dysphonia, globus, or chronic cough, is triggered by a sensory stimulus. ILS occurs when brainstem laryngeal controlling neuronal networks are held in a perpetual hyperexcitable state and therefore react inappropriately to sensory stimulation. Treatment can be directed most appropriately when the specific underlying causes are identified.

2.10 Summary

Voice problems are caused by any combination of the 4 etiological platform components, sometimes in association with other overlying pathologies. Identification of each of the etiological factors contributing to an individual's voice disorder is imperative for the most descriptive clinical profile to be developed and for the most effective management to be

ILS - Pathways to CNS Plastic Change

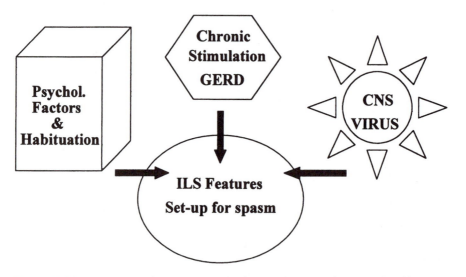

Figure 2–14. Hypothesized factors that may lead to development of the hyperirritable state.

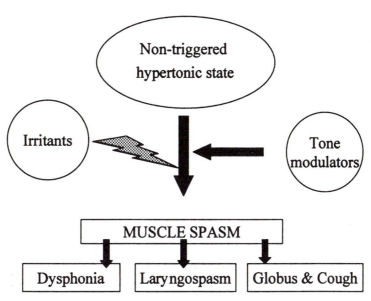

Figure 2–15. Mechanisms whereby symptoms may be triggered in the irritable larynx syndrome patient.

planned. A variety of classification paradigms may be adopted to help clinicians describe and label voice disorder types. Because the causes of voice disorders are by nature complex and multifactorial, it is typically necessary to employ more than one classification scheme to fully describe a clinical profile.

References

1. Ambalavanar, R., Tanaka Y., Damirjian, M., & Ludlow, C. L. (1999). Laryngeal afferent stimulation enhances Fos immunoreactivity in periaqueductal gray in the cat. *Journal of Comparative Neurology, 409*(3), 411–423.
2. American Joint Committee on Cancer, Manual for Staging of Cancer. (1992). *Larynx*, 4th Edition. Philadelphia: J.B. Lippincott Co.
3. American Speech-Language-Hearing Association. (1995). Position statement and guidelines for acoustics in educational settings. *ASHA, 37* (Suppl. 14), 15.
4. Bandler, R., Keay, K. A., Vaughn C. W., & Shipley M. T. (1996). Columnar organization of the PAG neurons regulating emotional and vocal expression. In P. J. Davis, & N. H. Fletcher (Eds.), *Vocal Fold Physiology: Controlling Complexity and Chaos* (pp. 137–152). San Diego: Singular Publishing Group, Inc.
5. Behbehani, M. M. (1995). Functional characteristics in the midbrain periaqueductal gray. *Progress in Neurology, 46*, 575–605.
6. Belisle, G., & Morrison, M. D. (1983). Anatomic correlation for muscle tension dysphonia. *Journal of Otolaryngology, 12*, 319–321.
7. Bouchayer, M., Cornut, G., Witzig, E., et al (1985). Epidemoid cysts, sulci, and mucosal bridges of the true vocal cord: A report of 157 cases. *Laryngoscope, 95*, 1087–1094.
8. Bradley, J. S. (1986). Speech intelligibility studies in classrooms. *Journal of the Acoustical Society of America, 80*, 846–854.
9. Brewer, D. W. & Briess, F. B. (1960). Industrial noise: Laryngeal considerations. *New York State Journal of Medicine*, June, 1737–1740.
10. Campbell, S., Reich, A., Klockars, A. J., & McHenry, M. (1988). Factors associated with dysphonia in high school cheerleaders. *Journal of Speech and Hearing Disorders, 3*, 175–185.

11. Carrive, P. (1993). The periaqueductal gray and defensive behavior: Functional representation and neuronal organization. *Behavioural Brain Research, 58,* 27–47.

12. Coderre, T. J., Katz, J., Vaccarino, A. L., & Melzack, R. (1993). Contribution of central neuroplasticity to pathological pain: Review of clinical and experimental evidence. *Pain, 52,* 259–285.

13. Cohen, S., Evans, G. W., Krantz, D. S., & Stokols, D. (1980). Physiological, motivational and cognitive effects of aircraft noise on children. *American Psychologist, 35,* 231–243.

14. Cohen, S., Krantz, D.S., Evans, G.W., Stokols, D., & Kelly S (1981) Aircraft noise and children: Longitudinal and cross-sectional evidence on adaptation to noise and the effectiveness of noise abatement. *Journal of Personality and Social Psychology 40,* 331–345.

15. Cooper, M. (1973) *Modern Techniques of Vocal Rehabilitation.* Springfield: Charles C. Thomas.

16. Curran, A. J., Barry, M. K., Callanan, V., & Gormley, P. K. (1995). A prospective study of acid reflux and globus pharyngeus using a modified symptom index. *Clinical Otolaryngology, 20,* 552–554.

17. Darley, F. L., Aronson, A. E., & Brown, J. R. (1969a). Differential diagnostic patterns of dysarthria. *Journal of Speech and Hearing Research, 12,* 246–267.

18. Darley, F. L., Aronson, A. E., & Brown, J. R. (1969b). Clusters of deviant speech dimensions in the dysarthrias. *Journal of Speech and Hearing Research, 12,* 246–267.

19. Darley, F. L., Aronson, A. E., & Brown, J. R. (1975). *Motor Speech Disorders.* Philadelphia: W.B. Saunders Co.

20. Davis, P. J., & Zhang, S. P. (1991). What is the role of the midbrain periaqueductal gray in respiration and vocalization? In A. Depauliis, & R. Bandler (Eds.), *The Midbrain Periaqueductal Gray Matter* (pp. 57–66). New York: Plenum Press.

21. DSM-IV (1994). *Diagnostic and Statistical Manual of Mental Disorders, 4th Edition.* Washington, D.C.: American Psychiatric Association.

22. Egger, J., Friedl, W., & Freidrich, G. (1990). Functional dysphonia: Personality and coping behavior in stressful situations. In H. G. Zapotoczky, & T. Wenzel (Eds.), *The Scientific Dialogue: From basic research to clinical intervention.* Amsterdam: Swets and Zeitlinger.

23. Froeschels, E. (1943). Hygiene of the voice. *Archives of Otolaryngology, 37,* 122–130.

24. Gill, C., & Morrison, M. D. (1997). Esophagolaryngeal reflex in a porcine animal model. *Journal of Otolaryngology, 27,* 76–80.

25. Gotaas, C., & Starr, C. D. (1993). Vocal fatigue among teachers. *Folia Phoniatrica, 45,* 20–129.

26. Green, G. (1988). The interrelationships between vocal and psychological characteristics: A literature review. *Australian Journal of Human Communication Disorders, 16*(2), 31–43.

27. Green, G. (1989). Psycho-behavioural characteristics of children with vocal nodules: WPBIC ratings. *Journal of Speech and Hearing Disorders, 54,* 306–312.

28. Hammond, T. H., Zhou, R., Hammond, E. H., Pawlak, A., & Gray, S. D. (1997). The intermediate layer: A morphologic study of the elastin and hyaluronic acid constituents of normal human vocal folds. *Journal of Voice, 11,* 59–66.

29. Harris, T. (1998). Laryngeal mechanisms in normal function and dysfunction. In T. Harris, S. Harris, J. S. Rubin & D. M. Howard (Eds.), *The Voice Clinic Handbook* (pp. 64–90). London: Whurr Publishers Ltd.

30. Heaver, L. (1958). Psychiatric observations on the personality structure of patients with habitual dysphonia. *Logos, 1,* 21–26.

31. Hetu, R., Truchon-Gagnon, C., & Bilodeau, S. A. (1990). Problems of noise in school settings: A review of literature and the results of an exploratory study. *Journal of Speech-Language Pathology and Audiology, 14,* 31–39.

32. Houtgast, T. (1981). The effect of ambient noise on speech intelligibility in classrooms. *Applied Acoustics, 14,* 15–25.

33. Houtgast, T., & Steeneken, H. J. M. (1984). A multi-language evaluation of the RASTI–method for estimating speech intelligibility in auditoria. *Acustica, 54,* 185–199.

34. Jansen, G., & Gros, E. (1986). Non-auditory effects of noise: Physiological and psychological effects. In L. Saenz, & R. W. B. Stephens (Eds.), *Noise Pollution.* (Chapter 8), New York: Wiley.

35. Jurgens, U. (1994). The role of the periaqueductal gray in vocal behavior. *Behavioural Brain Research, 62*, 107–117.

36. Kahane, J. C. (1981). Anatomic and physiologic changes in the aging peripheral speech mechanism. In *Aging: Communication Processes and Disorders*. New York: Grune & Stratton.

37. Ko, N. W. M. (1979). Responses of teachers to aircraft noise. *Journal of Sound and Vibration, 62*, 277–292.

38. Ko, N. W. M. (1981). Responses of teachers to road traffic noise. *Journal of Sound and Vibration, 77*, 133–136.

39. Koufman, J. A., & Blalock, P. D. (1982). Classification and approach to patients with functional voice disorders. *Annals of Otology, Rhinology and Laryngology, 91*, 372–377.

40. Lane, H., & Tranel, B. (1971). The Lombard sign and the role of hearing in speech. *Journal of Speech and Hearing Research, 14*, 659–672.

41. Lieberman, J., & Harris, T. (1993). The cricothyroid mechanism, its relation to vocal fatigue and vocal dysfunction. *Journal of Otolaryngology, 12*, 302–306.

42. Linville, S. E. (1996). The sound of senescence. *Journal of Voice, 10*(2), 190–200.

43. Long, J., Williford, H. N., Scharff, Olson, M., & Wolfe, V. (1998). Vocal problems and risk factors among aerobics instructors. *Journal of Voice, 12*, 197–207.

44. Loughlin, C. J., & Koufman, J. A. (1996). Paroxysmal laryngospasm secondary to gastroesophageal reflux. *Laryngoscope, 106*, 1502–1505.

45. Malmgren, L., Gacek, R., & Etzler, C. (1983). Muscle fibre types in the human posterior cricoarytenoid muscle: a correlated histochemical and ultrastructural morphometric study. In I. R. Titze, & R. C. Scherer (Eds.), *Vocal Fold Physiology: Biomechanics, acoustics and phonatory control* (pp. 41-56). Denver: Denver Center for the Performing Arts.

46. Mans, E.J., Kuhn, A.G., & Lamprecht-Dinnesen, A. (1992). Psychosomatic findings in patients with vocal cord contact granulomas: Initial results. *Head and Neck Surgery, 40*, 346–351.

47. Mattiske, J. A., Oates, J. M., & Greenwood, K. M. (1998). Vocal problems among teachers: A review of prevalence, cause, prevention, and treatment. *Journal of Voice, 12*, 489–499.

48. McGlone, R., & Hollien, H. (1963). Vocal pitch characteristics of aged women. *Journal of Speech and Hearing Research, 6*, 164–170.

49. McHugh-Munier, C., Scherer, K. R., Lehmann, W., & Scherer, U. (1997). Coping strategies, personality, and voice quality in patients with vocal fold nodules and polyps. *Journal of Voice, 11*, 452–461.

50. Milenkovic, P., Bless, D. M., & Rammage, L. A. (1991). Acoustic and perceptual characterization of vocal nodules. In J. Gauffin, & B. Hammarberg (Eds.), *Vocal Fold Physiology: Acoustic, Perceptual, and Physiological Aspects of Voice Mechanisms* (pp. 265–272). San Diego: Singular Publishing Group, Inc.

51. Morrison, M. D. (1997). A pathophysiological model of dysphonia. In *Proceedings of the XVI World Congress of Otolaryngology* (pp. 1649–1655). Bologna: Monduzzi Editore.

52. Morrison, M. D., & Morris, B. D. (1990). Dysphonia and bulimia: Vomiting laryngeal injury. *Journal of Voice, 4*, 76–80.

53. Morrison, M. D., Nichol, H., & Rammage, L. A. (1986). Diagnostic criteria in functional dysphonia. *Laryngoscope, 96*, 1–8.

54. Morrison, M. D., & Rammage, L. A. (1993). Muscle misuse voice disorders: description and classification. *Acta Otolaryngologica, 113*, 428–434.

55. Morrison, M. D., Rammage, L. A., Belisle, G., Nichol, H., & Pullan, B. (1983). Muscular tension dysphonia. *Journal of Otolaryngology, 12*, 302–306.

56. Morrison, M. D., Rammage, L. A., & Emami, A. J. (1999). The irritable larynx syndrome. *Journal of Voice, 13*(3), 447–455.

57. Morton, V. (1999, August). Dysphonia in the classroom—A double edged sword. Presentation at PEVOC—*Occupational Voice Problems*. Utrect, The Netherlands.

58. Nemec, J. (1961). The motivation background of hyperkinetic dysphonia in children: A contribution to psychologic research in phoniatry. *Logos, 4*, 28–31.

59. Newman, C., & Kersner, M. (1998). Voice problems of aerobics instructors: implications for preventative training. *Logopedics-Phoniatrics-*

Vocology Scandinavian University Press, 1401–1439.

60. Pekkarinen, E., & Viljanen, V. (1991). Acoustic conditions for speech communication in classrooms. *Scandinavian Audiology, 20,* 257–263.

61. Rameck, M. F., & Ferreira, L. P. (1999, August). Aerobics instructors: Vocal profile and vocal behavior. Presentation at PEVOC—*Occupational Voice Problems.* Utrecht, The Netherlands.

62. Rammage, L. A. (1992). Acoustic, aerodynamic and vibratory characteristics of phonation with variable posterior glottis postures. Doctoral dissertation, University of Wisconsin-Madison.

63. Rammage, L. A., Nichol, H., & Morrison, M. D. (1987). The psychopathology of voice disorders. *Human Communication Canada, 11,* 21–25.

64. Rammage, L. A., Peppard, R. C., & Bless, D. M. (1989). Aerodynamic, laryngoscopic and perceptual-acoustic characteristics in dysphonic females with posterior glottal chinks: a retrospective study. *Journal of Voice, 6,* 64–78.

65. Reimers, N. L., & Yairi, E. (1987). Effects of noise on vocal fatigue and vocal recovery. *Folia Phoniatrica, 39,* 104–112.

66. Russell, A., Oates, J., & Greenwood, K. M. (1998). Prevalence of voice problems in teachers. *Journal of Voice, 12,* 467–479.

67. Sapir, S., Atias, J., & Shahar, A. (1990). Symptoms of vocal attrition in women army instructors and new recruits: Results from a survey. *Laryngoscope, 100,* 991–994.

68. Sapir, S., Attias, J., & Shahar, A. (1992). Vocal attrition related to idiosyncratic dysphonia: Re-analysis of survey data. *European Journal of Disorders of Communication, 27,* 129–135.

69. Sapir, S., Keidar, A., & Mathers-Schmidt, B. (1993). Vocal attrition in teachers: survey findings. *European Journal of Disorders of Communication, 28,* 177–185.

70. Sargent, J. W., Gidman, M. I., Humphreys, M. A., & Utley, W. A. (1980). The disturbance caused to school teachers by noise. *Journal of Sound and Vibration, 70,* 557–572.

71. Sataloff, R. T., Rosen, D. C., Hawkshaw, M., & Spiegel, J. R. (1997). The three ages of voice: The aging adult voice. *Journal of Voice, 11*(2), 156–160.

72. Schmidt, C. P., Andrews, M. L., & McCutcheon, J. W. (1998). An acoustical and perceptual analysis of the vocal behaviour of classroom teachers. *Journal of Voice, 12,* 434–443.

73. Scott, S. (1999). *Types of Cerebral Palsy.* Lecture Handout, School of Audiology & Speech Sciences, University of British Columbia.

74. Smith, E., Gray, S. D., Dove, H., Kirchner, L., & Heras, H. (1997). Frequency and effects of teachers' voice problems. *Journal of Voice, 11,* 81–87.

75. Smith, E., Kirchner, H. L., Taylor, M., Hoffman, H., & Lemke, J. H. (1998). Voice problems among teachers: differences by gender and teaching characteristics. *Journal of Voice, 12,* 328–334.

76. Smith, E., Lemke, J., Taylor, M., Kirchner, H. L., & Hoffman, H. (1998). Frequency of voice problems among teachers and other occupations. *Journal of Voice, 12,* 480–488.

77. Sperry, E. E., & Klich, R. J. (1992). Speech-breathing in senescent and younger women during oral reading. *Journal of Speech and Hearing Research, 35,* 1246–1255

78. Titze, I. R., Lemke, J., & Montequin, D. (1997). Populations in the U.S. workforce who rely on voice as a primary tool of trade: A preliminary report. *Journal of Voice, 11,* 254–259

79. Toohill, R. J. (1975). The psychosomatic aspects of children with nodules. *Archive of Otolaryngology, 101,* 591–595.

80. Van Heusden, E., Plomp, R., & Pols, L. C. W. (1979). Effect of ambient noise on the vocal output and the preferred listening level of conversational speech. *Applied Acoustics, 12,* 31–43.

81. Wilson, J. A., Heading, R. C., Maran, A. G. D., Pryde, A., Piris, J., & Allan, P.L. (1987). Globus sensation is not caused by gastro-esophageal reflux. *Clinical Otolaryngology, 12,* 271–275.

82. Wilson, F. B., & Lamb, M. M. (1973). Comparison of personality characteristics of children with and without vocal nodules on Rorschach protocol interpretation. *Acta Symbolica, 5,* 43–55.

83. Winkworth, A. L., & Davis, P. J. (1997). Speech breathing and the Lombard effect. *Journal of Speech, Language and Hearing Research, 37,* 535–556.

84. Yano, J., Ichimura, K., Hoshino, T., & Nozue, M. (1982). Personality factors in the pathogenesis of polyps and nodules of the vocal cords. *Auris Nasus Larynx, 9,*105–110.

Recommended Reading:

American Joint Committee on Cancer, Manual for Staging of Cancer (1992). *Larynx*, 4th Edition, Philadelphia: J.B. Lippincott Co.

Darley, F. L., Aronson, A. E., & Brown, J. R. (1969a). Differential diagnostic patterns of dysarthria. *Journal of Speech and Hearing Research, 12,* 246–267.

Darley, F. L., Aronson, A. E., & Brown, J. R. (1969b). Clusters of deviant speech dimensions in the dysarthrias. *Journal of Speech and Hearing Research, 12,* 246–267.

DSM-IV:*Diagnostic and Statistical Manual of Mental Disorders*, 4th Edition, (1994). Washington: American Psychiatric Association.

Duffy, J. R. (1995*). Motor Speech Disorders Substrates, Differential Diagnosis, and Management.* St. Louis: Mosby.

Harris, T., Harris S., Rubin, J. S., & Howard, D. M. (1998). *The Voice Clinic Handbook*. London: Whurr Publishers Ltd.

Love, R. J. (2000). *Childhood Motor Speech Disabilities*, 2nd Edition. Boston: Allyn & Bacon.

Morrison, M. D., Rammage, L. A., & Emami, A. J. (1999). The irritable larynx syndrome. *Journal of Voice, 13*(3), 447–455.

CHAPTER

3

Medical Treatment of Voice Disorders

3.1 Introduction

Optimal medical management of a patient with a voice disorder requires accurate diagnosis. When hoarseness is accompanied by a clearly identifiable acute upper respiratory tract infection or follows excessive shouting at an athletic event, the diagnosis may be easy, but in other situations the causes and best treatment plan may be more elusive. The medical treatment discussions that follow in this chapter presuppose a full evaluation and clarification of the cause(s) of the voice disorder as outlined in Chapters 1 and 2. For the sake of uniformity, topics will be addressed in the same order that they were dealt with in the previous chapter, beginning with medical treatment for the four dysphonia platform components that were presented in the model.

3.2 Dysphonia Model Platform Components

3.2.1 Platform Component 1: Technique and Level of Vocal Skill–Muscle Misuse Factors.

Voice therapy for vocal technique problems are discussed in Chapter 4. Occasionally, the physician may play a role through the provision of manual therapy to the larynx and neck. Various techniques are used to assist in the reduction of muscular tension in the thyrohyoid region, as well as in hypopharyngeal constrictors. The approach employed in our clinic has been derived from Lieberman's techniques[25]. A detailed knowledge of the anatomy and physiology of the area is essential; for this reason, this part in dysphonia treatment usually is undertaken by an otolaryngologist because he or she has a thorough knowledge of the relevant anatomy. For example, it is essential to have a clear image of the relative location of the carotid arteries and other vital structures while performing deep manual therapy techniques around the larynx. Manual therapy is sometimes uncomfortable for patients, and it is important that they are in control and able to stop the process at any time. Our patients are told that the magic word is "stop." They say, and we do.

The techniques used for evaluation of muscle misuse by palpation of the larynx were described in Chapter 1. Manual therapy of the larynx is a natural extension of the palpation techniques. A full description is beyond the scope of this text; the interested reader is referred to Lieberman's chapter referenced above.

3.2.2 Platform Component 2: Lifestyle

Because the injurious effects of abuse on the vocal cords are associated primarily with lifestyle factors, it is through modification of lifestyle that healing can be achieved. For example, any assistance that the physician can provide toward the cessation of smoking is of utmost importance in helping patients rid themselves of a voice disorder. Smokers can be helped in various ways, including direct counseling, provision of nicotine patches, or medications such as Zyban® that curb the nicotine craving. Each physician should have at hand a list of resources that are available in the local community, such as self-help groups or stop-smoking programs.

It is in some people's nature to talk loudly and excessively for long periods of time in poor acoustic environments. For them to adjust their pattern of misuse and abuse involves alteration of lifestyle as part of their voice therapy program. Sometimes patients need to be reminded to get adequate rest, drink plenty of liquids, and avoid excessive amounts of caffeine, alcohol, or other dehydrating substances.

3.2.3 Platform Component 3: Psychological Factors

A detailed discussion of psychological management of patients with voice disorders is included in Chapter 5. A few comments in this section on medical treatment may be helpful to the general physician or otolaryngologist.

Once the physician has assured the patient that there is no structural abnormality such as tumor or infection in the larynx, it helps to point out that the voice disorder is caused by muscles being held too tightly in the laryngeal area and then to describe mechanisms whereby psychological factors bring this about. We usually explain that there is a network of nerve cells in the brain stem, a part of the brain not directly accessible to the conscious mind, which we think acts as if it contains a "muscle use" program not unlike a computer data file. This hypothesized computer program controls the manner in which muscle systems in and around the larynx are coordinated and their associations with the adjacent centres for basic emotions. We respond to the unexpressed negative emotions of anxiety, sadness, and anger by holding tension in the muscles of vocal expression. Additionally, almost everyone is aware that our bodies react to undue stress through generalized increase in muscular tension throughout the body. We point out the fact that the words "tense" and "uptight" are psychological words, as well as muscle words. This form of explanation is often a useful introduction to the potential benefits of further psychological exploration and counseling.

3.2.4 Platform Component 4: Gastroesophageal Reflux

It is useful to consider the treatment of gastroesophageal reflux (GER) on four levels of care as follows:

Level one consists of lifestyle changes that someone with reflux should adopt forever. In other words, these are the things that should be continued as preventive measures even in the absence of all reflux symptoms. Body weight should be kept as close to the optimum as possible. The head of the bed should be raised on blocks so that while the body remains straight, the shoulders are at a higher elevation than the hips, and the stomach contents will stay where they belong—particularly if the individual sleeps on his or her right side. Eating should be avoided for 3 hours before going to bed at night, and if this is not possible a mild antacid, such as Tums®, should be taken when retiring. The habit of lying down after a meal should be avoided. Excessive amounts of coffee or other caffeinated beverages should be avoided, as should excessive use of any of the foods that are known to increase reflux. Smoking should also be avoided. Both caffeine and nicotine are known to reduce the pressure in the lower esophageal sphincter.

Level two consists of everything that an individual can do to reduce reflux apart from taking prescription medications. Most of these measures are included in the patient handout such as that included in Appendix 3–1. Clinicians reading this book are welcome to copy this handout for distribution to their own patients. The dietary restrictions suggested in the handout are rather severe, and in some patients a simple avoidance of those foods that provoke symptoms may be sufficient.

The regular use of antacids is considered a part of level two care. Antacids work by neutralizing the gastric acid and thus increasing the pH in the stomach. They have a short duration of action of an hour or two and may inhibit the absorption of other drugs. There are some side effects of antacid use that must be taken into consideration, such as increased serum calcium levels with calcium carbonate antacids (may be good for osteoporosis but bad for kidney stones), constipation with aluminum containing compounds, or diarrhea with magnesium antacids.

Level three consists of the above lifestyle and diet factors plus the use of prescription medications to either reduce acid production or alter gastrointestinal motility. It has been our experience that reduction of stomach acid secretion is more effective than pharmacologic attempts to alter esophageal motility. There are two broad groups of medications to reduce stomach acid secretion, H2-receptor antagonists, and proton pump inhibitors. The chemical action of both groups is to inhibit the acid secretion of the parietal cells in the stomach lining, but each group works at a slightly different part of the production line. It is well recognized that proton pump inhibitor medications are more effective at acid reduction than are the H2 blockers. Consequently, in our clinic, we tend to begin treating the patient with proton pump inhibitor therapy. Each of the three drug groups involved in reflux treatment will be discussed briefly.

1. Proton pump inhibitors. There are three currently available agents in this group, omeprazole (Losec®), lansoprazole (Prevacid®), and pantoprazole (Pantoloc™). The proton pump inhibitor blocks the final common pathway of acid secretion from the gastric parietal cell. It is more effective when taken first thing in the morning than at nighttime[27]. When these drugs were first introduced, there was concern that long-term use would be dangerous, and various publications still suggest that treatment should be limited to a few months. Increasingly, clinical experience suggests that they are safe to take in the long term, and many patients with significant laryngeal problems of GE reflux have been on these medications for several years[34].

2. H2-receptor antagonists. Four currently available drugs in this group include cimetidine, ranitidine, famotidine, and nyzatidine. They all act to block the stimulation of gastric parietal cells by histamine[16]. They also reduce output of pepsin from the stomach. Apart from being somewhat less effective than proton pump inhibitors, these medications must be taken more than once a day. An important advantage is that they are currently less expensive.

3. Prokinetic drugs (motility modifiers). Drugs in this group include domperidone, metoclopramide, and cisapride. They may increase pressure in the lower esophageal sphincter. They may also increase gastric emptying. Although several studies have suggested that they are effective in treating GE reflux[31], they do not seem to be so effective in the management of reflux generated voice problems as do the acid reducing medications. They often are used in combination

with H2 blockers. It is felt that many of the head and neck symptoms associated with GE reflux are related to increased muscle tone in the larynx and hypopharynx; this class of drugs does not seem to have any direct effect on those muscles.

Level four care involves surgery. In a very small proportion of patients, reflux cannot be adequately controlled with lifestyle measures and drugs; these people may require a procedure to reduce GE reflux. A laparoscopic fundoplication can be performed whereby the upper part of the stomach is wrapped around the lower part of the esophagus to create a functional valve. Because it is still necessary to be able to vomit after the surgery, this closure cannot be too tight. The fundoplication procedure is not a perfect operation, but it can be helpful in those people with uncontrollable reflux.

To generalize, about 90% of people with laryngeal manifestations of GE reflux are eventually able to sustain control of the problem with lifestyle measures and periodic antacid use. Another 9% of patients will need prolonged or intermittent regular use of acid reducing drugs, and 1% are likely to be offered an antireflux operation.

3.3 Medical Therapy for Muscle Misuse Voice Disorders

Treatment of patients with muscle misuse voice disorders usually is shared between the speech-language pathologist, psychologist or psychiatrist, voice teacher, and other professionals. The reader is referred to Chapters 4, 5, and 7 for detailed discussions of intervention. The otolaryngologist's role is to ensure the absence of any structural factors—and to be sure that the patient understands this—as well as to treat concomitant conditions such as gastroesophageal reflux.

3.4 Structural–Organic Factors

3.4.1 Tumors

3.4.1.1 Laryngeal Papilloma (Recurrent Respiratory Papillomatosis)

As discussed in Chapter 2, papilloma is a warty growth that is caused by the human papilloma virus. Because the virus infects all of the intralaryngeal mucous membrane, it is not possible to remove all of the diseased tissue. Sometimes the body's immune system is able to totally eradicate the disease, and it may be that careful removal of all apparent papilloma permits this to occur more readily. In new adult laryngeal papilloma cases, every effort is made, over the first two or three surgical procedures, to achieve a papilloma-free larynx. If, after a few episodes, it seems that the patient is destined to suffer constant recurrence over the long term, the timing of repeat surgery is based more on the severity of symptoms rather than physical appearance of the larynx.

Careful CO_2 laser ablation of papilloma generally is accepted as the surgical procedure of choice. As with other surgical procedures for benign laryngeal disease, however, some surgeons are finding it equally effective, or even preferable, to use a selection of fine microsurgical instruments to dissect out the lesion. The objective is to remove the papilloma while causing as little trauma to the underlying connective tissues as possible, thus reducing postsurgical scarring. It is especially important to avoid injuring both vocal cords near the anterior commissure because the formation of a web at this site is the most frequent and significant complication of surgery for papilloma.

Zeitels and Sataloff have presented the case for subepithelial infusion of an adrenaline-saline solution under the papilloma, followed by careful microflap dissection and excision of all visible lesions in the larynx. They suggested that recurrence of papilloma is reduced with this technique, particularly when operating on new lesions[37].

Although repeated careful excision is the mainstay of papilloma treatment, there are other adjuvant therapies available. Indole-3-carbinol (I3C) is a chemical that is found in high concentrations in cruciferous vegetables and which may alter the growth pattern of laryngeal papilloma. I3C affects the body's estrogen metabolism by affecting the ratio of hydroxylation of estradiol. Usually, 400 mg per day are taken as a food supplement in capsule form[33]. Because laryngeal papilloma is a viral illness, antiviral therapies may be helpful. Application or injection of drugs such as cidofavir may slow down the recurrence rate of papilloma but has not been shown to have any permanent effect.

3.4.1.2 Squamous Cell Carcinoma

Most early vocal fold cancers can be treated effectively with radiation therapy or limited surgery, both of which result in high cure rates. T1 lesions (confined to the glottis and vocal folds with normal mobility) can be controlled in more than 90% of patients, but curability of late lesions drops dramatically and treatment may involve total laryngectomy. This book does not consider the treatment of cancer in the larynx in any detail, and the reader is referred elsewhere for this information.

Voice restoration following laryngectomy has evolved considerably since Blom and Singer[5] introduced the tracheoesophageal fistula technique in the early 1980s. It has become common practice to create the fistula tract through the back wall of the trachea and into the cervical esophagus at the time of laryngectomy and to use the fistula as access for the feeding tube in the early postoperative days. Before discharge from hospital, the feeding tube is withdrawn and the voice prosthesis inserted. Exhalation with an occluded tracheal opening forces the air into the pharynx, and it is vibration of the neopharyngeal walls that generates a new vocal tone. Having a readily accessible voice at the time of discharge from hospital is a great psychological boost to the new laryngectomee. Further details regarding postlaryngectomy speech rehabilitation are provided in Chapter 4.

3.4.2 Infection

Dysphonia associated with upper respiratory viral illness is temporary and not a major problem—unless the patient happens to be a professional voice user. Rest and extra hydration are the mainstays of treatment, but an urgent need for voice, such as for a concert, may lead to an array of treatment options including systemic steroids with antibiotic coverage. The following case illustrates this.

Case 3.1

Sandra Soprano is a 39-year-old diva who had a leading role in a local production of La Boheme. *On the day before the third of four performances, she developed a tickle in her throat and a minor but irritating cough. She felt generally tired and yet the demands of the performance gave her the energy to carry on. She managed to get through the role reasonably well, although some of her high notes were effortful, and she felt generally unwell the next morning. The pitch of her speaking voice had dropped a tone, and her throat was slightly sore. On examination, the nose, oral cavity, and pharynx were normal, but indirect laryngoscopy showed slightly pink and glistening vocal folds. Because the examiner had not seen this patient before, it was hard to say whether the examination was revealing features within the bounds of what might be considered normal for this individual. Of greatest concern, however, was a distinctly thickened and irritated tracheal mucosa visible between the vocal folds, and thus the diagnosis of laryngotracheitis, likely of viral cause, was entertained.*

Without further vocal demands, the treatment of the situation is easy, consisting of adequate hydration and rest. But Sandra was scheduled to sing again in 2 days to a sold-out house of 3000 opera fans. The understudy was poorly prepared but could sing the part from the wings leaving Sandra to walk through the staging. Sandra had no singing commitments for 3 weeks after the show (an important point) and wanted to carry on if at all feasible. It was therefore decided to reduce the inflammation and the risk of injury as much as possible, coupled with rest and adequate fluid intake, to allow Sandra to carry on. Treatment was started using prednisone 50 mg daily plus antibiotics to cover the possibility of opportunistic bacterial infection. Her usual good hydration habits were supplemented with steam inhalations. The prednisone was tapered off over 10 days. Guaifenesin was also used to thin secretions.

The day following her initial consultation, Sandra's speaking voice pitch seemed more normal, and she was feeling a little better although, as is usual in this situation, she felt a little "spacey." By performance day, the adrenaline rush, coupled with an extra careful and lengthy warm-up, carried her through.

This scenario is not uncommon, but in some instances, the laryngologist together with the singer must decide that to attempt such a "rescue" is not worth the risk. The degree of laryngotracheitis and the early response to treatment will help make this decision.

Bacterial laryngitis may follow viral illness as a superinfection but more commonly occurs with *Haemophilis influenzae, Staphylococcus aureus, Streptococcus pneumoniae,* or *Beta hemolytic streptococcus* being the most common offenders. Pain and fever may be severe with airway and swallowing difficulties generally overshadowing voice loss, although loss of voice is certainly a symptom. Treatment in adults involves the use of intravenous antibiotics, hydration, humidification, and possibly corticosteroids. Close observation is essential in case airway support is required.

Candida is the most common **fungal disease** of the larynx. A treatment that is effective in most cases is to use clotrimazole tablets as a lozenge, dissolved slowly in the mouth four times a day. Oral nystatin suspension used as a gargle does not seem to work as well, probably because it is washed away so quickly. An alternative is a single dose oral tablet of fluconazole (Diflucan™ 150).

Other fungal diseases are rare but do occur in the larynx. Examples include *Blastomycosis,*

Histoplasmosis, and *Coccidiodomycosis,* so-called "deep" mycotic infections. The disease often is confused with carcinoma or other types of infection, and a high index of suspicion is needed to get a diagnosis in some cases. Long-term treatment with antifungal agents, such as amphotericin B, is necessary to rid the larynx of the disease.

Other granulomatous infections include tuberculosis, leprosy, and scleroma. Long-term treatment with the appropriate drugs is required.

3.4.3 Chronic Noninfective Laryngitis

Over the past number of years, it has become increasingly clear that many patients suffering from nonspecific chronic laryngitis have **reflux** of gastric secretions into the larynx and pharynx. The typical diagnostic features have been described in Chapter 2. Treatment of these patients is the same as for other problems that result from GE reflux and is described in Section 3.2.4. Even if there is clear evidence of vocal abuse or misuse, it is important to concomitantly treat any underlying reflux. There have been a number of studies that have confirmed resolution of the symptoms of chronic laryngitis through GE reflux therapy alone[17].

Although extremely common, reflux is obviously not the only causative factor in chronic non-infective laryngitis. **Autoimmune disorders** such as systemic lupus erythematosis, dermatomyositis or scleroderma may affect the vocal folds and the voice. In these disorders, a collection of gritty nodular tissue may form in Reinke's space and cause the mucosa to adhere to it. There are often several of these thickenings lined up along the superior surface of the vocal cord, and they have been referred to as "bamboo nodes." If the voice is severely affected and mucosal wave greatly damped, the lesions can be removed at microlaryngoscopy. An incision is made in the mucosa along the superior surface of the cord, just lateral to the lesion. The mucosa is then elevated from the node and the inflammatory tissue is removed from the underlying vocal ligament with fine cup forceps. Fibrin glue may be used to assist with adherence of the mucosa to the lamina propria, and the cord is injected with a hydrocortisone solution.

Amyloidosis is a disorder of protein metabolism in which "amyloid" proteinaceous material is deposited in the larynx, usually in the submucosal tissue of the false vocal cords of the supraglottic larynx. Laryngeal amyloidosis is not associated with generalized amyloidosis and simultaneous occurrence in other areas is rare. The voice effect of amyloid is usually the result of damping of vocal fold vibration by the masses in the false cords and laryngeal ventricles. Treatment is usually by laser excision of the false vocal folds and the disease contained in them. It is not necessary to achieve a surgical margin around the deposit, and even if some tissue remains behind, the disease may remain quiescent for many years. Long-term follow-up is essential.

Allergic laryngitis seems to be a relatively small problem in laryngology practice when one considers the huge extent of allergy problems elsewhere in the respiratory tract. Clearly, allergy can lead to some edema and erythema in the larynx, but generally in association with more severe symptoms in the nose or lower airways to the point that treatment of the larynx is done in passing. Singers who have laryngeal allergy problems generally are helped by seasonal use of antihistamine medications. If allergy is suspected to be a significant factor in a patient with a voice disorder it may be important to undertake allergy testing either by way of radioallergosorbent serum tests or skin testing. Vocal fold edema may result from allergy; it may also contribute to additional misuse and abuse effects[22].

Medical management of unusual laryngeal inflammatory disorders such as Wegener's granulomatosis, sarcoidosis, mucosal pemphigoid, epidermolysis bullosa, or relapsing polychondtitis may be complex. Usually the voice aspects are less important than airway problems. They are not discussed here.

3.4.4 Lesions Due to Misuse and Abuse

Vocal Nodules

Abnormally high levels of shearing stress on the vocal folds as a result of loud persistent abusive voice use, especially in the absence of good vocal technique, will cause injury. This often takes the form of nodular thickening at the middle of the vibrating portions of the cords, usually bilateral and symmetrical. The lesions are situated in the superficial layer of the lamina propria, or Reinke's Space. Because they do not affect deeper structural layers, normal vocal fold mobility and a full mucosal wave are typically still visible during laryngostroboscopy. The cause is behavioral, and so is the treatment in most cases. This includes avoidance of vocal abuse and correction of technical misuses. Sometimes the nodules are so large that additional laryngeal effort is required to adduct the vocal folds and generate a vocal tone, resulting in even more trauma. Only when the nodules seem to be getting in the way of further progress in voice therapy should one consider surgical removal.

Unilateral firm vocal nodules are usually the result of a distinct episode of vocal trauma, and surgical excision is the rule rather than the exception in these cases. Should the decision be made to remove vocal nodules, it is important to be delicate and conservative. There is no role for "stripping" in surgery for benign vocal fold disease. Whether to use "cold steel" instruments or the CO_2 laser for removal of excess tissue depends on the surgeon's preference and may be made on a case by case decision. The object is to minimize scar tissue in the healing process, and therefore a technique that leaves mucosal edges closely applied to each other will usually be best. The following case illustrates a common scenario.

Case 3.2

Betty Belter, aged 23 years, has always taken lead roles in school and community theatre productions. She is outgoing and attractive with a naturally pleasing singing voice. She is socially active, enjoying the company of others in nightclubs where she sometimes works as a hostess to help augment her daytime salary. Betty's regular work as a receptionist is vocally demanding, and she is frequently hoarse by the end of a stressful working day. She smokes a pack of cigarettes a day, as does her boyfriend. Incidentally, the relationship with her boyfriend seems to be coming apart.

Betty was encouraged to get involved with a rock band that a group of friends was starting up in which she would, of course, be the lead singer. She now complains of the loss of much of her upper vocal register and is concerned about the degree of breathiness in her voice. Her hoarseness persists even after a few days rest. Singing lessons have been suggested, but her friends warned her that lessons would ruin her natural voice.

The fleshy, sessile, almost polypoid nodules seen in Betty's larynx are noted to accompany a characteristic isometric muscle misuse, identified by increased paralaryngeal muscle tension and an abnormally open posterior glottic chink on stroboscopy. The misuse combined with voice abuse and cigarette smoking all contribute to her voice difficulty. (Figure 3–1).

Primary management of this problem includes behavioral modification, counseling, direct voice therapy, and smoking cessation. Should it become necessary to consider "trimming" the vocal nodules, the procedure should be in combination with the primary treatments and consist of a conservative reduction of polypoid tissue while retaining as

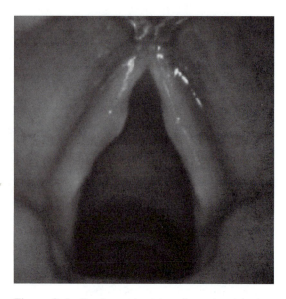

Figure 3–1. Sessile, moderately soft vocal nodules in a 23-year-old female singer.

full a mucosal cover as possible. A more widespread "stripping" would result in the problem illustrated in Section 3.4.5.

Reinke's edema and polypoid degeneration are removed by way of an incision along the superior surface of the vocal fold. The mucosa is elevated as a small flap allowing the myxoid tissue that makes up the polyp contents to be teased out with a suction tip or fine cup forceps. After the tissue has been cleared away, the mucosa is returned to its position covering the underlying vocal ligament, and any excess mucous membrane is trimmed with fine microscissors. A layer of fibrin glue between the mucosa and ligament may provide additional stability.

There are numerous excellent texts and video demonstrations of the instruments and techniques used in microlaryngeal phonosurgery[7,8,18]. The reader is directed to one of those sources for detailed guidance. Postoperative instructions are given to the patient as a handout, as shown in Appendix 3–2.

Abuse-related Vocal Fold Hemorrhage

Treatment of this situation may be best described through an example case.

Case 3.3

*Beryl Belcher, aspiring 28-year-old pop singer,
suddenly lost her voice following an evening of
effortful singing. Examination shortly after the
episode revealed a diffuse subepithelial hemorrhage along the entire length of the right vocal
fold (Figure 3–2). Total voice rest was recommended, and the hematoma resolved, leaving
only a bright red nodular mass on the superior
surface of the cord, consistent with the diagnosis
of an organized hemorrhagic nodule.*

*Because it has been shown that vocal fold
telangiectasia and microhemorrhages often are
associated with the repeated vomiting of bulimia
nervosa, the subject was broached, and it was determined that Beryl had been bulimic between the
ages of 16 and 18. Careful microcauterization of
the vascular anomaly stopped the occurrences of
bleeding.*

Subepithelial hemorrhage of the vocal fold
is an infrequent but important serious event
that can put a singing career on hold. Micro-
laser vaporization or microcauterization of
any small telangiectatic vessels, particularly
in a singer who has already had one bleed,
may prevent it. A period of absolute voice rest
is essential after a bleed. If the hematoma is at
all bulky, it may be advisable to evacuate it
surgically.

3.4.5 Laryngeal Trauma

The treatment of voice disorders associated
with scarring and mucosal tethering following vocal fold stripping can be difficult. These
dysphonias are often unresponsive to voice
therapy, and injection of the folds with substances such as teflon is generally not helpful.
The use of collagen to inject the vocal folds
submucosally is still being evaluated but may
hold some promise. The best approaches to
reducing vocal fold stiffness with voice
therapy are discussed in Chapter 4, Section
4.6.1. The following case illustrates the problems encountered due to excessive removal of
vocal fold mucosa at surgery.

Case 3.4

*Gravel Gerty Green arranged a visit to her doctor
because she became tired of being called "sir" on
the telephone. Her church choir leader suggested
that she move from the alto to the tenor section,
and she wanted to know if there was anything
that could be done to raise the pitch of her voice
back to its previous level. Consequently, a laryngoscopy and removal of edematous vocal fold
mucosa was performed. Four months later, her
voice had not yet recovered, remaining squeaky,
strained, and breathy in spite of a number of
voice therapy sessions postoperatively.*

*Stroboscopic videolaryngoscopy showed that
both vocal folds were stiff, and the mucosal wave
was damped, more severely on the right side than
the left. There appeared to be an area towards the
anterior end of the fold that lacked bulk and was
less pliable on strobe exam (Figure 3–3).*

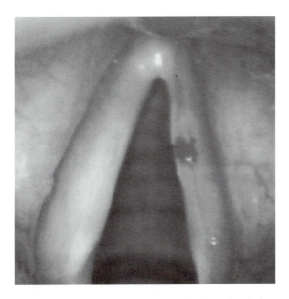

Figure 3–2. Posthemorrhagic telangiectatic lesion
(varix) on the right vocal fold.

As demonstrated by Gerty's case, when
stripping leaves areas bared of mucosa, re-

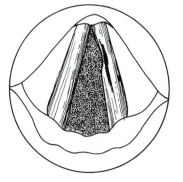

Figure 3–3. A stiff, indented scar is noted on the anterior half of the right vocal fold. This is the result of tethering of mucosa following stripping of polypoidal disease.

generating glottic mucosa may become densely adherent to the underlying lamina propria and simply not vibrate well. It may slowly soften with time, but persistent dysphonia is difficult to treat. Submucosal injections of collagen have been shown to be helpful in some cases[15,32].

3.4.6 Contact Ulcer and Granuloma

Because of the strong positive relationship with GE reflux, the treatment of contact granuloma of the larynx focuses on control of reflux with concomitant voice therapy in well-motivated individuals. The reflux relationship with laryngeal granuloma has been documented by many authors in the past[9,24,30,36]. Compliance in voice therapy has been a problem in this group of patients, and Jaroma's series showed that only 41 % participated in a voice therapy program[23].

The cornerstone of GE reflux treatment in patients with laryngeal granuloma remains the reduction of acidity of gastric secretions using proton pump inhibitors. Details of antireflux therapy were described in Section 3.2.4. For granulomas to heal, the antireflux

therapy must be continued for a long time. The usual practice in our clinic is to make a video recording of the larynx for comparative purposes and then place the patient on proton pump inhibitor therapy for 3 months, along with other general antireflux measures. At the end of this time, the patient returns for a follow-up videolaryngoscopy. Sequentially, over a number of examinations, the granuloma generally is seen to slowly disappear. There have been a number of recent studies that support this management strategy for the treatment of vocal process granuloma[13,19, 35]. In those cases where reflux treatment and voice therapy are not adequate to clear the granuloma, additional measures may include:

1. Botulinum toxin injection: This is used in a manner similar to treatment for adductor spasmodic dysphonia, in the assumption that a period of time with reduced posterior glottic closure pressures will facilitate healing (see Section 3.5.2).
2. Corticosteroid injection: This is not a first-line therapy, and is usually not very helpful.
3. Surgical excision: Surgical removal sometimes is done to confirm the pathological diagnosis, but in most cases the diagnosis is so evident that it is not required. Removal with CO_2 laser or cold knife excision may be offered in large lesions that have obstructive symptoms, but the recurrence rate is high unless combined with maximum reflux therapy.

The following case is a typical example.

Case 3.5

Larry Litigator spends much of his day in the courtroom. He loves his work. He also loves black coffee and late-night Mexican dinners. His coworkers have begun to complain about his constant throat clearing, and he finds that the amount of effort to keep talking all day has greatly increased.

The most obvious sign seen on laryngoscopic examination is a heaped up granular lesion overlying the medial surface of the left arytenoid cartilage (Figure 3–4). The vocal folds look normal, but stroboscopic assessment demonstrates excessive medial compression, evidenced by a prolonged closed phase of the vibratory cycle. As in Larry's case, contact granulomata frequently are associated with chronic gastroesophageal reflux, together with a muscle misuse voice disorder. Antireflux management results in a slow resolution of the granuloma. Larry also attends a group voice therapy program that targets the needs of occupational voice users and has been gratified by his increased ability to perform in court.

3.4.7 Intracordal Cysts and Sulcus Vocalis

Special sets of microlaryngeal surgical instruments have been developed to permit cysts to be delicately dissected free. An inci-

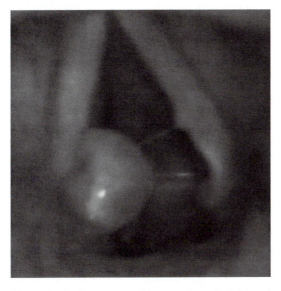

Figure 3–4. Contact granuloma overlying the left vocal process.

sion is made along the superior surface of the vocal fold in the direction of the fold, just through the mucous membrane that is then elevated medially towards the free edge of the vocal fold, exposing the cyst. Because the deep aspect of the cyst is very adherent to the lamina propria below it, great care must be taken to peel it away without breakage. If the cyst does rupture, the surgeon must decide whether to try to remove all of the cyst lining with some surrounding fibrous tissue or to stop the surgery and come back to try another day after the cyst has reformed.

Surgical treatment of vocal fold sulci in which a strip of mucosa is densely adherent to the free edge of the fold, is difficult and several less-than-satisfactory techniques have been tried and discarded. This is particularly true for sulcus vergeture in which the opening of the sulcus is wide, and there is little in the way of pliable mucous membrane that can be elevated around it. If the sulcus is surgically excised down to the underlying vocal ligament, it frequently will leave scar tissue in such a way that the clinical voice problem may be no better. On the other hand, if the sulcus is a mucosally lined sac and there is sufficient mucous membrane around it, an incision can be made around the sulcus opening, the mucosa elevated, and the sac excised. This leaves enough mucous membrane so that the wound can be closed and the creation of additional scar tissue averted.

Whether there is an intracordal cyst, an open sulcus vergeture, or a pitlike sulcus vocalis, that portion of the sulcus mucosa in the depth of the lesion is always densely adherent to the middle layer of the lamina propria. This part of the sulcus must be meticulously removed and any overlying pliable mucous membrane assiduously protected[6]. Following excision of the sulcus or cyst, the vocal cord frequently is injected with corticosteroid to reduce inflammation and scar tissue formation. As with other surgery for benign vocal lesions, patients are given instructions about postoperative voice care, as provided in Appendix 3.2.

3.4.8 Transgender Laryngeal Surgery

3.4.8.1 Thyroid Cartilage Reduction

Many male-to-female transgender patients come to the voice clinic with the request for a "tracheal shave," by which they mean reduction in the prominence of the Adam's apple. The whole larynx can be big and account for much of the prominence, but in most people the prominence is the projecting upper forward angle of the thyroid cartilage. The procedure of thyroid cartilage reduction involves exposing the front of the larynx through a horizontal incision about 1 inch long over the prominent area. After dividing the superficial fascia and platysma muscle horizontally, the strap muscles of the larynx are separated in the midline to expose the thyroid cartilage. A scalpel is used to incise the external thyroid perichondrium along the upper margin of the cartilage, and the perichondrium is then elevated. Most of the upper front half of the thyroid cartilage can be removed with scalpel, drill or rongeur. Bone has often replaced much of the cartilage (this gradually increases with age), and the surgeon may need to use a drill. The main restrictions in cartilage removal concern the anterior commisure area where the vocal cords attach and the anterior arch of the cricoid cartilage. It is most important to preserve and protect the region of thyroid cartilage midway between the notch and the lower margin, which is where the vocal cords attach to the inner surface. After the thyroid cartilage has been reduced, the cricoid may be the largest prominence. It is helpful to point it out to the patient ahead of time and explain that it cannot be made smaller.

3.4.8.2 Cricothyroid Approximation for Pitch Elevation

Ishikki first described this procedure as one of a number of types of thyroplasty, or laryngeal framework surgery, to increase the vocal pitch[21]. Approximating the cricoid and thyroid cartilages results in a stretching pull on the vocal cords by tilting the back part of the cricoid and arytenoids backward and the front end of the cords (where they attach to the inner thyroid cartilage) forward. The procedure is done under local anesthesia with a similar exposure as for the thyroid cartilage reduction. Local anesthesia permits the operator to listen to the voice while closing the cricoid space, thus "tuning" the vocal pitch to some degree. It is necessary to make the cricothyroid sutures a bit tighter than what seems correct during surgery because there is always a degree of release over a few days.

The cricothyroid approximation mimics the action of the cricothyroid muscles. Although singers skillfully learn to use this muscle to sing in the high registers with a minimal amount of strain, approximation of the cricothyroid space surgically, with permanent suture material, enforces the voice user to speak in a falsetto range. If effective, it should make it impossible to speak in modal register because the vocal folds are unable to relax into that register. Many transgender voice users can learn to speak in a higher modal pitch range or falsetto register through voice therapy. (Voice therapy techniques for transgender patients are discussed in Chapter 4, Section 4.6.3.) The advantage of surgical intervention is the impossibility of slipping into the male pitch range during spontaneous vocalizations or when fatigue or distraction catch the speaker off-guard.

3.4.8.3 Laser-Assisted Anterior Commissure Plication

There are several reasons why a cricothyroid approximation may not be successful in achieving the desired pitch elevation. Sometimes the thyroid cartilage is so soft that the sutures do not hold adequately, and when they pull out in the postoperative period (or sooner), then the effect is lost. In a few people, the vocal folds are not stretched even with a fully closed cricothyroid space, probably because there is a structural variation that precludes it. In this situation, one may try to increase the pitch by shortening the length of the folds instead of stretching and tightening them. One way of shortening the vibrating segment is to create a web anteriorly (Figure 3–5). Although this raises the pitch, it also tends to affect voice clarity by adding some breathiness or huskiness and may reduce vocal power, particularly in noisy environments. The larynx is viewed through an operating laryngoscope using a microscope coupled to a CO_2 laser. The mucous membrane lining of the anterior quarter of the folds is vaporized with the laser following which the denuded folds are sewn together

with an absorbable suture, utilizing endoscopic needle driver and knot tier.

Because inappropriate pitch is only one feature of communication that may influence gender perception, surgical intervention is ideally coupled with a speech therapy program that provides insight and training in achieving other important goals, such as gender-appropriate resonance, articulation, syntax, and vocabulary. Details are provided in Chapter 4.

3.5 Neurological and Neuromuscular Disorders

3.5.1 Vocal Fold Paralysis

Unless there are factors present that require more urgent treatment, the common approach to treatment of unilateral recurrent laryngeal nerve paralysis is to wait for 6 to 9 months for spontaneous recovery to occur. If aspiration of liquids puts respiratory health at risk or if the voice is urgently required for some reason, a procedure to medialize the paralyzed vocal cord is considered. If spontaneous recovery is anticipated, then a procedure without permanent ill effects will be used, such as injection of gelfoam paste, fat, or bovine collagen. Each of these will resolve to the point of not having any adverse effects if the vocalis recovery is complete. Because transcutaneous collagen injection is easily done in the clinic and offers a quick resolution of symptoms, if only for a short time, it may become the norm to do this as a temporary measure in most patients.

If symptoms persist after passage of the generally accepted spontaneous recovery time, then some form of surgical procedure will be offered to the patient. There are advantages and disadvantages for each of the surgical methods of voice augmentation for unilateral recurrent laryngeal nerve paralysis. There is no single best method, and each clin-

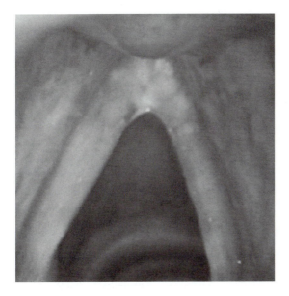

Figure 3–5. Shortening the vibrating segment by web formation.

ical situation must be considered on its own merits. Forms of surgery include vocal cord injection, medialization through external placement of a laryngeal implant, or selective muscle reinnervation.

3.5.1.1 Vocal Cord Injection

A common surgical technique is to inject **teflon paste** into the tissues of the paralyzed vocal fold. Arnold originally introduced this technique in 1962[1]. Augmentation by teflon injection may be done in the operating room via direct laryngoscopy or in the clinic transcutaneously. There is a consensus that the voice results may not be as good in the long term as with other techniques, but this treatment still has great value, particularly for quick rehabilitation of patients with mediastinal metastatic carcinoma.

The problem with teflon injection is that it is easy to do, but difficult to do well. The teflon incites a foreign body inflammatory reaction, and it may be necessary to remove the teflon many years later. The glottis is not as evenly medialized as with thyroplasty, and voice quality may not be as good[11]. Good results with teflon injection demand good placement technique. The teflon must be deeply placed in the vocalis muscle and on the glottal plane (Figure 3–6). Problems are more likely to occur if the material is placed too superficially, too high or too low (Figure 3–7).

Other materials can be injected into the vocal cord to achieve temporary medialization while waiting for spontaneous recovery. **Gelfoam paste** is made by mixing one gram of Gelfoam powder with 5 cc of saline. The paste is rolled into a "worm," loaded into the teflon injector syringe, and injected in a manner similar to teflon.

Fat may be harvested from the abdominal area by open dissection or liposuction. Open excision may be preferable because the fat globules can be teased apart and cleaned

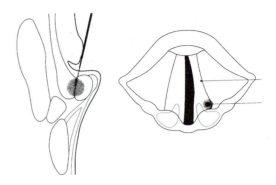

Figure 3–6. Correct placement of teflon for augmentation of the paralyzed vocal fold. From *Phonosurgery* (p. 128), by C. N. Ford and D. M. Bless, 1991, New York: Raven Press. Copyright 1991 by Raven Press. Reprinted with permission.

with saline before loading into the injector, whereas suctioned fat may be more prone to tissue damage and earlier reabsorption. Because much of the tissue bulk will be reabsorbed, it is necessary to overinject by 50% to 100%. Because the reabsorption is variable, the results are difficult to predict.

Bovine collagen injection has the advantage of being easier to inject in the clinic than gelfoam or teflon. It passes easily through a 27-gauge needle and is injected in the same manner as Botox for spasmodic dysphonia. The laryngeal image is observed on a monitor during the injection. This technique, as well as collagen injection for Parkinson's disease hypophonia, has been described by Berke[2]. The technique and results using the indirect laryngoscopy approach has been described by Remacle[32] and by Ford[14,15].

3.5.1.2 Laryngeal Framework Surgery (Thyroplasty)

Isshiki, Okamura, and Ishikawa[20,21] have described two types of **thyroplasty** that are very effective in rehabilitating vocal paralysis. Vocal fold medialization can be achieved via

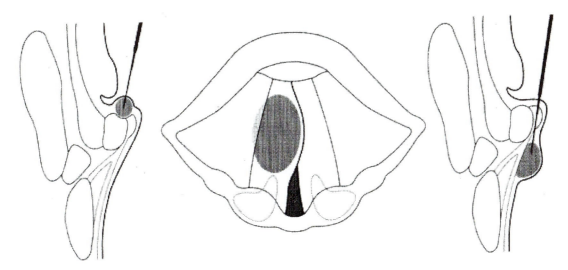

Figure 3–7. Incorrect teflon injection location. From *Phonosurgery* (p. 129), by C. N. Ford and D. M. Bless, 1991, New York: Raven Press. Copyright 1991 by Raven Press. Reprinted with permission

an external neck incision and subperichondrial insertion of a silastic block prosthesis through a window cut into the thyroid cartilage (Figures 3–8–3–11). This medializes the cord in much the same way as teflon adds bulk to the deep laryngeal tissues, but without the associated stiffness or inflammation. It also is reversible or "tuneable" in that the prosthesis may be removed or exchanged for one of another size.

The advantages of medialization thyroplasty are that it is well tolerated and safe. There is minimal inflammatory reaction and a stable result. Because the implant is outside the perichondrium, it can be removed and replaced if necessary, so the procedure is reversible and tunable. Disadvantages of medialization thyroplasty include the need for an open operation (scar) and an overnight stay to watch the airway. A problem that affects the results of medialization thyroplasty is difficulty in getting good posterior closure.

Isshiki has also described a technique for **arytenoid adduction** that involves attaching a suture on the muscular process of the arytenoid and passing it forward to an anchor point in the anterior thyroid cartilage[21]. Suture tension can be adjusted to stretch and medialize the vocal fold. Although more difficult to perform, this technique gives excellent voice results in selected cases. The arytenoid adduction procedure has some advantages, such as putting the paralyzed cord on a stretch without bulk, which may make it vibrate better. It may close the posterior commisure more effectively than medialization. Disadvantages are that it is a more difficult operation and the results are more difficult to "fine tune."

Zeitels recently added two further modifications to the arytenoid adduction procedure. One is to close the posterior commissure more completely by moving the body of the arytenoid cartilage toward the midline and anchoring it to the cricoid[38]. The second stretches the vocal fold by subluxation of the cricothyroid joint and fixing the thyroid cartilage in a more anterior position relative to the cricoid[39]. Further innovations in thyroplasty surgery are anticipated.

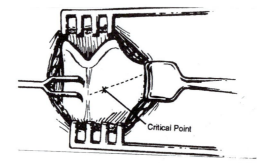

Figure 3–8. Exposure of the larynx for medialization thyroplasty.

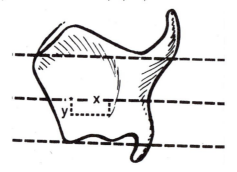

Figure 3–9. Location of the thyroid cartilage window. X – horizontal line from the midpoint between the thyroid notch and the lower cartilage margin. Y – approximately 1 cm posterior to the anterior cartilage angle.

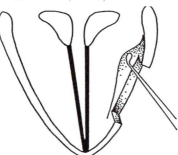

Figure 3–10. Subperichondrial elevation of the thyroplasty prosthesis pocket.

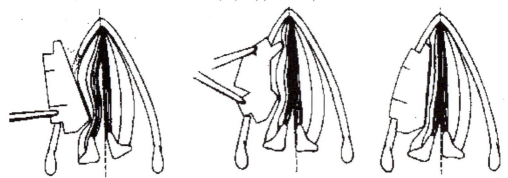

Figure 3–11. Insertion of the thyroplasty prosthesis.

3.5.1.3 Neuromuscular Reinnervation

Reinnervation procedures are based on the hypothesis that reinnervated muscle will have increased bulk and tone and therefore vibrate more effectively and with a restored mucosal wave. A nerve crossover procedure between the ansa cervicalis and the recurrent nerve, as described by Crumley, lzdebski, and McMicken[10], may be the best way to do this (Figure 3–12). An ideal patient is one that has lost the recurrent nerve in the chest because of aortic arch surgery. The procedure may be combined with fat or gelfoam injection for interim benefit.

3.5.2 Dystonia and Tremor

Medical therapy for the voice problems associated with dystonia are directed toward release of the spasmodic muscular tension associated with the disease or diseases in-volved. There was little otolaryngologists could do to help patients with spasmodic dysphonia until Dedo[12] discovered in the early 1970s that section of one recurrent laryngeal nerve was accompanied by relief of the dysphonia in a significant proportion of patients. Because of relatively high recurrence rates and the evolution of botulinum toxin therapy for this disorder, section of the recurrent laryngeal nerve now is seldom performed. Botulinum toxin (Botox®) injections were introduced for treatment of spasmodic dysphonia by Blitzer and Brin[4], and although these injections provide miraculous relief for many patients, they are associated with some problems, not the least of which is the need to return for repeated injections several times each year. Some patients are frustrated by the need for repeated treatment, as well as the several days that the voice is weak and breathy after the injection. Berke recently described a more selective denervation-

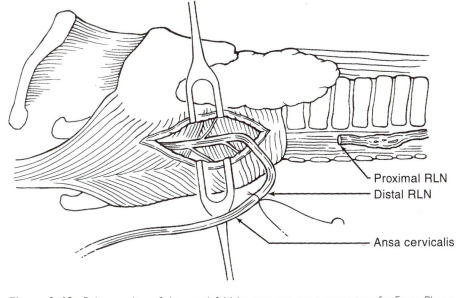

Figure 3–12. Reinnervation of the vocal fold by ansa-recurrent nerve transfer. From Phono-surgery (p. 209), by R. L. Crumley, 1991, New York: Raven Press. Copyright 1991 by Raven Press. Reprinted with permission.

reinnervation procedure that may offer promise for patients who wish to have something permanently fixed[3]. The key feature of this procedure is that the vocal cords are immediately reinnervated by a nerve that takes its origin from a different part of the brain than that which is affected by the dystonia.

Botulinum toxin is manufactured by the bacteria, *Clostridium botulinum*, and is an extremely potent toxin that blocks the transmission of nerve signals at the motor endplate. It does not directly treat dystonia but produces a partial paralysis so that the vocal cords cannot become spasmodic even though the brain is telling them to do so. Botox® simply relieves symptoms. Its effects predictably wear off after 3 or 4 months. This is the time it takes the nerve endings to resprout and make new connections to the muscle fibers.

Dystonic muscle spasm is one type of movement disorder that affects the larynx and voice. Tremor is the other. Although botulinum toxin is effective at releasing the spasm, it is not of any help to the tremor. Essential tremor may respond to medical treatment with beta-blockers such as propranolol. Voice therapy strategies for spasmodic dysphonias and benign essential tremor are discussed in Chapter 4, Section 4.6.

3.5.2.1 Adductor Spasmodic Dysphonia

Following a full medical, neurologic, psychological, and voice pathology evaluation the patient with adductor spasmodic dysphonia will likely be offered botulinum toxin therapy. In our clinic, this procedure is done under EMG guidance transcutaneously. Our usual initial dose is 1.5 units for female patients and 2 units in each vocal cord for male patients. The patient is told that he or she may expect the voice to become weak and breathy within about 12 hours, and this side effect will become maximal in about a week. Recovery takes place in the subsequent few

days or week. During the time that the voice is breathy, the patient needs to avoid drinking liquids quickly to avoid aspiration. Drinking through a straw might help if the problem is severe, but usually it is only a matter of being attentive to the possibility. After the injection, each patient is given a diary card and asked to rate their own voice twice a month. We use a scale on which *1* is the worst their voice has been and *10* is what they would consider to be a normal voice. If possible, the patient returns in about 8 weeks for a follow-up laryngeal examination and voice recording. Determination of their response to the first Botox® injection helps with the decision about what the dose should be the next time. Those patients who live farther away are asked to contact us for a return visit when they begin to note the voice tightening up again and the numbers on their diary card begin dropping. If the degree of breathiness has been a distressing problem for the patient, a decision may be made to use unilateral injections of botulinum toxin subsequently. This sometimes reduces the duration of side effects but may slightly diminish the quality of voice during the good phase[26]. Adjunctive voice therapy in individuals having Botox® injections for adductor spasmodic dysphonia is described in Chapter 4, Section 4.6.2.2.

3.5.2.2 Benign Essential Tremor and Spasm-Tremor Combinations

Unfortunately, persons with essential voice tremor do not receive the same dramatic relief from botulinum toxin injections as those with dystonic spasm, even though the spasm component in patients with mixed tremor-spasm can be helped. The tremor component is often relieved by beta-blockers such as propranolol in doses that can be gradually increased up to 40 mg four times daily (maximum 160 mg per day). In our experience, about one third of patients with benign essential vocal tremor receive sufficient relief with botulinum toxin injections that they wish to continue with them. About one third find them entirely unhelpful, and the other third are in the middle. If there is a spasmodic quality to the tremor, most patients are given the opportunity to try the Botox®, knowing that the effect will wear off and they will return to where they were before.

3.5.2.3 Abductor Spasmodic Dysphonia (Posterior Cricoarytenoid)

Botulinum toxin injected into the posterior cricoarytenoid (PCA) muscle for abductor spasmodic dysphonia is not nearly as effective as it is for the adductor variant of the disorder. Our initial technique involved rotating the larynx and directing the injection needle posterior to the thyroid lamina into the muscle behind the cricoid cartilage. We found this difficult, and the results were difficult to reproduce even when they did work well. More recently, we have been employing the transluminal technique. A long, teflon-coated electromyographic (EMG) injection needle is passed into the subglottic lumen above the anterior cricoid arch and angled laterally and slightly superiorly to abut the posterior cricoid lamina. The needle is then passed through the posterior cricoid plate and into the PCA muscle. The patient is asked to sniff, and correct placement in the muscle is confirmed by brisk EMG muscle activity with this exercise. The two PCA muscles are treated sequentially 2 months apart. This treatment regimen is moderately successful in some patients but still does not give the level of satisfaction achieved with vocalis muscle injections for adductor spasmodic dysphonia.

3.5.2.4 Dysphonia With Other Forms of Dystonia (eg, Meige's Syndrome)

Botulinum toxin therapy for other dystonia syndromes around the head and neck is similar to that for adductor spasmodic dysphonia. It is interesting to note that other dystonia components sometimes improve when the vocal cords have been treated. Occasionally it is necessary to inject Botox® into other muscles around the head and neck at the same time as the vocal cord injections. In time, the otolaryngologist treating spasmodic dysphonia becomes an artist in the use of botulinum toxin for treating regional dystonia.

3.5.2.5 Adductor Laryngeal Breathing Disorders (Vocal Cord Dysfunction)

The clinical situation in a patient with a laryngeal breathing disorder may suggest that several processes are going on simultaneously. Treatment accordingly may be drawn from a menu of possibilities including: reflux therapy, inhalation therapies, psychotropic medications, endotracheal intubation, tracheotomy, voice therapy, biofeedback, psychotherapy, botulinum toxin injections, physiotherapy, massage therapy, acupuncture, or laryngeal manipulation. If the "irritable larynx syndrome" hypothesis described in Chapter 2 is correct[29], the question becomes whether the process can be reversed. If the hypothesized neuro-plastic change in brainstem nuclei is due to repeated noxious stimulation, then perhaps repetitive "normal" stimuli, as may occur with voice therapy exercises, can encourage readaptive change. Because multiple causes are likely, multiple treatments may be advised.

Episodic laryngospasm due to reflux usually responds well to aggressive antireflux therapy. Although measures such as bed elevation, diet control, weight loss, and antacid use may be helpful, it is generally appropriate to initially achieve symptomatic control with proton pump inhibitor medications. The use of 20 mg of omeprazole twice daily, lansoprazole 30 mg, or pantoprazole 40 mg daily taken in the morning usually will bring symptoms under control after a number of weeks, but the dosages may occasionally need to be increased. Long-term control may require continued use of these medications and possible consideration of laparoscopic fundoplication.

The etiology of vocal cord dysfunction (VCD) is not known, although it is often felt to be psychogenic. In the absence of treatable GE reflux, the mainstays of treatment in these patients is a combination of voice therapy and psychotherapy. The adductor movement is usually less evident when breathing in through the nose than through the mouth. It is generally felt that this is related to the presence of a nasal-laryngeal reflex and is useful information in helping patients to learn how to break out of attacks. They are asked to "sniff" many times through the day, as often as they think of it, in the anticipation that the abductor reflex will be more accessible during an attack. Persistent inspiratory stridor with observable paradoxical vocal cord movement on inspiration may respond to botulinum toxin injection. A somewhat higher dose than that used for spasmodic dysphonia, in the range of 3 to 5 units per vocal cord every 3 months, may be effective.

Voice therapy approaches include techniques for reducing strain on the phonatory mechanism and are discussed in Chapter 4, Section 4.6.8. While recognizing the stridor as real, the therapy is directed toward appropriate breathing strategies and adjusting general and laryngeal postures.

Psychiatric therapy is best used in a team approach, as these patients generally do not do well with insight therapy. Associated psychiatric conditions include depression, obsessive-compulsive disorder, adjustment reaction, borderline personality, passive-dependant personality, or somatization. As with muscle misuse voice disorders, the patients have difficulty expressing anger, fear, or sadness. It is important to inform the patient that the nature of the disorder is known and that they will not die of respiratory obstruction. Showing them a videorecording of their larynx is helpful in getting the message across. They should be reassured that with time and treatment, they will get better. The aim is to allow patients to retain many of their psychiatric symptoms without needing to use airway obstruction as part of their coping syndrome. It is useful to deal with this in a limited paradigm and brief psychotherapy format rather that in long-term insight-oriented dynamic therapy.

Even though vocal fold dysfunction in the absence of reflux or dystonia may be psychologically based and tracheotomy should not be necessary, there are cases in which the psychological base is difficult to discern. When these patients become acclimatized to a permanent valved tracheotomy tube, some return to full normal activity without evidence of psychiatric disturbance.

3.5.2.6 Parkinson's Disease

The drug and neurological management of Parkinson's disease is beyond the scope of this book, but it should be pointed out that voice therapy can be quite useful in increasing vocal power and projection, thus delaying the onset of the typical voice of hypokinetic dysarthria. This is discussed in Chapter 4, Section 4.6.2. Surgical augmentation of the vocal cords in severe Parkinsonian hypophonia may be helpful in selected cases. Transcutaneous injection of collagen may be a useful adjunct to voice therapy in some patients with Parkinson's disease[2].

3.5.3 Other Motor Speech Disorders

Medical therapy in the voice clinic for patients with neurologic diseases such as amyotrophic lateral sclerosis, multiple sclerosis, myasthenia gravis, or muscular dystrophy usually involves assorted attempts at alleviating complications and disturbing side effects. Generally treatment is directed toward helping with problems of swallowing, aspiration, or drooling.

3.6 Voice Disorders in the Elderly

Most age-related voice changes result from natural physiological degenerative processes. So how should patients for whom these changes are a problem be treated? Should we coax them into accepting their "old voices" and help them reduce their compensatory muscle misuses and maximize vocal performance? Should we offer dissection or suction removal of submucosal tissue of Reinke's edema for early polypoidal degeneration? Often the elderly patient needs only to be reassured that the changes they are detecting in their voice do not represent any life-threatening illness. In some cases, helping them to understand why things are changing as they are is all the treatment that is needed. The treatment plan clearly depends on a team decision, with the patient leading the team. We will outline the primary aspects of the treatment program.

3.6.1 Changes Due to Normal Aging

In men, the loss of muscle bulk, slackened fibrous tissue, and thinned vocal folds results in a higher pitched, thinner, reedy vocal tone. In women, thickening of loose tissue under the vocal fold lining results in deeper pitch. This effect is worsened by smoking.

Conservatism in surgery should be the general rule when managing elderly patients with voice disorders, particularly when treating patients with polypoidal degeneration. If altering voice use through a voice therapy program has not been successful, and the voice problem is severe enough then reduction in the amount of polypoidal degenera-

tion may be warranted. This entails removal of the Reinke's space edema tissue only, with maintenance of the epithelial cover. It can be accomplished by making an incision laterally along the superior aspect of the vocal fold and reflecting the mucosal flap medially toward the free margin. Cup forceps, alligator forceps, or suction can then be used to ease the gelatinous polypoidal tissue away from the underlying deep layers of the lamina propria. Mucosa can then be draped back over the vocal fold. Fibrin glues (such as Tisseel) can be helpful in keeping the mucosa in place.

3.6.2 Unsuccessful Compensatory Voice Use

Attempts to compensate for age-related changes result in vocal strain. Men tend to drive the pitch down to what they feel is normal. Women try to drive the pitch upward to avoid being addressed as "sir" on the telephone. The vocal strain, effort, and fatigue may cause more difficulty than the original vocal cord change. Therapy for voice disorders in the elderly frequently is focused on reducing the muscular misuses that accompany attempts by the patient to compensate for the changes that have occurred. The therapy program may be directed toward encouraging the upward adjustment of vocal pitch in the elderly man with thinning vocal folds, coupled with any necessary alterations of respiratory support and resonance. In women, it may consist of encouraging them to accept a deeper vocal pitch and to develop an easier, more relaxed style of laryngeal muscle use. This is discussed in greater detail in Chapter 4, Section 4.6.6.

3.6.3 Psychopathology

Counseling by the laryngologist and the speech-language pathologist and a direct voice therapy program make up a major portion of the management of psychological components of the dysphonia. The reassurance and attentive care that patients receive during this process cannot help but have positive therapeutic effects. In some cases, however, where associated anxiety, depression, or both is a major causative factor in dysphonia, management may be more difficult without assistance from a psychologist or psychiatrist.

Sometimes voice disorders in elderly people reflect their general social situations. They may find themselves living alone with little opportunity to use their voices except on the telephone. In persons for whom this lifestyle reflects a major change or is clearly undesirable to them, we encourage and support them in altering this social situation to permit more frequent, direct voice use and better mental health.

3.6.4 Miscellaneous Causes of Dysphonia in the Elderly

Stiffness in the joints of the larynx, neck, shoulders, and elsewhere makes it important that vocal technique be optimal. Vocal skills learned in earlier years may no longer work because the instrument has changed.

Dryness may affect the elderly larynx more than in younger people because salivary tissue is somewhat less effective. Some older people also restrict water intake because of problems with urination. To keep the body well hydrated, it is necessary to drink about eight glasses of noncaffinated, nonalcoholic beverages daily.

About 10% of people suffer with **GE reflux** symptoms caused by inflammation in the larynx and reflex tightening of laryngeal muscles. Control of reflux is extremely important for singers. Ninety percent are able to achieve control with lifestyle measures (see Appendix 3.1), but the remaining 10% require long-term use of prescription medications.

Age-related **hearing problems** may cause difficulty in one of two ways. Often a person to whom the patient frequently speaks has a hearing problem, making it

necessary for the patient to speak more loudly. Hearing loss in the speaker or singer results in inadequate voice feedback and more vocal strain. A good hearing aid may be helpful.

Prescription drugs also may cause voice problems. Consider the following:

➤ Blood pressure pills may aggravate reflux due to their action on the smooth muscle of the lower esophagus.
➤ Nonsteroidal antiinflammatory drugs are irritating to the stomach and further the affects of reflux.
➤ Diuretics (eg, lasix, hydrodiuril) may have a systemic drying effect.
➤ Inhalers used to treat asthma or chronic bronchitis may irritate the larynx or promote a laryngeal yeast infection.
➤ Blood thinners (Aspirin, Coumadin) may increase the chance of a vocal cord hemorrhage during strenuous singing.
➤ Antihistamines exert a drying effect on the larynx.

To maintain good vocal function into the later years, **youth and flexibility must give way to wisdom and skill.**

3.7 Summary

As with any therapeutic process, appropriate medical treatment of the patient with a voice disorder requires accurate diagnosis(es). This chapter discussed the treatment processes involved in management of the four major platforms that are felt to underlie dysphonia. Particular attention was given to the treatment of gastroesophageal reflux. General information was provided about treatment philosophies for organic disease states affecting the larynx, such as papilloma, carcinoma, and infections. Case studies were included for viral laryngitis, vocal nodules, abuse-related vocal fold hemorrhage, postsurgical vocal fold scarring, and contact granuloma. Evolving surgical procedures for management of less usual conditions, such as sulcus vocalis and intracordal cysts, were discussed, as were options for the management of the male to female transgender patient.

There have been a number of advances in treatment of vocal fold paralysis during recent years. Teflon injection has largely given way to thyroplasty in its various forms. Other laryngeal "injectibles" plus nerve-transfer procedures continue to develop. This chapter provided an overview of management options for the patient with a paralyzed or immobile vocal cord.

Medical and surgical treatment for spasmodic dysphonia and associated forms of laryngeal dystonia were discussed, including techniques for the use of botulinum toxin. Finally, comment was offered regarding the treatment of special voice problems in the elderly.

Medical treatment is often undertaken in association with voice therapy, psychological intervention, and vocal performance rehabilitation. Details regarding these management approaches are provided in the following chapters.

References

1. Arnold, G. E. (1962), Vocal rehabilitation of paralytic dysphonia. *Archives of Otolaryngology, 76,* 358–368.
2. Berke, G. S., Gerratt, B., Kreiman, J., & Jackson, K. (1999). Treatment of Parkinson hypophonia with percutaneous collagen augmentation. *Laryngoscope, 109,* 1295–1299.
3. Berke, G. S., Blackwell, K. E., Gerratt, B. R., Verneil, A., Jackson, K. S., & Sercarz, J. A. (1999). Selective laryngeal adductor denervation-reinnervation: A new surgical treatment for adductor spasmodic dysphonia. *Annals of Otology Rhinology and Laryngology, 108,* 227–231.
4. Blitzer, A., Brin, M. F., Fahn, S., & Lovelace, R. E. (1988). Localized injections of botulinum toxin for the treatment of focal laryngeal dystonia (spastic dysphonia). *Laryngoscope, 98,*193–197.
5. Blom, E. D., & Singer, M. (1979). Surgical prosthetic approaches for post-laryngectomy voice restoration. In R. L. Keith & F. L. Darley (Eds.), *Laryngectomee Rehabilitation.* Houston: College-Hill.
6. Bouchayer, M., Cornut, G., Witzig, E., Loire, R., Roch, J. B., & Bastian, R. W. (1985). Epidemoid cysts, sulci, and mucosal bridges of the true vocal cord: A report of 157 cases. *Laryngoscope, 95,*1087–1094.
7. Bouchayer, M., & Cornut, G. (1994). *Phonosurgery for Benign Vocal Fold Lesions.* (videotape). London: 3 Ears Company Ltd.
8. Bouchayer, M., & Cornut, G. (1991). Instrumental microsurgery of benign lesions of the vocal folds. In C. N. Ford, & D. M. Bless (Eds.), *Phonosurgery: Assessment and Surgical Management of Voice Disorders.* (pp. 143–165) New York: Raven Press.
9. Cherry, J., & Maarguiles, S. L. (1968). Contact ulcer of the larynx. *Laryngoscope, 78,* 1937–1940.
10. Crumley, R. L., Idzebski, K., & McMicken, B., (1988). Nerve transfer versus teflon injection for vocal fold paralysis: A comparison. *Laryngoscope, 98,* 1200–1203.
11. D'Antonio, L. L., Wigley, T. L., & Zimmerman, G. J. (1995). Quantitative measures of laryngeal function following Teflon injection or thyroplasty type I. *Laryngoscope, 105,* 256–262.
12. Dedo, H. H., (1976). Recurrent laryngeal nerve section for spastic dysphonia. *Annals of Otology, Rhinology and Laryngology, 85,* 451–459.
13. Emami, A. J., Morrison, M. D., Rammage, L. A., & Bosch, D. (1999). Treatment of laryngeal contact ulcers and granulomas: A 12 year retrospective analysis. *Journal of Voice, 13(4),* 612–617.
14. Ford, C. N., Bless, D. M. (1986). A preliminary study of injectable collagen in human vocal fold augmentation. *Otolaryngology Head and Neck Surgery, 94,* 104–112.
15. Ford, C. N., & Bless, D. M. (1986). Clinical experience with injectable collagen for vocal fold augmentation. *Laryngoscope, 96,* 863–869.
16. Goodman, L. S., & Gillman, A. G. (1990). *The Pharmalogical Basis of Therapeutics* (8th ed., pp. 899–904). New York: Pergamon.
17. Hanson, D. G., Kamel, P. L., & Kahrilas, P.J. (1995). Outcomes of antireflux therapy for the treatment of chronic laryngitis. *Annals of Otology, Rhinology and Laryngology, 104,* 550–555.

18. Harris, T. (1998). Phonosurgery—the cutting edge. In T. Harris, S. Harris, J. S. Rubin, & D. M. Howard, D. M. (Eds.), *The Voice Clinic Handbook*. (pp. 286–302) London: Whurr Publishers.

19. Havas, T. E., Priestley, J., & Lowinger, D. S. G. (1999). A management strategy for vocal process granulomas. *Laryngoscope, 109*, 301–306.

20. Isshiki, N., Okamura, H., & Ishikawa, T. (1975). Thyroplasty type I (lateral compression) for dysphonia due to vocal fold paralysis or atrophy. *Acta Otolaryngologica, 80*, 65–73.

21. Isshiki, N. (1989). *Phonosurgery—Theory and Practice*. Tokyo: Springer-Verlag.

22. Jackson-Menaldi, C. A., Dzul, A. I., & Holland, R. W. (1999). Allergies and vocal fold edema: A preliminary report. *Journal of Voice, 13*, 113–122.

23. Jaroma, M., Paarinen, L., & Nuutinen, J. (1989). Treatment of vocal cord granuloma. *Acta Otolaryngologica, 107*, 296–299.

24. Koufman, J. A. (1991). The otolaryngologic manifestations of gastroesophageal reflux disease: A clinical investigation of 225 patients using ambulatory 24-hour pH monitoring and an experimental investigation of the role of acid and pepsin in the development of laryngeal injury. *Laryngoscope, 101*, (Suppl. 53).

25. Lieberman, J. (1998). Principles and techniques of manual therapy: applications in the management of dysphonia. In T. Harris, S. Harris, J. S. Rubin, & D. M. Howard (Eds.), *The Voice Clinic Handbook* (pp. 91–132). London: Whurr Publishers.

26. Maloney, A. P., & Morrison, M. D. (1994). A comparison of the efficacy of unilateral versus bilateral botulinum toxin injections in the treatment of adductor spasmodic dysphonia. *Journal of Otolaryngology, 23*, 160–164.

27. Mohamed, A. H., & Hunt, R.H. (1994). The rationale of acid suppression in the treatment of acid related disease. *Ailmentary Pharmacology & Therapeutics, 8*(Suppl.1), 3–10.

28. Morrison, M. D., & Morris, B. D. (1990). Dysphonia and bulimia: Vomiting laryngeal injury. *Journal of Voice, 4*, 76–80.

29. Morrison, M. D., Rammage, L. A., & Emami, A. J. (1999). The irritable larynx syndrome. *Journal of Voice, 13*, 447–455.

30. Olson, N. R. (1991). Laryngopharyngeal manifestations of gastroesophageal reflux disease. *Otolaryngologic Clinics of North America, 24* (5), 1201–1213.

31. Ramirez, B., Richter, J. E. (1993). Promotility drugs in the treatment of GE reflux disease. *Ailmentary Pharmacology & Therapeutics, 7*(1), 5–20.

32. Remacle, M., Marbaix, E., Hamoir, M., Bertrand, B., & van den Eeckhaut, J. (1990). Correction of glottic insufficiency by collagen injection. *Annals of Otology, Rhinology & Laryngology, 99*, 438–444.

33. Rosen, C. A., Woodson, G. E., Thompson, J. W., & Hengesteg, A. P. (1998). Preliminary results of the use of I3C for recurrent respiratory papillomatosis. *Otolaryngology, Head and Neck Surgery, 118*, 810–815.

34. Spencer, C. M., & Faulds, D. (1994). Lansoprazole: A reappraisal of its pharmacodynamic and pharmacokinetic properties, and its therapeutic efficacy in acid-related disorders. *Drugs, 48*, 404–430.

35. Wani, M. K., & Woodson, G. E. (1999). Laryngeal contact granuloma. *Laryngoscope, 109*, 1589–1593.

36. Ward, P. H., & Berci, G. (1982). Observations on the pathogenesis of chronic nonspecific pharyngitis and laryngitis. *Laryngoscope, 92*, 1377–1382.

37. Zeitels, S. M., & Sataloff, R. T. (1999). Phonomicrosurgical resection of glottal papillomatosis. *Journal of Voice, 13*, 123–127.

38. Zeitels, S. M., Hochman, I., & Hillman, R. E. (1998). Adduction arytenopexy: A new procedure for paralytic dysphonia with implications for implant medialization. *Annals of Otology, Rhinology and Laryngology, 107*, (Suppl. 173).

39. Zeitels, S. M., Hillman, R. E., Desloge, R. B., & Bunting, G. A. (1999). Cricothyroid subluxation: A new innovation for enhancing the voice with laryngoplastic phonosurgery. *Annals of Otology, Rhinology and Laryngology, 108*, 1126–1131.

Recommended Readings:

Ford, C. N., & Bless, D. M. (1991). *Phonosurgery: Assessment and Surgical Management of Voice Disorders*. New York: Raven Press.

Harris, T. (1998). Drugs and the pharmacological treatment of dysphonia. In T. Harris, S. Harris,

J. S. Rubin, & D. M. Howard (Eds.). *The Voice Clinic Handbook* (pp. 266–285). London: Whurr Publishers.

Harris, T. (1998). Phonosurgery—the cutting edge. In T. Harris, S. Harris, J. S. Rubin, & D. M. Howard (Eds.), *The Voice Clinic Handbook* (pp. 286–302). London: Whurr Publishers.

Lieberman, J. (1998). Principles and techniques of manual therapy: applications in the management of dysphonia. In T. Harris, S. Harris, J. S. Rubin & D. M. Howard *The Voice Clinic Handbook* (pp. 91–132). London: Whurr Publishers.

Olson, N. R. (1991). Laryngopharyngeal manifestations of gastroesophageal reflux disease. *Otolaryngologic Clinics of North America*, 24 (5), 1201–1213.

APPENDIX 3–1

PATIENT HANDOUT FOR THROAT PROBLEMS AND GASTROESOPHAGEAL REFLUX

Stomach contents are normally acidic and are generally kept in the stomach by a valve at the lower end of the esophagus. **Reflux** is the term used when stomach acids come back up into the esophagus or throat. **Symptoms** result from direct acid irritation, or reflex tightening of throat muscles.

The **sense of a lump in the throat**, called globus, may result from chronic reflux laryngitis or from increased tension in the upper esophageal opening behind the voice box. The resulting **increase in secretions** in the throat leads to **habitual throat clearing**. These increased secretions may be mistaken as **postnasal drip** or "phlegm." A person with **nighttime reflux** will frequently waken with a sore, irritated throat and a gravely voice. Muscle tension in the larynx may lead to **vocal difficulty, trouble swallowing**, and, in severe cases, to **choking spells and airway obstruction. Heartburn**, the typical symptom of reflux, may not be present when the throat is affected.

Treatment is directed at keeping the stomach contents where they belong and neutralizing them when reflux is likely to occur. The following are suggested lifestyle changes that may reduce reflux.

➤ Obesity promotes reflux. Try to achieve an optimal weight.

➤ Avoid tight clothing around the midsection of the body or stooping after meals.

➤ Use abdominal breathing. Let your abdomen expand with each breath in.

➤ Elevate the head of your bed on blocks, 4 to 6 inches. Extra pillows are not as effective. Do not eat for 3 hours before lying down.

Antacids may be used to neutralize stomach acids and should be taken half an hour after each meal and at bedtime. Examples include TUMS®, Maalox, Mylanta™, Gaviscon®. Acid production can be blocked by medications, some of which can be purchased over the counter without a prescription (eg, Pepcid AC®). **Prescribed drugs** such as H2 blockers (eg, cimetidine or ranitidine) are taken twice daily with meals, and proton pump inhibitors (eg, Losec®, Prevacid® or Pantoloc™) are usually taken once a day in the morning.

Additional factors that may improve symptoms of reflux:

➤ Eat small meals, up to six times each day.

➤ Caffeine and nicotine increase reflux. Stopping the use of these addictive chemicals will help to relieve the reflux symptoms.

➤ Avoid foods that cause heartburn such as tomatoes, spicy foods, and citrus fruits. Some fruit juices are irritating as well as acid producing.

➤ Include protein with each meal and reduce your fat intake. (See the section on diet that follows.)

➤ Although throat lozenges may temporarily reduce symptoms, they cause more reflux. Avoid chewing gum, cough drops, and mouthwashes.

Antacid, Antireflux diet

Type of Food	Allowed	Avoid
Beverage	skim milk, non-cola drinks, noncarbonated beverages, herb teas	whole milk or cream, citrus juices, alcohol, caffeine, carbonated beverages
Breads/cereals	enriched white, whole-wheat, or rye bread; soda or graham crackers, hot and dry cereals	egg breads, sweet rolls, doughnuts, waffles, high-fat granola-type cereals, pancakes
Cheese	low-fat cottage cheese, cheese made from skim milk	cheese from whole milk, processed cheese
Dessert	fruit, fruit ices, gelatin desserts, angel food cake, popsicles, homemade cakes, pies, pudding made with skim milk	chocolate, peppermint, coconut, high-fat desserts, high-fat cakes, pies, ice cream, nuts
Eggs	I egg daily	more than I egg daily
Fats	3 teaspoons equivalent daily (eg, 3 tsps butter or oil)	fried foods and gravy
Fruit	all except those under "avoid".	avocado, grapefruit, oranges, lemons, limes, pineapple
Nuts	none	all
Miscellaneous	salt, mild spices, herbs, flavoring	peppermint, spearmint, curry, pepper, hot spice, chili, horseradish, olives
Potatoes and other starches	white or sweet potatoes prepared with no more than the allowed fat, macaroni, rice, noodles, spaghetti	potato chips, deep fried foods
Soup	chicken or beef broth, soups made from allowed foods	cream soups made with whole milk, cream, or animal fat
Sweets	honey, jam, jelly, sugar, marshmallows	chocolate, coconut, nuts, hard candy, chewing gum, cough drops, lozenges
Vegetables	all are allowed except tomatoes	fried vegetables, tomatoes

Note. From: *The Management of Voice Disorders* (p. 230), by M. Morrison, L. Rammage, et al., 1994, San Diego: Singular Publishing Group Inc. Copyright 1994 by Singular Publishing Group Inc.

APPENDIX 3.2

POSTOPERATIVE INSTRUCTIONS

PROVINCIAL VOICE CARE RESOURCE PROGRAM
Linda A. Rammage, PhD, S-LP(C), Director

PACIFIC VOICE CLINIC. INC
Murray D. Morrison, MD, FRCSC, Director

WWW.PVCRP.COM

4th floor, Willow Pavilion
Vancouver Hospital
805 West 12th Ave
Vancouver, BC
V5Z 1M9

Phone: (604) 875-4204
Fax: (604) 875-5382

Post Operative Patient Instructions:

1. VOICE REST: For the first 48 hours following surgery you are to be on voice rest. This means that you are not to use your voice unless it is absolutely necessary and, when it is necessary, restrict your speaking to no more than 5 minutes within any 1 hour period. Any talking should be soft, in a quiet environment and in the middle of your vocal range where it is easier to speak without strain. Do not engage in vocal throat-clearing or coughing. **DO NOT WHISPER.** Use a notepad, "magic slate" or other writing tool to communicate your needs. Cancel all social engagements. Stay at home and get plenty of rest and hydration. You can determine whether you are adequately hydrated by observing your urine: it should be pale in colour. If it is dark you should increase your intake of non-caffeinated, non-alcoholic beverages.

2. RESTRICTED VOICE USE: For the week following 48 hours of voice rest, use your voice normally. When speaking you should be close enough to your listener to touch his/her shoulder. Do not engage in throat-clearing or coughing. **DO NOT WHISPER.** Do not speak outside, in groups, in a vehicle, aeroplane or any other noisy environments, such as restaurants. Any voice use should be soft, in a quiet environment and in the middle of your vocal range where it is easiest to speak without strain. During this period be sure you are adequately hydrated by drinking at least 8 glasses of non-caffeinated, non-alcoholic beverages daily.

3. PRUDENT VOICE USE: For the next 2 weeks, before you return for your follow up exam, you have few restrictions on your voice use. Observe common sense rules of vocal hygiene. Avoid vocally abusive activities: yelling, cheering, screaming, throat-clearing, coughing, loud or prolonged laughing/crying. Continue to speak in the middle of your vocal range, avoiding extremes in pitch and loudness. Whenever possible, be within arm's length of your listener. **DO NOT WHISPER**. If you are speaking in a group larger then 20, outside or in a noisy environment, use a vocal amplification system. Maintain adequate hydration. If you experience vocal fatigue or strain, contact your speech pathologist for further instructions.

Adapted from: Bless, D.M.(1992) University of Wisconsin Hospital and Clinics, Madison.

CHAPTER

4

Approaches to Voice Therapy

4.1 Purpose of Therapy

The purpose of a voice therapy program varies from patient to patient. In most cases, the intent is to improve vocal communication and in some cases to normalize voice function, that is, to restore function so that the vocal profile falls within an accepted normal range. When pathogenesis includes irreversible or degenerative organic pathology, voice therapy may be initiated to maintain the current level of function as long as possible and reduce ineffective compensatory behaviors. When surgery or other medical intervention is selected as the primary management approach, preoperative voice therapy may be undertaken to eliminate vocal abuses and to provide models for optimizing postoperative voice. Postoperative therapy programs are designed to facilitate patients' adaptation to structural changes and to optimize results of medical-surgical procedures with technical fine-tuning.

In an ideal world of health care, the primary purpose of voice therapy programs for occupational and professional voice users would be to prevent dysphonias arising from the 4 primary dysphonia platform components discussed in the previous chapters.

An important aspect of the voice therapy program is diagnostic therapy, which ideally commences during the interdisciplinary evaluation period. (See Chapter 1).

4.2 Factors Influencing Selection and Success of Therapy Programs

Voice therapy programs may consist primarily of relatively short-term **symptomatic** techniques or may encompass long-term **comprehensive** rehabilitation strategies. Sometimes **holistic** approaches are used to augment specific therapy exercises. The choice of approaches and the duration of the program depends on clinical, personal and economic factors. In general, individuals experiencing muscle misuse or psychogenic voice disorders with gradual onset, long-term, and consistent symptoms require longer, more comprehensive treatment protocols than those whose onset was sudden, with short-term or intermittent symptoms.

Patients who have experienced gradual dysphonia onset are more likely to demonstrate generalized muscle misuse during speech and nonspeech activities. Further, considerable adaptation may take place during a gradual onset, and an individual comes to accept the sounds and sensations of his or her disordered voice production as normal, if not desirable. At this point, a muscle misuse voice disorder is habituated and a patient's awareness of muscle tension is compromised, as is the ability to correct inappropriate behaviors.

Presence of a primary or secondary organic component may complicate prognosis and influence the choice of therapy techniques. If a long-standing lesion, such as a fibrotic nodule, is present in the larynx, compensatory behaviors may have developed and been reinforced as part of an individual's day-to-day coping strategies. The same may hold true for organic tremor, laryngeal dystonia, or other neurological or systemic diseases. In cases where medical or surgical intervention is indicated, preoperative voice therapy may be introduced to reduce vocal abuses and inappropriate compensatory behaviors, such as incoordinate breathing, increased glottal resistance, or splinting in the jaw and tongue. Most patients with long-standing muscle misuse dysphonias benefit from a comprehensive voice rehabilitation program either as the primary treatment or following medical-surgical intervention, assuming no psychological issues compromise motivation to effect voice changes.

The physical aspects of vocal rehabilitation programs are dependent on the principles of **motor learning**. These have been well established, and attention to relevant aspects of the principles governing acquisition of motor skills is essential to ensure appropriate outcomes in voice therapy. Simply stated, conditions that assist in motor learning include an understanding of the purpose and expected sensory result of a simple movement pattern, observations of individuals producing the correct movement pattern, observations of individuals learning the movement pattern, repeated "rehearsals" of the movement pattern, and use of sensory feedback to correct inappropriate responses and confirm appropriate responses[1,2,66,67].

The principles of motor learning highlight the importance of accessing feedback channels to assist in motor learning. These include the auditory, visual, and tactile-kinesthetic processing systems. Other prerequisites to successful therapy include adequate attention skills to process instructions, the use of feedback signals to change one's motor speech behaviors, and adequate memory for retrieval of information critical to effective practice and behavior changes.

Additional factors that may influence therapy selection and prognosis include hearing impairment, other sensory deficits, external support (both emotional and economic), impact of the dysfunction on one's life and unresolved psychological conflicts, or presence of a psychiatric disorder.

4.3 Symptomatic Therapy

The term **symptomatic therapy** implies that therapeutic techniques are selected to target a particular set of physiological signs or symptoms of a voice disorder. A list of facilitation techniques used commonly for treating patients symptomatically is listed in Chapter 1, Section 1.9. In some cases, we anticipate that correction of a primary sign or symptom of dysphonia will result in more generalized positive behavior changes, such as reduction of muscle tension during speech (as demonstrated in the case example below), or more dynamic speech patterns (such as following appropriate application of the Lee-Silverman voice therapy program for hypokinetic dysarthrias)[56–61].

Case 4.1

Kamal ("Stretch"), is a 15-year old, second-generation Indo-Canadian who is the tallest person in his family's history. He grew 14 inches in the past year, thus acquiring the nickname from his astonished, traditionally short, stocky family. He now looms a grand 6-foot, four inches but recently people have been making fun of his high-pitched, childish voice. Some of his peers refer to it as a "baby" voice. He confesses he has been embarrassed, not only about his high voice and its sudden breaks to a "low noise that is too loud," but also about his rapidly changing physical stature. People seem to expect a great deal of him now that he's so tall, and they find his high quiet voice a contradiction to his adultlike physique. The one positive outcome of his growth spurt has been a successful trial for the intramural basketball team, which he reports with pride. Shy by nature, Kamal is starting to spend more time with boys his size, and they sometimes overlook his "different" voice.

A principal sign of adolescent transitional voice disorder (ATVD) is use of falsetto register and a resultant speaking pitch that is too high for the age and gender of individuals such as Kamal. It may be adopted once the larynx has reached its full adult size because of its similarity to the prepubertal speaking pitch an individual is accustomed to feeling and hearing. Our voice assessment reveals that Kamal is speaking in falsetto register with a mean speaking f_0 of 310 Hz. During videostroboscopic examination, he is seen to damp the posterior one third of his vocal folds with tight approximation of the arytenoid cartilages, and the typical vibratory pattern for falsetto is identified. Examination using the flexible fiber-optic laryngoscope reveals an associated anteroposterior compression and a high larynx position. Diagnostic therapy demonstrates a lower larynx position and more appropriate vocal fold posturing following throat clearing, but he cannot sustain modal register phonation. He can produce a glottal fry register, which is associated with a lowered larynx position. Psychogenic etiologies are often suspected in ATVD, and habituated misuse of laryngeal and paralaryngeal muscles is common. The psychiatrist has determined that Kamal feels burdened by the sudden change in expectation by peers, teachers, family members, and strangers for him to behave like an adult, when, as he states, "I'm only a kid!" Fortunately, his recent success in basketball has generated some optimism for the future. In summary, Kamal's etiological profile includes significant contributions from psychological and muscle misuse platforms.

Appropriate counseling is undertaken with Kamal and his family, friends, and teachers. Once this counseling has helped Kamal understand and adapt emotionally to the physical changes that are taking place, and encouraged others to adopt more realistic expectations of Kamal, he is ready for voice therapy. Based on our observations during diagnostic therapy, symptomatic therapy is introduced to facilitate use of a more appropriate pitch by eliciting and extending use of glottal fry register. Although the final therapeutic goal is to help him find his baritone modal register for speech, Kamal, like many patients, is better able to produce extreme patterns of phonation, such as glottal fry, more readily than normal patterns. The first stage of therapy focuses on maximizing various visual, acoustic, and kinaesthetic aspects of the falsetto-glottal fry contrast using tactile feedback (his fingers placed over the thyroid lamina bilaterally) and a real-time computer program that demonstrates graphically the varying pitch and spectral features of falsetto and glottal fry. Initial successful behavior changes then are expanded and shaped into closer approximations of "normal." In this case, lower pitched modal register phonation is achieved using continued tactile and visual feedback by allowing the glottal fry to get "louder" (this tends to effect the desired changes in vocal fold postures and vibratory patterns to yield modal register). Because modal register is a more natural speaking mode, we expect that consistent use of the lower pitch results in Kamal's use of more relaxed and efficient speech behaviors.

To facilitate the carry-over of the more appropriate pitch to daily use, Kamal invites trusted individuals, one at a time, to attend his therapy session and to witness and assist him in using his "real" voice. In the final session, his therapist and best basketball buddy accompany him to McDonalds to try the voice out on strangers, which is to be followed by a "debut" performance at basketball practice, with his friend assisting with the transition.

Symptomatic therapy may take on one of several formats depending on the classification scheme and physiological theories held by the clinician and biofeedback instruments available in the clinic. In the ATVD case outlined above, auditory feedback might be used primarily to effect pitch-production changes using the clinician's voice or a musical instrument as a model. For a patient like Kamal, who is more successful with kinaesthetic and visual input, "feeling" the vibrations and application of a dedicated device for visual feedback of f_0 are employed to reinforce approximations to a target pitch range. Using the same patient profile, a different clinician may note an elevated laryngeal posture during phonation and choose a facilitation technique to adjust posture as a symptomatic approach. Manual pressure on the larynx or postural adjustments to the head and neck might be used initially to establish a lowered larynx position before and during phonation. Assuming the same patient has a clinical profile that includes long-standing muscle misuse (perhaps in association with chronic anxiety), the clinician might decide that a comprehensive long-term therapy program is more appropriate in association with psychological intervention if necessary. An example of a comprehensive voice rehabilitation program is outlined in the next section.

A symptomatic approach to therapy for individuals exhibiting specific muscle misuses is provided by Harris[34]. One example is application of Inspiraton-Expiration (inhalation phonation followed by exhalation phonation associated with the inspiration sensation) to reduce anteroposterior compression. In Chapter 1, we discussed the utility of this technique to improve the view of the vocal folds during laryngoscopic evaluation in cases of anteroposterior compression. This physiological approach to voice therapy assumes that transnasal fiber-optic videolaryngoscopy is frequently or simultaneously available to provide visual feedback about the appropriateness of the technique(s) chosen.

Manual massage to specific muscle groups identified as hypertonic is another symptomatic approach to voice therapy. This technique is discussed in Chapter 3, and specific techniques are provided by Lieberman[34]. It is critical that the clinician performing laryngeal massage and manipulation be thoroughly familiar with the anatomy of structures in and around the larynx and be competent with the manipulation techniques, both to maximize effectiveness and to avoid injury to the patient. The speech-language pathologist may require special postgraduate training to reach the necessary competency levels for this type of therapy.

Symptomatic therapy may be planned to effect changes in specific physiological measures associated with certain types of laryngeal dysfunction. Examples of symptomatic therapy goals for selected voice disorders are provided in Table 4–1. This symptomatic approach needs to be undertaken with a degree of clinical wisdom and discretion. It is tempting for the novice voice clinician to prescribe stereotyped programs of therapy based on the diagnostic label associated with a speech and voice disorder, for example, "Parkinson's disease". The underlying assumption in this approach is that the primary physiological features contributing to dysphonia can be predicted and thus treated, based on our knowledge of a particular disease process. Once a comprehensive assessment, including diagnostic voice therapy, has been completed, this assumption may be rejected. The most appropriate program of therapy needs to be determined by considering an individual's full clinical profile, including functional levels for all four etiological platforms (lifestyle, technique, psychological factors, and reflux), as well as the signs and symptoms generated by any overlying disease process.

4.4 Comprehensive Voice Rehabilitation Programs

Many of the voice patients seen in an interdisciplinary voice clinic are "occupational voice users," for example, teachers, business execu-

Table 4–1. Physiological measures targeted in the treatment of selected voice disorders. From *Voice Care in the Medical Setting* (p. 45), by D. L. Koschkee and L. A. Rammage, 1997, San Diego: Singular Publishing Group, Inc. Copyright 1997, by Singular Publishing Group, Inc. Reprinted with permission.

MEASURES	LARYNGEAL PATHOLOGIES							
	PD	VN	VFS	RLN	HAD	FR	MTD	SD
Increase f_0		●					●	●
Decrease f_0			●	●		●		
Increase f_0 Range	●	●	●		●	●	●	
Increase SPL	●		●	●		●		●
Decrease SPL		●			●			
Increase SPL Range	●		●	●		●		
Increase Airflow Rate					●			●
Decrease Airflow Rate	●	●		●		●	●	
Increase Sub-Glottal Pressure	●					●		
Decrease Sub-Glottal Pressure		●			●			●
Increase Air Volume	●							
Increase Phonatory Stability	●		●	●		●		●
Increase Glottal Closure	●		●	●		●	●	
Decrease Vocal Fold Hyperadduction		●			●		●	●
Decrease Supraglottal Compression		●			●		●	●
Increase Mucosal Wave			●	●		●		
Increase Amplitude of Vibration	●		●	●	●	●		●

Pathology Code Legend:

PD = Parkinson's Disease

VN = Vocal Nodules

VFS = Vocal Fold Scarring

RLN = Recurrent Laryngeal Nerve Paralysis

HAD = Hyperadducting Dysphonia/Lateral Compression

FR = Falsetto Register in ATVD

MTD = Muscle Tension Dysphonia/Laryngeal Isometric

SD = Adductor Spasmodic Dysphonia

tives, attorneys, swimming and aerobics instructors, clergy, vocational instructors, customer representatives, counselors, and media personnel. These individuals have heavy vocal demands, depend on their voices to conduct their jobs, often in difficult social-emotional and acoustic environments, yet rarely have training in voice care and vocal technique. Professional voice users, that is individuals who rely on vocal performance as a source of income, also occupy a high proportion of the voice clinic population. Because many aspiring professional voice users may need to supplement their income from vocal performance with other jobs, they also may experience occupational voice problems. This seems particularly likely based on our observations that individuals who like to perform and entertain seek, or are sought in, primary or secondary occupations that involve interacting extensively with people, particularly in lively environments. How many of us have been served by the charismatic waiter who informs us he or she is or is going to be a singer or actor?

Case 4.2

Tess is a 27-year-old primary school teacher. She teaches music half-time for her school and shares a first grade class with another teacher. She started teaching as a TOC (teacher-on-call) after she graduated 4 years ago and considers herself fortunate to have found a full-time permanent job after the first year. Tess reports a history of voice problems that goes back to high-school, where she was a cheerleader. She used to "lose her voice" for a day or so after a particularly high-energy game with loud cheering. Through her university years, she occasionally experienced a similar voice loss after a loud party, or an evening in the bar. She admits to being a "party animal" still, but not so much as she was in her early 20s. (She has a steady boyfriend and he keeps her "on a short leash.") Since she started teaching, including her in-class practical teacher-training period, Tess has had increasing problems with her voice. At first the hoarseness didn't bother her; in fact people used to compliment her on her "Marilyn

Monroe" voice. Since she started teaching music, however, it has become embarrassing to miss the high notes when singing. She also is experiencing throat discomfort when she talks and sings, which gets so bad by the end of the day that she takes several pain killers. The days that she teaches music all day are the worst for her voice. Tess informs us the music class is treated like "recess" by the students in her school, and they are difficult to control. When she is teaching a new song or instructing the junior band, she finds she often has to vocalize over a whole class of "noise-makers." Her throat feels most comfortable after a good night's sleep. Tess is reportedly healthy and physically active. She plays on a women's field-hockey team and a volleyball team. She likes to sing in the car, but finds it sometimes causes too much pain now. She is "prone" to headaches and neck and shoulder tension. She is a self-professed "talkaholic," and the prospect of losing her voice permanently is extremely distressing to her. Her concern about losing her job has lead her to reduce the amount that she uses her voice in social situations over the past few weeks. This seems to have eased the discomfort somewhat, but she is worried about her dysphonia.

During the interview, we note several postural misuses: jaw jut, anterior neck tension, and a forward sitting pose with exaggerated lordosis. The hypertonicity in Tess's suprahyoid muscles is not only palpable but also visible because of her extended jaw posture. Her thyrohyoid muscles are also hypertonic, and her cricothyroid visor is "closed." Her eyebrows are chronically adducted, and she looks anxious. Her voice is moderately breathy, and the pitch is focused at the base of her physiological f_0 range. Occasional phonation breaks are noted. Her physiological f_0 range is below expected norms, and even with simultaneous lip trilling to minimize laryngeal tension, the maximum f_0 is 620 Hz. Tess's rate of speech is excessive: over 8 syllables per second. Asked whether she considers herself to be a "fast talker, a slow talker, or a moderate-speed talker," she replies, "I'm a motor-mouth . . . I've been trying to talk slower when I teach, but it's very difficult." Tess's scores on the State-Trait Anxiety Inventory are high for both subscales[76]. During videolaryngostroboscopy, we note anteroposterior compression, an elevated larynx position, a *large posterior glottal chink, and moderately sized bilateral nodules. Vocal fold vibratory movements appear symmetrical, and the mucosal wave is normal.*

Tess's voice problem is addressed at the lifestyle, technical and psychological levels. She is referred for a more comprehensive evaluation with the clinic psychiatrist based on her high State-Trait Anxiety Inventory scores, her reports of anxiety, and her "chronically worried" visage. Behavioral intervention must include a consideration of strategies to minimize vocal abuse, vocal overuse, and a comprehensive voice therapy program. Tess will need to consult with her friends, family, and close colleagues to explore lifestyle changes that will allow her to have appropriate amounts of vocal rest and minimize voice use in unfriendly acoustic environments. She will consult a more experienced music teacher whom she has befriended to get advice on behavior modification in the classroom. She will speak to the principal about improving the profile of music class, so the other teachers can help her effect an attitude change among students. Because she does not have formal training in singing technique, Tess will interview some singing teachers to find one who can help her rehabilitate and train her singing voice. She will participate in the upcoming comprehensive group-therapy program for occupational voice users described below. She may require some additional intensive syllable prolongation therapy to slow her speaking rate.

Occupational voice users typically present with symptoms and signs of vocal abuse and overuse, muscle misuse, dysphonia, somatic complaints, and sometimes primary or secondary anxiety or depression. As busy professionals, some individuals may rely heavily on caffeine, have poor dietary habits, conduct business in noisy environments and on the run, and use alcohol or recreational drugs to relax. These lifestyle features may contribute further to poor vocal health by adding dehydration, anxiety, reflux laryngitis, and vocal abuse to the etiological profile. Clearly, successful vocal rehabilitation with occupational

voice users needs to address problems at each of the relevant etiological platforms. The methods presented here also serve as a useful outline for preventative programs, the ultimate health care goal for this particularly susceptible population. Most individuals respond well to a group therapy format for comprehensive voice rehabilitation. The group therapy approach has the advantages of saving time and money for the health care system and the patient, and of providing a supportive venue for self-motivation, motor learning, problem solving, desensitizing, and carry-over of techniques through peer monitoring and role-playing exercises.

Comprehensive voice management ideally involves interdisciplinary program coordination. The speech-language pathologist, who typically directs the vocal rehabilitation program, may call on the physical therapist or posture specialist, the psychiatrist or psychologist, the singing teacher or voice coach, and the otolaryngologist as required.

For individual education and practice of new motor skills, each patient is provided with a copy of the manual, *Vocalizing with Ease: A Self-Improvement Guide*, which outlines our comprehensive vocal rehabilitation program[63]. This manual was developed as a guide for such therapy programs, but is also used extensively as a self-help information guide (See Figure 4–1 for a contents list).

The essential components of a comprehensive voice rehabilitation program for occupational voice users are discussed below.

4.4.1 Education

Education includes basic information on speech physiology, vocal health issues, and responses of the system to psychological and physical stressors. Hydration is a critical issue for many occupational voice users, who may think their 8 cups of coffee constitutes the daily fluid requirement. For many occupational voice users who communicate extensively in

TABLE OF CONTENTS

iii

Figure 4–1. Table of contents from *Vocalizing with Ease: A Self-Improvement Guide* (p. iii), by L. A. Rammage, 1996, Vancouver: Pacific Voice Clinic. Copyright 1996, by L. A. Rammage. Reprinted with permission.

acoustically unfriendly environments, education regarding meeting or classroom management and appropriate and regular use of vocal amplification devices provides basic vocal survival strategies. Although education and self-awareness are ongoing processes, the core information set is presented early to allow for peer support and problem solving to develop throughout the program.

4.4.2 Problem Solving

Problem solving is learned for making the necessary adjustments to lifestyle and environmental conditions that are contributing to vocal abuse and postural misuse. Stress management practice incorporates relaxation, voice breaks, time management (Figure 4–2), work delegation, and so forth. This is an

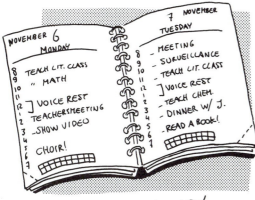

SCHEDULE YOUR VOICE USE!

If you can't avoid back-to-back vocal "performances", plan your presentation carefully to allow for appropriate turn-taking, pauses, and non-vocal activities. Remember, people absorb information better if they are stimulated through a variety of input channels, and if they are directly involved in a meeting or class, rather than passive information "sponges".

If you feel your presentation or teaching strategies could use some polishing, consider participating in a course on public speaking, teaching techniques, or meeting management. Effective presentation tactics are designed to help you impart information efficiently while maximizing your audience's attention and participation. Once you are a skilled public speaker, you will be able to economize on vocalizing time and effort.

Figure 4–2. Sample schedule for time management, including voice rest. From *Vocalizing with Ease: A Self-Improvement Guide* (p. 26), by L. A. Rammage, 1996, Vancouver: Pacific Voice Clinic. Copyright 1996, by L. A. Rammage and M. Haijtink. Reprinted with permission.

ongoing component of the program. Initially topics are introduced by the clinician(s), but later on, patients often raise issues as they become more aware of external and internal factors contributing to optimal or inappropriate voice use.

4.4.3 Relaxation Training

Relaxation training includes programs such as Jacobson's Progressive Relaxation[40] or other cognitive or image-based exercises. Individuals are guided in a process of awareness and reduction of muscle tension in specific regions of their bodies. The supine position often is used for the initial portion of the self-awareness process to minimize habitual postural tension. To help patients recognize and contrast the sensations associated with intentional hypercontraction of muscle sets, an isometric exercise may be used initially, followed by relaxation. Input on cognitive aspects of relaxation responses may be provided by the psychiatrist or psychologist. This is an ongoing learning process but ideally is introduced as one of the earliest rehabilitative activities.

4.4.4 Alignment-Posture Training

Alignment-posture training includes basic principles of proper alignment for the whole body to reduce muscle misuses and ensure freedom of the respiratory, phonatory, resonance, and articulatory systems. Theoretical perspectives such as the Alexander Technique[6] and the Feldenkrais method[28] guide the training program, and a specially trained instructor may be engaged to train patients in a particular method. A physical therapist specializing in problems of the back and neck can provide valuable information in the group-therapy format and may be used as a referral source for individuals experiencing specific chronic symptoms of postural misuse or disease. Figure 4–3 demonstrates some basic aspects of alignment training.

It is virtually impossible to experience coordination between the respiratory and phonatory systems for voice onset activities if the abdomen is held tightly; similarly, passive jaw mobility during phonation cannot be established if the head is chronically retracted on the neck. Therefore, balanced posture is a prerequisite to more focused therapy activities. Because specific relaxation training and optimal voice use depends on balanced posture, this training is introduced early in the therapy program[68].

4.4.5 Specific Relaxation Exercises

Specific relaxation exercises are introduced based on individual needs, although presentation of each exercise set in a group therapy setting can be a useful way to facilitate observation and learning. Because each patient will have strengths and weaknesses, a peer-learning situation can be created with appropriate patient grouping. Commonly, patients require training in relaxation of the abdomen, shoulders, neck, face, jaw, tongue, and pharynx. Tension-reduction strategies may incorporate visual and kinesthetic feedback and cognitive imaging. In addition, biofeedback devices may be useful in early training stages.

Flexibility and independent movement of articulators during speech is an ultimate goal for many of the specific relaxation protocols. This ensures that articulatory postures and movements do not impose undue postural constraints on the larynx during phonation or minimize resonance potential. These

---

Good posture provides us with a nice-looking and nice-feeling body. It also ensures maximum freedom for all the body's moving parts: head, neck, shoulders, elbows, wrists, finger joints, breathing system, legs...

Maximum freedom of body parts gives us potential for flexibility and power when we perform physical activities like talking. Good posture is dynamic: a constantly adjusting system that improves mobility, *not* a set of positions. Good posture makes vocalizing EASY!

Now let's begin applying some principles of natural, dynamic body posture:

Use your mirror to "back up" your observations: As you stand, your head, neck and back are *aligned:* an imaginary line passes through your body from the crown of the head through the back of the neck and centre back...

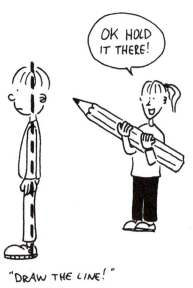

Figure 4–3. Principles and exercises for optimizing alignment. From *Vocalizing with Ease: A Self-Improvement Guide* (pp. 38, 39, 41, 45), by L. A. Rammage, 1996, Vancouver: Pacific Voice Clinic. Copyright 1996, by L. A. Rammage and M. Haijtink. Reprinted with permission.

HELIUM-HEAD:

Pretend your head is a helium balloon. It is attached to the rest of the body by a very delicate string that is the neck and spine. Let the light helium gas draw your head up off your neck-string, to provide the spine-lengthening effect. If a gentle breeze comes up, you will feel your helium-head float about in space.

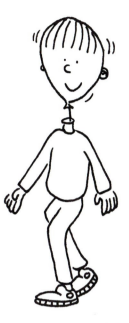

EASY WALKING:

You can also use gravity in upright positions, standing or sitting, to relax the body and free individual body parts: feel the effect of gravity on your shoulders, arms, legs, and breathing equipment. Take your body for a little walk using the imaginary suspension rope (or helium) to release your head and lengthen your spine, and using gravity to keep your arms and legs free and mobile.

HIGH ON HELIUM!

DO THE "V" THING:

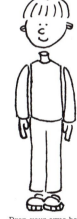

To banish the homo slouchus within, start with your helium-head floating upward; arms dropped at your sides.

With your head still floating up and away from the neck, slowly raise your arms from the sides of your body, palms facing the ceiling. Raise them to the sides of your head, until your arms form a "V" with the palms of your hands facing each other.

Drop your arms back to the sides of your body. Feel the natural expansion across your chest: more room to breathe. Repeat several times.

Figure 4–3 (continued)

The forward pivot is the first step in changing position from sitting to standing or standing to sitting. It will take some awareness and practice to accomplish these motions without "jaw-jut". Remember, the action begins with a release of the head from the neck and natural lengthening of the spine: the crown of the head dictates the upward and forward direction of movement: don't let the jaw take over!

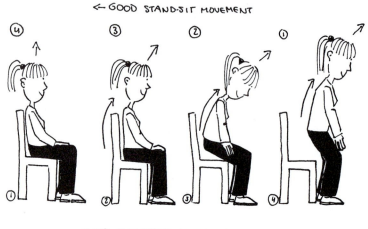

Figure 4–3 (continued)

exercises may be introduced before phonation exercises; however, they are continued throughout the program in association with exercises for voice onset and extension of phonation. Some sample exercises for specific relaxation are provided in Figure 4–4.

4.4.6 Coordinated Voice Onset

Coordinated voice onset exercises are introduced to maximize voice onset control and power while minimizing extraneous voice-onset gestures in the larynx, such as hyperadduction leading to glottal attacks or hypoadduction leading to breathy onsets. Examples of traditional voice onset exercises for hyperadducting behaviors include use of simulated *yawn-sigh*; or imagined insertion of the glottal fricative /h/ in word or phrase-initial positions.

Most patients respond well to a voice onset technique that uses spontaneous vocalizations: /hm/ ("Hm!"), as in the affirmative /m hm/, which can be elicited with a good clinical model in virtually everyone and lends itself well to the current theories of speech-breathing control. We call this type of production a **coordinated voice onset** (CVO; see Figure 4–5). The CVO approach is based on several important theoretical assumptions for optimizing vocal efficiency and power. First, Titze has presented evidence that the greatest vocal power can be achieved when the vocal folds are "spread apart slightly."[85] The almost-imaginary /h/ preceding voice onset during spontaneous utterances such as "Hm!" or "Huh!" helps the voice user meet this ideal prephonatory glottal width condition. Second, phonation threshold pressures are minimal when the ideal prephonatory

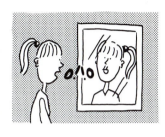

a.

SKELETON-SUSPENSION:

Imagine your skeleton is suspended from the crown of the head. Gravity helps your torso, arms and legs fall away from the head in a natural alignment: your body grows taller because of the gentle upward pull from the suspension force.

As your head is gently pulled upward, it is released from the top of your neck. Prove this by gently shaking it in a "no" gesture. Imagine you are drawing a 2 centimetre horizontal line with your nose. Make the movement small and loose and confine it to your head. The big neck muscles should not be assisting.

As your head is gently pulled upward, make a teeter-toter movement with it: like nodding "yes". Imagine you are drawing a 2 centimetre vertical line with your nose. As with "no", the "yes" gesture is very small and free. It confirms that you have liberated your head from your neck and spine.

LIBERATE YOUR LIPS:

The lips form one of your important speech articulators. Their freedom to move is influenced by several areas in the face. A static "position" of the lips, in turn, can restrict other speech functions, like jaw movement. If your face gets stuck in the "social smile" position, your lips will be stiff, and your speech nasal and indistinct. We need to banish the "stiff upper lip" to vocalize with ease.

Using your mirror, gently whisper "O". The upper lip should be stretched forward, like a half-open umbrella, your jaw dropped. Allow your body to breathe through the "O", leaving your jaw hanging, and your tongue lying on the floor of your mouth.

To release tension in lip muscles, close them loosely, and blow air between them so they vibrate and flutter in the breeze. See how long you can keep your lips vibrating in the airflow.

b.

Do the following exercise frequently to remind your monitors what free lip movements feel like during speech (use a mirror):

Gently vocalize the sound sequence: **"OO-EE-OO-EE-OO-EE-OO-EE ..."**

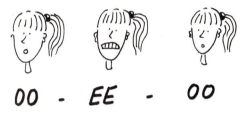

Keep your voice flowing through the transition from "oo" to "ee". Make sure your lips pucker forward for "oo" and spread back for "ee". Start with slow repetitions, then increase the rate so you are changing sounds at the rate of normal speech.

c.

NEW LANGUAGES:

1. **PLUTONIAN:** AnAnAnAnAnAnAnAnAnAnAnAnAnA....
↓↓↓↓↓↓↓↓↓↓↓↓↓↓↓

(say the "A" vowel like "ah"; the arrows mean your jaw drops for each new "ah")
(use your regular speech speed, or about 4 syllables/second)
(don't cheat by articulating "n" with your tongue tip: you will create "n" automatically when the jaw carries your tongue-mass to the roof of your mouth!)

2. **VENUTIAN:**

SIDE VIEW

FRONT VIEW

(let gravity be responsible for the jaw drop on each "ah")
(don't cheat by articulating "v" with lower-lip movement: you will create "v" automatically when the jaw carries your lower lip up to your upper teeth!)

3. **MARTIAN:** AdAdAdAdAdAdAdAdAdAdAdAdAdAdAd...
↓↓↓↓↓↓↓↓↓↓↓↓↓↓↓

4. **URANIAN:** AsAsAsAsAsAsAsAsAsAsAsAsAsAsAs...
↓↓↓↓↓↓↓↓↓↓↓↓↓↓↓

e.

The jaw is capable of several types of movements. When we eat, it may move forward and back, up and down, and side to side. **When we use the jaw for talking or singing, the main movement is a down and up movement, with the jaw pivoting within its joints, like a door pivoting on its hinges.**

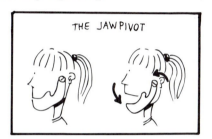

THE JAW PIVOT

The jaw joint is located directly in front of the ear hole. Place your fingers flat on the sides of your face to feel the area over the jaw joint. It will become evident if you gently push your jaw forward a few millimetres: your fingers will feel a slight bulging over the joint. This bulge should not be evident when you are talking. Instead, your face should stay flat when your jaw is moving for speech.

d.

GRAVITY AND THE TONGUE:

In its rest position, when we are not talking, singing, eating or doing other acrobatic maneuvers with the tongue, it should lie flat on the floor of the mouth, like a rug. Gravity helps the tongue assume the rug position on the mouth's floor.

Let your jaw fall free under the influence of gravity. The tongue falls down with the jaw. Let your tongue rest lazily on the floor of your mouth, so it touches the back edges of all your bottom teeth. Enjoy breathing through your relaxed open mouth and throat: feel the air flowing freely over the lazy tongue. If your tongue starts to feel too long and wide for your mouth cavity, let it slide forward and rest on your bottom teeth and lips as you enjoy breathing through your open mouth and throat.

This indulgence in relaxation may bring on some yawns. Enjoy them, but protect your jaw from opening too wide! Then let your tongue return to its relaxed rug-like position on the floor of your mouth, resting against your lower teeth...

THE TONGUE ASSUMES THE RUG POSITION

f.

Figure 4–4. Exercises for specific relaxation and mobility; (**a**) head and neck, (**b**) lower face, (**c**) lips, (**d**) jaw, (**e**) jaw, (**f**) tongue, (**g**) tongue, (**h**) tongue. From *Vocalizing with Ease: A Self-Improvement Guide* (pp. 38, 59, 61, 64, 68, 71), by L. A. Rammage, 1996, Vancouver: Pacific Voice Clinic. Copyright 1996, by L. A. Rammage and M. Haijtink. Reprinted with permission.

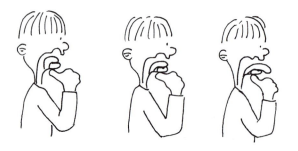

" HANGING OUT THE RUG "

g.

Figure 4–4. (continued)

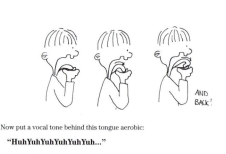

AND BACK!

Now put a vocal tone behind this tongue aerobic:

"HuhYuhYuhYuhYuhYuh..."

Let the tongue do all the work. *(Keep your jaw still and passive! Your vocal tone should flow freely through your open throat and mouth as you free the base of your tongue-rug by rolling it.)*

h.

glottal width condition is met during phonation in lower pitches, as in modal register, which is typically elicited during CVO productions[85]. Third, phonation initiated during spontaneous utterances such as "Hm!" are typically associated with lung volumes near the resting expiratory level. We discuss in Chapter 8 some mechanical advantages that may accrue by initiating phonation at lower rather than higher lung volumes: voice users may experience greatest flexibility for inspiration and expiratory activities near the resting expiratory level[35], and glottal posture may be most independent of respiratory mechanics at lower lung volumes[37,38,81,82]. Fourth, acoustic pressures are large in the frontal resonators during production of nasal consonants, so the greatest opportunity is presented for patients to achieve the desired kinaesthetic feedback when the onset phoneme is a nasal one such as /m/[85].

The majority of patients immediately acknowledge kinesthetic awareness of lower thoracic-abdominal muscle activity when they employ a coordinated voice onset. Flexible endoscopy has revealed a reduction in magnitude of posterior glottal chinks in patients with laryngeal muscle misuse while they are employing this technique. It may contribute to more efficient voice production in patients with isometric muscle misuse dysphonias, as demonstrated by this laryngoscopic sign, as well as to reduced mean phonatory flow rates and breathy perceptions[62,64].

The coordinated voice onset has also been used successfully to optimize voice onset strategies in individuals with spasmodic dysphonias and for a variety of organic problems leading to incompetent glottal closure. Once the basic onset technique is established, it can be extended to train use of respiratory support for sustained sounds, intensity dynamics, and then speech phrases.

4.4.7 Resonance Enhancement

Resonance enhancement exercises are introduced to improve vocal tone, clarity, and power. Patients are trained to maximize vocal resonance, initially by attending to kinesthetic sensations associated with sympathetic vibration of the vocal tract resonators (Figure 4–6). Nasal phonemes or vowels associated with high tongue postures (/i/; /u/) often are used to facilitate the kinesthetic learning because of the distinct resonance sensations associated with the large acoustic pressures in the nasal cavities or front of the oral cavity during these sounds[85]. Lessac's "Y-buzz" exercise is an example of a resonance-training

Find a rhythm to repeat CVO that suits your current energy level:

"hm!(RR) hm!(RR) hm!(RR) ..."

*(remember: **RR** means "Respiratory Release" that is, the immediate natural release of abdominal muscles, allowing the breath-tide to flow in quickly between sounds).*

Start with a rate of about three repetitions per second. You will know when your repetition rate matches your current adrenalin level, because the CVO system will seem to be self-perpetuating: (and you will not gasp for air after several repetitions). In fact, once you submit your body to the spring-like actions of CVO-RR-CVO-RR, you will feel as though you could continue responding in this way indefinitely, or at least until the cows come home.

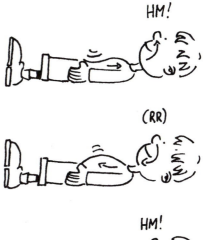

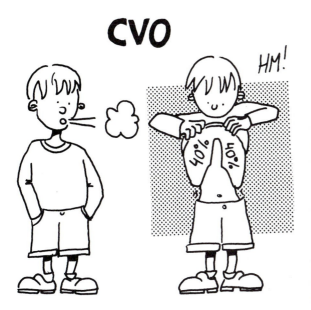

CVO ON YOUR FEET:

The CVO response is equally effective in upright positions: sitting or standing, assuming you apply principles of healthy posture as you vocalize.

Practice CVO while sitting or standing in front of a full-length mirror: Notice the absence of activity in your upper body during CVO (no head, neck, jaw, face or shoulder movements). If you're not wearing lots of bulky clothing, you will be able to see the CVO-RR activity in your abdomen.

You have just rediscovered one of your most important vocal functions. Enjoy and be proud of yourself!

Figure 4–5. Coordinated voice onset technique. From *Vocalizing with Ease: A Self-Improvement Guide* (p. 52), by L. A. Rammage, 1996, Vancouver: Pacific Voice Clinic. Copyright 1996, by L. A. Rammage and M. Haijtink. Reprinted with permission.

technique that helps individuals associate particular facial postures with specific resonance sensations to enhance vocal power and achieve desirable voice quality features[47]. The kinesthetic awareness achieved in the initial exploratory exercises is used as a reference for sensations that can be present during all other vowels and nonnasal voiced phonemes and, in essence, during running speech. Relaxed articulatory movements of the jaw, tongue, and lips are incorporated to facilitate maximum oral resonance sensations in a variety of sound sequences and then during speech. Attention may be drawn to the relationships between perceived resonance and vocal power and the corresponding activity of the respiratory muscles which, in a sense, feed the vocal tract resonators by ensuring continuous air flow through the glottis.

4.4.8 Vocal Flexibility

Vocal flexibility exercises are introduced to establish rapid pitch and intensity changes without muscle misuse. This stage of training targets effective intonation and linguistic stress in speech and provides basic technical drills for pitch and register dynamics during singing. Initially, general and specific relaxation exercises are combined with "vocal eases" often used in singing pedagogy, such as glissandos during lip and tongue trills and siren imitations (Figure 4–7). Patients are encouraged to apply the techniques to pitch and intensity dynamics during speech and may use information from the clinician, each other, or instrumental feedback to confirm dynamic range increases. Simultaneous production of a specific upper vocal tract effect (lip bubbling, tongue trilling, voiced fricative production, finger buzzing, or frontal resonance monitoring) is always introduced in association with vocal flexibility exercises for f_0 range extension, to ensure that inappropriate compensatory pitch-changing strategies are not used. This type of technique is prescribed as a laryngeal stretching exercise for

use during all vocal warm-up activities. It is also used frequently in the treatment of vocal fold stiffness and scarring.

4.4.9 Prosody and Phrasing

Prosody encompasses the overall fluency, rhythm, rate, and timing issues that contribute to speech that is meaningful, socially appropriate, and intelligible. Two primary issues have a large impact on prosody: rate of speech and phrasing. Individuals with muscle misuse voice problems frequently also exhibit excessively fast speaking rates, poor phrasing skills, and inappropriate speech-breathing patterns. Individuals with excessively fast speaking rates may benefit from rate-reduction strategies used extensively in intensive stuttering treatment programs. Slow (vowel) prolongation or speech using Delayed Auditory Feedback devices both have been demonstrated to improve speech fluency and reduce speaking rate[22,36,71].

Because appropriate phrasing also can have a positive impact on speech-breathing and speaking rate, it is an important activity in comprehensive therapy programs. Phrasing can be presented as both a physical and a linguistic activity. Physically, phrasing is represented by one expiratory speech limb, preceded and followed by appropriate inspiratory activity. Grammatically, phrasing is defined as a sequence of words that together represent a concept. Hixon et al. have provided evidence that speech-breathing is regulated in part by linguistic phrasing codes[35].

Strategies that allow grammatical phrase boundaries to dictate speech-breathing patterns are used to improve communication at both cognitive and physical levels. The CVO extended to various lengths can be presented as an example of physical phrasing. Serial speech sequences, poetry, and speech sequences with predictable carrier phrases can be used to implement grammatically regu-

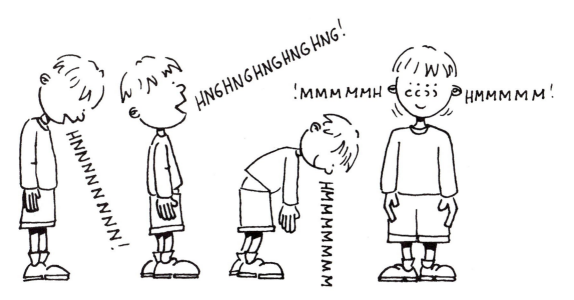

Figure 4–6. Exercises for resonance enhancement. From *Vocalizing with Ease: A Self-Improvement Guide* (p. 73), by L. A. Rammage, 1996, Vancouver: Pacific Voice Clinic. Copyright 1996, by L. A. Rammage and M. Haijtink. Reprinted with permission.

lated physical phrasing early in therapy. Intermediate stages may include reading script with phrase boundaries marked directly onto the manuscript and reciting simple instructions with highly predictable language. Phrasing during natural discourse is the final challenge and requires careful attention to technique at both cognitive and physical planning levels.

4.4.10 Generalization

Generalization of appropriate motor skills to speech, to vocal performance, or both is the ongoing process of applying these newly acquired techniques to real-life situations. Ideally, patients incorporate new behaviors during day-to-day communication at each stage of rehabilitation, so the final stage of therapy can focus on troubleshooting in difficult situations. For example, early in the program, techniques are trained for establishing balanced posture, and these are practiced intensively until the optimal behaviors predominate in everyday activities and become automatic. Balanced posture then becomes a

prerequisite for good speech and singing while other techniques are being learned or applied concurrently. In the group-therapy format, peer review and role-playing serve as useful practice activities for generalization. Ultimately, each individual needs a method to monitor his or her vocal performance on an ongoing basis. The clinician may participate by means of on-site evaluation or by reviewing videotapes of a patient communicating or performing in typical situations. Vocal performers are encouraged to recommence or continue an appropriate vocal pedagogical program.

4.4.11 Practice, Practice, Practice!

The most common concern expressed by patients participating in a vocal rehabilitation program is difficulty finding time to practice and incorporate appropriate techniques into their busy lives. If patients understand the principles of motor learning, they often can refine their vocal warm-up regimens so that simple rehearsals of vocal techniques become part of their daily routines. We emphasize the need to interrupt inappropriate motor behaviors frequently throughout the day, replacing them with more appropriate behaviors, and receiving the expected feedback about the response correctness immediately. Each patient is expected to use vocal warm-up and cool-down regimens daily. These activities may be selected on an individual basis from the repertoire of techniques employed successfully during the rehabilitation program. The vocal warm-up is advocated as a long-term daily commitment for occupational and professional voice users.

4.5 Holistic Therapy

Certain types of holistic therapy may complement symptomatic or comprehensive therapy programs. Holistic programs include strategies for general relaxation, such as Jacobson's Progressive Relaxation[40] and cognitive imaging techniques, programs to improve flexibility and alignment (such as the Alexander Technique[6]), yoga, Pilates, or the Feldenkrais method[28], and more speech-specific holistic techniques such as the Accent Method[30,46,73], Froeschel's chewing method[29], the Yawn-Sigh technique[48], and Vocal Function Exercises[79]. The clinician directing a voice therapy program needs to have some familiarity with each approach to offer appropriate advice about their potential benefit for improving voice function.

One popular holistic voice therapy program that may be used to improve voice function is the Accent Method[30,46,73]. In this program, coordination between speech-breathing and phonation is regulated by varying prosodic aspects of vocal productions at progressively higher levels of physical and linguistic demand. As timing, syllabic, and intonational stress are varied, attention is drawn to the respiratory muscle activity that generates these prosodic changes during simple vocal play, followed by more complex sound sequences and ultimately speech phrases. When the target prosodic

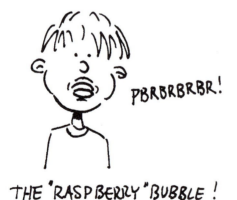

a.

Press your upper and lower lips together lightly (like for "p"). Keeping them together, blow air between your lips, so you get a "raspberry bubble". (Don't despair if at first this seems impossible. There will be other options for you if the bubble doesn't emerge).

Now turn your vocal motor on lightly during your raspberry-bubble:

"pbrbrbrbrbrbrbrbr..."

(remember to keep your lips together and your breath-flow steady: use your abdominal muscles to activate and sustain the flow; stop for a refill when you run out of air)

Figure 4–7. Exercises for increasing range, flexibility, and intonation; (**a**) lip bubbling, (**b**) the vocal siren. From *Vocalizing with Ease: A Self-Improvement Guide* (pp. 78, 82), by L. A. Rammage, 1996, Vancouver: Pacific Voice Clinic. Copyright 1996, by L. A. Rammage and M. Haijtink. Reprinted with permission.

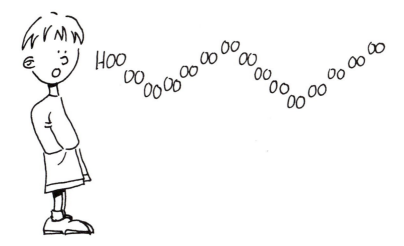

Try the vocal siren on some other sounds now. Keep the tone light but buzzy and piercing like a real siren:

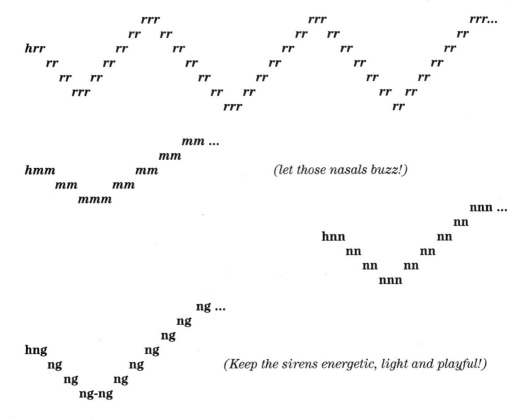

(let those nasals buzz!)

(Keep the sirens energetic, light and playful!)

b.

Figure 4–7 (continued)

patterns are modeled by the clinician immediately before a patient attempts them, it is important to monitor the vocal pitch and loudness level used by the patient because imitation of inappropriate pitch or loudness ranges by a patient with a compromised voice can lead to further muscle misuse.

4.6 Therapy for Special Voice Disorder Populations

4.6.1 Interdisciplinary Management for Patients with Structural-Organic Disorders: Optimizing Function

Many individuals with primary organic voice disorders may benefit from voice therapy in conjunction with other medical-surgical treatments or as a primary intervention approach. Because all patients consulting the voice clinic undergo a comprehensive voice evaluation as described in Chapter 1, including diagnostic therapy, it should be clear when voice therapy is indicated as an adjunct to medical-surgical treatment.

4.6.1.1 Therapy in Conjunction With Phonosurgery:

When the evaluation results in recommendation for medical-surgical intervention, the primary goals of preoperative therapy include reduction of vocal abuses and muscle misuses identified during evaluation and elimination of ineffective compensatory behaviors that have developed in the presence of organic disease. Postoperatively, therapy focuses on techniques that facilitate adaptation to medical-surgical changes, and that optimize the effectiveness of the primary treatment. Patients may benefit from therapy in conjunction with a number of medical-surgical procedures including surgical removal of vocal fold nodules, polyps, cysts, papillo-

mas and other benign or neoplastic lesions, surgical augmentation of vocal folds (by injection of collagen, fat, teflon or other inert substances), or by thyroplasty procedures, botulinum toxin injections (typically for spasmodic dysphonias or vocal cord dysfunction), thyroplasty procedures to modify pitch (typically cricothyroid approximation for raising pitch in treatment of gender dysphoria), nerve anastomosis or other micronerve surgery, radiation treatment for cancers, and partial and total laryngectomy. The role of the speech-language pathologist in laryngectomee rehabilitation will be discussed in a separate section in this chapter.

To select the most appropriate therapy facilitation techniques to optimize postsurgical results, the speech-language pathologist needs to be familiar with laryngeal anatomy and physiology and with the basic goals and procedures of the various phonosurgical techniques. Review of Chapters 3 and 8 and recommended readings should provide clinicians with the necessary information.

To vibrate in a way that produces the most efficient, powerful and periodic sound source, the vocal folds need to meet certain structural and mechanical criteria. First, they need to be able to adduct sufficiently to interrupt the airflow so the self-oscillatory pattern can be initiated and sustained, but not adduct so tightly that vocal fold vibration is effortful or impossible. Second, the vocal folds need to be flexible enough to vibrate readily in complex ways to produce a rich harmonic spectral pattern. This latter condition assumes that the multilayer structure in the vocal folds is preserved and muscle tone is normal. Third, the vocal folds need to be symmetrical enough in their structures that they can move synchronously. Finally, the medial vibrating edges of the vocal folds need to be relatively straight or at least to have relatively smooth symmetrical contours along the primary vibrating portions. Phonosurgical procedures and other medical treatments for voice disorders are designed to meet these structural-mechanical conditions as best possible. In some cases, structural or neurological deficits may determine that only one vocal fold will vibrate, in which case the surgical goal may be to create sufficient approximation, stability, and smoothness of the immobile vocal fold to facilitate optimal function in the mobile fold. Voice therapy is introduced to refine the surgical results by attempting to meet optimal vocal fold vibratory conditions as closely as possible. This may be done in one of two ways: by applying physiological-symptomatic approaches, as described in a previous section or by optimizing overall vocal technique to ensure that inappropriate muscle misuses are not interfering with the desired postsurgical result. In the latter case, a comprehensive vocal rehabilitation program as described in this chapter may be useful.

Case 4.3

Peppy Loma is a 23-year-old lab technician who has experienced voice problems since she was a young child. She has had approximately 15 surgical procedures to remove papillomatosis that obstructed her airway as a child. The most recent operation was 2 years ago. She is seen in the voice clinic by the otolaryngologist and speech-language pathologist for an initial evaluation, complaining that her voice has been getting progressively hoarser and her speech more effortful over the past 6 months. Her speaking voice is indeed moderately breathy and harsh, her pitch and loudness ranges very limited, and phonation breaks are intermittent. Her voice onsets are characterized by breath holding and glottal attacks, and we see signs of muscle misuse in neck muscles and a tendency toward jaw jut posture. Her teeth are worn, and she confesses to being a nocturnal grinder. Her jaw movements are minimal, and suprahyoid and thyrohyoid muscles are hypertonic during speech. Her speech-breathing pattern is characterized by minimal abdominal displacement on inspiration, initiation of phonation around 70% vital capacity, and large lung volume excursions. Her videolaryngostroboscopic evaluation reveals that the right vocal fold is largely obstructed from view by

papillomatosis, and the left vocal fold is stiff (reduced mucosal wave and amplitude). Vocal fold closure is incomplete because of the irregular edge of the right vocal fold and bilateral stiffness. Lateral compression of the ventricular folds is noted during phonation, and most dramatically during voice onsets.

Peppy's etiological profile is completed by examining the four etiological platforms, and this suggests that multiple postural and muscle misuses in combination with some anxiety about her long-term vocal status are contributing to symptom formation, in combination with her primary organic pathology. Diagnostic voice therapy suggests that Peppy is able to recognize and correct certain muscle misuses with specific models and directions, but her voice quality does not improve with any facilitation techniques. She is provided with some preliminary posture and relaxation training to reduce muscle misuse in her abdominal muscles, neck, jaw, and tongue. The long-term prognosis for voice function is discussed with her with respect to the various etiological platforms and relevant treatments. She is offered an appointment with the team psychiatrist to discuss her apprehensions further, but she declines. She states that she feels reassured that a combined surgical and therapy intervention plan will offer her the best chance of a long-term functional voice.

Surgical intervention is scheduled to remove papilloma with a CO_2 laser. Because the papilloma does not extend to the anterior commissure, we are not anticipating problems with a postsurgical web. Peppy is provided with our standard postoperative voice use instructions (see Appendix 3–2). During her postsurgical review, diagnostic therapy is again undertaken; it is determined that, in addition to responding well to the posture and relaxation techniques, she now is able to produce significantly clearer voice when she uses a coordinated voice onset and extends it to humming. She recognizes the abdominal muscle activities associated with CVO, and the resonance sensations associated with humming and is able to reproduce these effects without modeling. She is provided with further guidelines for avoiding vocal abuse and overuse and a vocal warm-up routine based on her diagnostic therapy results: CVO while monitoring suprahyoid muscle activity and balanced head-neck posture *and extended humming to reinforce resonance. Because she has taken a 6-week leave from work, she is able to follow the clinician's advice to use her voice minimally when she is not practicing vocal techniques. During a second postsurgical therapy session, relaxed jaw movements during phonation are added to her vocal warm-up routine, and she is able to apply these immediately to serial speech productions. Because she is not a good lip-triller, she is provided with some initial instruction to practice the lip-trilling without voice. Some mild postsurgical edema is still evident on videostroboscopic evaluation, so we confine our vocal activities to those that require minimal laryngeal effort.*

At a 2-month postoperative evaluation, there is no sign of postsurgical edema or erythema, so her voice therapy program is expanded to include techniques that improve flexibility and minimize effects of postsurgical scarring: lip trilling with vocal tone in a gradual glissando. The glissando range is initially narrow but increases over the course of several months. On her return to work, Peppy demonstrates improved head-neck posture, is consistently aware of the abdominal muscle contribution to speech, can feel oral-nasal resonance when she remembers to attend to it, and continues to work on jaw relaxation during speech. She has expressed an interest in attending a comprehensive voice rehabilitation program, which will reinforce her good vocal technique and provide a group setting for learning and practicing a broader repertoire of appropriate communication strategies.

4.6.1.2 Therapy for Vocal Fold Stiffness and Scarring

An inevitable result of any surgical procedure is some degree of stiffness from scarring, which can cause adynamic vocal fold segments and tethering of the vocal fold mucosa to the underlying layer structures. Modern phonosurgical techniques are designed to minimize postsurgical scarring, so therapy may focus more on optimizing vocal technique in these cases. The more aggressive the surgery, the more likely scarring will occur. In some cases, such as Peppy's above, surgery must be aggressive to ablate invasive or obstructive lesions such as papillomas and carcinomas. Sometimes scarring occurs in the larynx as a result of prolonged intubation. Other types of scar tissue are congenital, as in many cases of sulcus vocalis. We are optimistic that surgeons are no longer creating extensive iatrogenic scarring by "stripping" vocal fold mucosa to remove nodules and polyps.

When the vocal folds are stiff from scar tissue or other structural abnormalities, certain therapy techniques may be useful in improving functional vocal status and the acoustic results of phonation. Some therapies may even serve to expedite scar softening.

Among the techniques that have been advocated to restore vocal fold mobility are use of lip and tongue trills, glottal fry, loud voice use, and vocal fold stretching with pitch elevation. Massage and stretching are techniques commonly used in physical therapy for resolution of scar stiffness in other regions of the body. Vocal activities that promote large vocal fold excursions during vibration, such as loud phonation or phonation simultaneous with lip trilling, may effectively "massage" the vocal folds. Trilling effects also have the advantage of minimizing supraglottal constriction[16]. A series of vocal function exercises may be helpful to restore balance and flexibility of the laryngeal mechanism. These exercises as described in the literature involve vowel prolongation and pitch glissandos at low intensities[79]. A pitch sweep simultaneous with lip or tongue trilling may serve the purpose of stretching and massaging and is used extensively in this clinic to treat vocal fold stiffness. Glottal fry is associated with a syncopated irregular vocal fold vibratory "pattern" and may also play a role in selectively massaging vocal fold tissue.

In addition to therapy techniques thought to soften scar tissue and improve vocal fold mobility, vocal rehabilitation for vocal fold stiffness may need to include more comprehensive programs such as the one outlined in this chapter or holistic programs such as the Accent Method[30,46,73].

4.6.2 Therapy for Neurogenic Voice and Speech Problems (Motor Speech Disorders)

Voice therapy is often useful to individuals suffering voice dysfunction due to neurogenic diseases, both as a primary treatment mode and in conjunction with medical-surgical management. Even in the presence of permanent vocal fold incompetence or asymmetry or of muscle weakness in respiratory, articulatory, or resonance mechanisms, optimal use of the various systems involved in voice production can result in improved functional communication.

Voice problems may be a component of most of the motor speech disorders identified in the traditional classification schemes outlined in Chapter 2. In children with cerebral palsies, therapy for the dysphonia components of motor speech disorders typically is incorporated into activities targeting overall communication goals. Treatment of young children with CP often requires a multidisciplinary approach. Typically, postural, motor control, and developmental cognitive-linguistic issues need to be addressed as a prerequisite to specific speech and voice therapy exercises. An individual with cerebral palsy may be well into the teen or adult years before intervention for specific voice symptoms is a priority or a possibility. Symptomatic therapy guidelines for the corresponding dysarthria types may then be applied as appropriate, or more comprehensive voice and speech therapy programs may be initiated.

Voice problems associated with acquired motor speech disorders—apraxias and dysarthrias—may be treated symptomatically or in more comprehensive voice and communication rehabilitation programs, depending on individual considerations. As is the case with all voice and speech disorders, it is critical to incorporate therapy strategies that target relevant dysfunctional areas on all etiological platforms, not just those associated with the motor speech disorder that has been

diagnosed. For a comprehensive review of treatment of motor speech disorders, the reader is referred to current literature in the recommended reading list at the end of this chapter.

Therapy approaches will now be presented for neurogenic voice problems that are most commonly encountered in the Voice Clinic.

4.6.2.1 Apraxia

Apraxia of speech is frequently associated with difficulty in initiating phonation. At its most extreme, apraxic patients may be mute. In some cases, finding strategies for initiating phonation is a critical first step in therapy. Common approaches to therapy to improve voluntary control over phonation include physical prompting such as sudden abdominal pressure; digital touch or pressure over the larynx; use of a cervical artificial larynx; and elicitation of laughter, coughing, yawning or other vocal gestures that are typically reflexive. Other strategies include use of semantic carrier phrases, singing or chanting, pairing meaningful gestures with automatic speech, and serial speech[24]. Many standardized programs have been introduced to improve voluntary control and fluency in individuals with apraxia of speech, and these are described in detail in current texts on motor speech disorders.

4.6.2.2 Dysarthrias

The diversity of effects on voice and speech of the many dysarthrias are outlined in Chapter 2. Duffy has provided a summary table that exemplifies symptomatic treatment for the spectrum of dysarthrias (see Table 4–2)[24]. Therapy programs should be planned to address specific neurogenic speech effects, as well as individual etiological components contributing to communication breakdown.

Flaccid Dysarthria (Lower Motor Neuron—Vocal Fold Paralysis). One of the most commonly encountered motor speech

Table 4–2 Treatment approaches and their relationship to various dysarthria types

Approach	Flaccid	Spastic	Ataxic	Hypokinetic	Hyperkinetic	Unilateral UMN
Behavioral	+	+	+	+	+	+
Respiration	+	+	+	+	−	−
"5 for 5" respiratory tasks	+	+	+	+	−	−
Pushing-pulling exercise	+ +	−	−	−	−	−
Supine-reclining postures	+	+	−	−	−	−
Manual push on abdomen	+	−	−	+	−	−
Inhale more deeply	+	+	−	+	−	−
Speak at onset of exhalation	+	+	+	+	−	−
Inspiratory checking	+	−	+	+	−	−
Neck breathing	+ +	−	−	−	−	−
Glossopharyngeal breathing	+ +	−	−	−	−	−
Maximum vowel prolongation	+	+	+	+	−	−
Controlled exhalation tasks	+	+	+	+	−	−
Terminate speech earlier during exhalatory cycle	+	+	+	+	−	−
Optimal breath group	+	+	+	+	−	−
Increase sentence length	+	+	+	+	−	−
Increase vocal strain	+	−	−	+	−	−
Shorten fricative duration	+	−	−	−	−	−
Shorten phrases	+	+	+	+	−	−
Phonation	+	+	−	+	+	−
Relaxation, massage	−	+	−	−	+	−
Turn head during speech	+ +	−	−	−	−	−
Lateralize thyroid cartilage	+ +	−	−	−	−	−
Head back, increased pitch, deep breath	−	+	−	−	−	−
Effort closure techniques	+ +	−	−	+ +	−	−
Abrupt glottal attack	+ +	−	−	+ +	−	−
Intense, high-level phonatory effort	+ +	−	−	+ +	−	−
Breathy onset	−	+ +	−	−	+ +	−
Speak at onset of exhalation	+	+	+	+	−	−
Continuous voicing of consonants	−	−	−	−	+ +	−
Optimal breath group	+	+	+	+	−	−
Resonance	+	+	−	+	−	−
Blowing-sucking exercise	+	+	−	−	−	−
CPAP	+ +	−	−	−	−	−
Supine positioning	+	+	−	−	−	−
Occlude nares	+	+	−	−	−	−
Exaggerate jaw movement	+	−	−	+	−	−
Increase loudness	+	+	−	+	−	−
Reduce pressure consonant duration	+ +	−	−	−	−	−

Table 4–2 (continued)

Approach	Dysarthria Type					
	Flaccid	Spastic	Ataxic	Hypokinetic	Hyperkinetic	Unilateral UMN
Articulation	+	+	+	+	+	+
Strengthening exercises	++	−	−	−	−	+
Relaxation exercise	−	+	−	−	+	−
Stretching	+	+	−	+	−	−
Biofeedback	+	+	+	+	+	+
Sensory tricks	−	−	−	−	++	−
Conservation of strength	+	+	−	+	−	−
Exaggerate consonants	+	+	+	+	−	+
Integral stimulation	+	+	+	+	−	+
Phonetic placement	+	+	+	+	−	+
Phonetic derivation	+	+	+	+	−	+
Minimal contrasts	+	+	+	+	−	+
Alternative place, manner, voicing strategies	+	+	−	−	−	−
Intelligibility drills	+	+	+	+	+	+
Referential tasks	+	+	+	+	+	+
Rate	+	+	+	+	+	+
Rate reduction	+	+	+	+	+	+
Hand or finger tapping	+	+	+	+	−	+
Rhythmic or metered cuing	−	+	+	+	−	+
Visual feedback	+	+	+	+	+	+
Modify pauses	+	+	+	+	−	+
Identify first letter on board	+	+	+	+	+	+
Prosody & naturalness	+	+	+	+	+	+
Breath group duration	+	+	+	+	+	+
Modify syllable duration and pause time	+	+	+	+	+	−
Across breath group tasks	+	+	+	+	−	−
Chunk by syntactic units	+	+	+	+	−	−
Contrastive stress tasks	+	+	+	+	+	+
Referential stress tasks	+	+	+	+	+	+
Prosthetic	+	+	+	+	+	−
Abdominal binders and corsets	++	−	−	−	−	−
Expiratory board or paddle	++	−	−	+	−	−
Vocal intensity controller	+	+	−	+	−	−
Vocal amplifier	+	+	−	+	−	−
Artificial larynges	++	−	−	−	−	−
Palatal lift	++	+	−	−	−	−
DAF	−	−	−	++	−	−
Pacing board	−	−	−	++	−	−
Metronome	−	−	−	++	−	−
Bite block	+	−	−	−	++	−
Nose clip or nasal obturator	+	+	−	−	−	−

(continued)

Table 4–2 (continued)

Approach	Dysarthria Type					
	Flaccid	**Spastic**	**Ataxic**	**Hypokinetic**	**Hyperkinetic**	**Unilateral UMN**
Jaw sling	++	−	−	−	−	−
Neck brace or cervical collar	+	−	+	−	+	−
Medical-surgical	+	+	−	+	+	−
Medialization laryngoplasty	++	−	−	+	−	−
Teflon or collagen injection	++	−	−	+	−	−
Recurrent laryngeal nerve resection	−	−	−	−	++	−
Botox injection	−	−	−	−	++	−
Pharyngeal flap	++	+	−	−	−	−
Neural anastomosis (VII-XII)	+	−	−	−	−	−
Pharmacologic	+	+	−	+	+	−
Artane (trihexyphenidyl)	−	−	−	−	+	−
Dantrium (dantrolene sodium)	−	+	−	−	−	−
Elavil (amitriptyline)	−	+	−	−.	−	−
Haldol (haloperidol)	−	−	−	−	+	−
Inderal (propanolol)	−	−	−	−	+	−
Klonopin (clonazepam)	−	−	−	+	+	−
L-Dopa (levodopa)	−	−	−	++	−	−
Librium (chlordiazepoxide)	−	+	−	−	−	−
Lioresal (baclofen)	−	+	−	−	+	−
Lithane, Eskalith (lithium carbonate)	−	−	−	−	+	−
Mestinon (pyridostigmine bromide)	++	−	−	−	−	−
Mysoline (primidone)	−	−	−	−	+	−
Neptazine (methazolamide)	−	−	−	−	+	−
Reserpine	−	−	−	−	+	−
Sinemet (carbidopa-levodopa)	−	−	−	++	+	−
Tegretol (carbamazepine)	−	−	−	−	+	−
Valium (diazepam)	−	+	−	−	−	−
Xanax (alprazolam)	−	−	−	−	+	−

+, may be appropriate; ++, uniquely appropriate but not necessarily for all patients; −, contraindicated, rarely necessary, or uncertain; *CPAP,* continuous positive airway pressure; *DAF,* delayed auditory feedback; *UMN,* upper motor neuron.

From *Motor Speech Disorders: Substrates, Differential Diagnosis and Management* (pp. 405–407), by J. R. Duffy, 1995, St. Louis: Mosby Year Book, Inc. Copyright 1995, by Mosby Year Book, Inc. Reprinted with permission.

disorders in voice clinics is unilateral paralysis of a vocal fold due to injury of the ipsilateral recurrent laryngeal nerve. This typically results in a flaccid vocal fold that often is positioned away from the glottal midline. The unaffected vocal fold is unable to make complete contact with the paralyzed fold, and voice production is subsequently associated with high airflow rates, breathy voice, reduced pitch and loudness ranges, high pitch, and occasionally diplophonia. Surgical techniques often are used as primary treatment for augmenting or repositioning the paralyzed vocal fold once the anticipated spontaneous recovery period has passed. Common phonosurgical procedures are described in Chapter 3.

Voice therapy may play a role for the patient with unilateral vocal fold paralysis during the spontaneous recovery waiting period (typically 9–12 months), as a primary treatment approach, or as an adjunct to phonosurgery.

During the spontaneous recovery period, or when voice therapy is used as the primary rehabilitation approach, symptomatic techniques may be used to facilitate vocal fold adduction. Common approaches include forced adduction techniques (phonating while pushing, pulling, lifting weights, holding the breath, glottal attacks), application of lateral pressure to the thyroid lamina (usually on the paralyzed side, but sometimes on the non-paralyzed side), and turning the head to the right or left, whichever produces best voice[13,49,50]. Stemple, Glaze, and Gerdeman have suggested that the effectiveness of vocal fold adduction exercises depends on "the degree of vocal fold gap," with prognosis for improvement being most favorable if a "light touch closure" is evident during the videostroboscopic evaluation[79]. McFarlane et al have reported success in treating patients with vocal fold paralysis using three specific techniques to improve vocal fold adduction as the primary treatment modality: lateral digital pressure to the thyroid cartilage; "half-swallow boom," and head turned to the side[49,50].

When therapy is initiated during the spontaneous recovery waiting period, it may not always be advisable to elicit forced vocal fold adduction behaviors that may need to be extinguished later if spontaneous recovery occurs. We have found that patients typically achieve improved glottal closure when they target a low pitch or attempt to imitate glottal fry phonation. In the low-pitched glottal fry posture, the vocal fold margins are thick, and anteroposterior contraction may assist in achieving closure, particularly in the anterior portions of the vocal folds, which may have "touch" closure. Encouraging the patient to target a low-pitched, quiet voice may minimize air wastage and noise and optimize communication attempts. A high-quality vocal amplification system paired with these techniques may augment communication further and allow a vocally active person to maintain work and social activities during the waiting period.

Another important role of voice therapy in the patient with unilateral vocal fold paralysis is ensuring that inappropriate muscle misuses are not adopted as compensatory strategies during communication. Comprehensive evaluation and frequent follow-up assessments will allow the clinician to identify and extinguish these behaviors, as adjustments in vocal technique are made. Vocal amplification systems should be introduced whenever physical limitations threaten appropriate application of vocal techniques or functional communication.

When the site of lesion in the vagus nerve is above the pharyngeal branch, hypernasality may accompany the dysphonia because of an incompetent velopharyngeal valve. If hypernasality is caused by unilateral impairment and is mild, it often is treated successfully with voice therapy alone. Strategies may include optimizing jaw and tongue postures and movements to improve oral resonance; use of glottal fry, which is associated with constriction in the nasopharynx[8]; use of biofeedback devices to monitor and reduce transnasal airflow; and direct velar stimulation techniques. In more severe cases, nasality can cause significant reductions in intelligibility, and prosthetic management or pharyngoplasty may be necessary to manage the incompetent velopharyngeal valve.

Spastic Dysarthria. Individuals with spastic dysarthria typically have harsh tense (strained-strangled) voice qualities, low pitch, compromised pitch and loudness ranges, and often hypernasality, in addition to imprecise articulation and slow speaking rates. The vocal folds are hyperadducted, and anteroposterior compression is common. Techniques for voice problems related to upper motor neuron disease are typically incorporated into the speech therapy program. Whereas stretching of peripheral articulators may be useful to reduce hypertonicity, it is difficult to conduct and monitor any effects of stretching laryngeal muscles. General or specific relaxation exercises may be useful in treating individuals with spastic dysarthrias, but specific effectiveness data does not exist. Diagnostic therapy may be used to investigate the usefulness of training including speech-breathing strategies, voice onset strategies, increased airflow during phonation, elevated and varied pitch, phrasing, reduced speech rate, and enhanced oral resonance. Additionally, Dworkin and Culatta advocated desensitization of hyperactive gag reflexes in individuals with spastic dysarthrias when prosthetic management of hypernasality is being considered[25].

Hypokinetic Dysarthria (Associated with Parkinson's Disease or Parkinsonian Features). Dysarthria associated with Parkinson's disease (PD) is typically characterized by irregularities in speaking rate (especially rushes of speech); reduced speech intelligibility due to rigidity and reduced dynamics in articulator muscles; breathy, weak, sometimes harsh voice due to rigidity and bowing in the vocal folds; monotonicity and monoloudness; sometimes tremor or tremolo; and often short breath groups due to rigidity in respiratory muscles and glottal incompetence. As with any progressive neurological disease, individuals may also experience fatigue, depression, anxiety, and side effects from medications, all of which can compromise communication. The neuromuscular effects of PD may affect esophageal motility and contribute to swallowing problems or gastroesophageal reflux. Because reflux can cause reflexive hypertonicity in the larynx, this may contribute further to voice impairment. Clearly, contributing factors at all etiological levels need to be considered in treatment planning.

The stage of the PD typically will influence treatment priorities and choices. Individuals in early stages of PD may benefit from comprehensive voice and speech therapy programs that introduce effective communication strategies at all levels of function, including maintenance of optimal posture, natural speech-breathing tactics, relaxation of specific articulator muscles, resonance enhancement, and application of intonation and phrasing strategies that complement appropriate speech-breathing and other techniques. Vowel prolongation techniques used frequently for stutterers may help control and reduce speaking rate. When PD patients present themselves to the voice clinic at later disease stages, their communication complaints often are quite specific, such as, "My wife says she can't hear me even when she's right beside me!"

Case 4.4

Theo is 72 years old, and he was diagnosed with Parkinson's disease 7 years ago. Initially the disease seemed primarily to affect his stability when he stood for extended periods, and his writing became cramped and difficult to read. He continued to enjoy his retirement as best possible, spending lots of time on the golf course, singing in the church choir, and chairing meetings for several community organizations. Over the past 2 years, his mobility and physical stamina have deteriorated significantly. Additionally, he has noted that speaking is increasingly effortful, and all too frequently people ask him to repeat what he has said, complaining that he mumbles. Sometimes people appear to ignore him altogether when he talks, or worse, they make inappropriate responses because they don't understand what he said, but don't want to embarrass him by admitting it. He has stopped singing and often "misses" committee meetings. He is becoming increasingly frustrated and withdrawn because of his communication experiences, and he always leaves his wife to answer the phone now. His neurologist recently adjusted his medication, but he has not noticed any improvement in his speech. He has a constant sensation of a "lump" in his throat, and he clears it frequently, which makes his voice louder for a few seconds. He has been using a lot of antacid after meals in the past few months. His wife contributes the observation that he often chokes when he eats, but he denies this symptom. He contributes the opinion that his wife is hard-of-hearing, but she denies this.

Theo's speech is characterized by reduced articulatory dynamics and intelligibility, low vocal intensity, breathy monotone voice, and short breath groups. He overstraightens his neck during speech, retracting his jaw. Jaw movements are minimal during speech, although he can imitate a model for jaw drop on each syllable at his typical speaking rate. His torso is somewhat collapsed, and inspiratory movements in the abdomen are almost imperceptible. His voice is indeed louder when he coughs, clears his throat, shouts, and uses a coordinated voice onset model on "Hm!" His esophageal manometry and pH studies reveal an incompetent lower esophageal sphincter, a hiatal hernia, and excessive reflux. The voice care team concludes that Theo has significant factors contributing to his throat and speech complaints on the gastroesophageal reflux, psychological, and vocal technique platforms, in addition to the direct effects of PD. Additionally, he has mild presbycusis. His wife's audiogram suggests a degree of hearing loss that warrants a hearing-aid evaluation. He spends additional time with the voice clinic psychiatrist expressing anxiety and distress over his increasingly dependent physical status and discussing ways that he can reclaim some personal autonomy and seek opportunities to continue contributing to society.

Theo is keen to hear about reflux treatments to reduce his annoying throat symptoms and therapy programs that will help him regain control of communication situations. Following a brief individual therapy program to correct postural misuse, and initiate jaw relaxation exercises (which he does well) Theo is enrolled in an intensive group-therapy speech program for individuals with Parkinson's Disease, based on the Lee-Silverman approach[56–61]. In this program, he learns to use his speech-breathing mechanism more effectively when he shouts at progressively higher functional levels. Some of the other therapy group participants are instructed to "push" or "pull" with their arms to close their vocal folds and make louder sounds, but Theo successfully applies the abdominal sensations he became aware of when he learned about coordinated voice onset on "Hm!" At first he feels as though his voice is always unacceptably loud when he uses his "shouting" voice, but the cali-

bration portion of the therapy program helps desensitize him to his kinaesthetic and acoustic reactions and realize that awareness of these sensations tells him he is "doing it right." He finds it easier to reproduce and accept his louder voice after using the computer program on some productions to monitor his vocal intensity level he says he can "see the intensity level in my head as it was on the computer screen, before I start the sound." He also learns to increase his pitch range using the computer program and his own kinaesthetic awareness for feedback. After the first week, he recognizes changes in people's responses to his speech: fewer requests to repeat himself, attention without distressed looks, and specific appropriate responses. This provides the motivation to persevere with the 3-week intensive program and to practice daily on his own. The informal results of Theo's success are supported by improved objective measures for vocal intensity, intonation, and even intelligibility. One common outcome of the Lee Silverman voice therapy approach is an increase in articulatory dynamics in association with higher effort levels in respiratory and phonatory mechanisms[57,58].

Theo celebrates completion of his voice therapy program by attending a committee meeting after his last therapy session and proudly showing off his better speech. His committee members are suitably impressed and happy to have him back with his previous optimistic demeanor. Theo explains that he will have to continue practicing daily and that he will attend "booster" voice therapy sessions to maintain the positive speech behaviors as long as he is able to. He is making inquiries about purchasing a portable amplification system for speech in difficult environments and for conversations with his many hearing-impaired communication partners who refuse to admit they need hearing aids.

Hyperkinetic Dysarthrias: Organic Vocal Tremor (Benign or Familial Essential Tremor). Organic tremor of the larynx is a rhythmic fluctuation of intensity, frequency, or both, of approximately 5 Hz (see Figure 1–11). It may exist on its own or be associated with tremor in other articulators, the head, or the hands. It often is observed in association with laryngeal dystonias (spasmodic dysphonias). Associated tremors or vocal spasms may influence the choice of treatment approaches. When vocal tremor exists on its own or is the predominant dysarthric symptom, some voice therapy approaches may be helpful in increasing laryngeal stability, minimizing inappropriate compensatory strategies, or both. Voice therapy may be undertaken in conjunction with medications such as propranolol or botulinum toxin injections. Details about medical approaches to treatment are provided in Chapter 3.

A common compensatory response to organic vocal tremor, and the psychogenic tremolo associated with stage fright, is pitch lowering, increased medial compression of the vocal folds, and anteroposterior or lateral compression of supraglottal structures. These compensatory behaviors, which represent a subconscious attempt to stabilize the vocal system, may serve to intensify symptoms of effort and dysfluency. The most successful behavioral change often is realized when such compensatory responses are replaced with relaxation techniques, increased pitch, and reduced intensity or effort. Dworkin and Meleca advocate an elevation in f_0 of approximately 50 Hz[26]. Visual feedback with a software program or oscilloscope may be useful in establishing the appropriate target pitch. Additional techniques that have been reportedly successful in minimizing tremor symptoms include chanting, bracing the larynx manually, and using an elastic neckband to stabilize the larynx[26]. When vocal tremors are severe, prognosis for improvement is guarded, and a multidisciplinary approach is recommended.

Hyperkinetic Dysarthrias: Dystonia (Focal Laryngeal Dystonia or Spasmodic Dysphonia). Spasmodic dysphonias may have etiological components that encompass the four etiological platform components. The individual etiological profile does not seem to determine the combination or severity of typical

symptoms: tense, strained voice quality, hyperadducting or hypoadducting phonation breaks, pitch breaks, hyperadducting or hypoadducting delayed voice onsets, and a sensation of laryngeal effort during speech.

Speech-voice therapy for patients experiencing spasmodic dysphonias may be undertaken as a primary or secondary treatment. Primary therapy programs are those that focus on behavioral management techniques as the first or dominant symptom reduction strategy. Secondary speech therapy is used as an adjunct to other surgical, medical, or psychological treatment programs to enhance the primary treatment.

Primary voice therapy is generally intensive and long term, lasting from 6 months to 2 years, with daily, biweekly, or weekly sessions and intensive daily practice. As with all disorders, diagnostic therapy is undertaken initially to determine a patient's ability to alter spasmodic dysphonia symptoms under controlled conditions and to specify technical approaches that may be useful in achieving symptom reduction before a voice therapy program is recommended as the primary treatment approach. Because the pathogenesis of spasmodic dysphonia may include primary or secondary psychological components, an interdisciplinary management program is often advantageous, and psychiatric evaluation and treatment may be a prerequisite to successful voice therapy[4]. Primary voice therapy is most successful with patients who have minimal associated tremor, for whom psychological conflicts have been resolved, and in whom symptoms are incipient.

The long-term voice therapy program encompasses holistic or symptomatic protocols (or both) that reduce primary symptoms of laryngeal hypervalving or hypovalving, and secondary symptoms that exacerbate communication attempts, such as respiratory overloading and incoordination, head retraction, facial tension and grimacing, jaw and tongue splinting, pitch lowering, avoidance, and linguistic editing. Various types of biofeedback (acoustic software, electromyography, videolaryngoscopy, electroglottography, aerodynamic measures) may be used to supplement motor learning. Many aspects of behavioral management may resemble those used for treating speech fluency disorders; the intensity of therapy and drills is equally important so that changes in motor behavior are integrated into speech. Examples of holistic techniques that may be used in voice therapy include the following:

➤ Accent Method[30,46,73]
➤ Alexander Technique[6]
➤ Progressive Relaxation[40]
➤ Chewing Approach[29] (*Do not use in individuals with TMJ dysfunction*)
➤ Yawn-sigh[48]

Symptomatic techniques that may be used include the following:

➤ Continuous voicing or prolongation (primarily for abductor spasmodic dysphonia)
➤ Coordinated voice onset or lowered lung volumes[63]
➤ Easy voice onset or breathy voice
➤ Forward or neutral tongue positioning
➤ Forward resonance focus or humming
➤ Inhalation phonation[70] (*Do not use if paradoxical vocal fold movements are present*)
➤ Passive jaw movements[48,63]
➤ Pitch register therapy[5]

Selection of symptomatic techniques is guided by specific phonatory characteristics of an individual's dysphonia, especially the primary nature of laryngeal spasms, whether adductory or abductory, as well as secondary features that need to be targeted.

Secondary voice therapy is an important adjunct to medical-surgical intervention techniques. Voice therapy techniques may be trained before medical-surgical intervention to help patients reduce secondary behavioral

symptoms before treatment. Preoperative or postoperative voice therapy (or both) using approaches such as those listed above may enhance and prolong the effects of primary medical-surgical treatments such as botulinum toxin injections, or may be used to facilitate transition through the acute breathy voice stage immediately posttreatment. For patients who have had botulinum toxin injections, recurrent laryngeal nerve sectioning, or other surgical procedures to treat spasmodic dysphonia, adjunctive therapy may be undertaken to optimize communication in the presence of chronic postsurgical vocal fold weakness, asymmetry, or other post-surgical symptoms[39]. Details regarding medical-surgical approaches to treating spasmodic dysphonia are provided in Chapter 3.

Case 4.5

Allen's first comment when he visited the voice clinic was, "I'm afraid I'm going to have to change my name . . . Every time I try to say it, it gets stuck in my throat, and I have to push and it still won't come out, and I feel so mortified I want to fall through a hole in the floor and disappear!" Allen's first recognition of his voice problem occurred following a cold 10 months ago. He does, however, remember having a humiliating experience in high school when his voice would not come out as he stood at the front of the class, terrified, to give a mandatory oral presentation. He equates the sensation he feels most of the time now in his throat to a sensory memory from that earlier incident. When he was preparing for his first job interview after trade school, Allen remembered the humiliating voice block in high school and approached his doctor to request a "relaxation pill" to get him through the interview. Propranolol was prescribed, and he survived the interview but didn't get the job. He started using the drug regularly whenever he felt jittery about a job interview or a social situation. He contracted the cold soon after starting his current job. He is convinced that his frequent use of the "relaxation pill" is responsible for his voice problem and that the voice problem is "punishment" for a drug dependency. Coworkers and clients are starting to comment on his tense, choppy voice, and he is afraid he may lose his job, which is the first one he has really liked since graduating. He spends a lot of time on the phone marketing a new product, and he dreads the experience because his voice is "always worse on the phone." The only times his voice is predictably normal are when he talks to his dog or when he sings in the car.

Allen's speech is dysfluent because of frequent adductory vocal fold spasms. He uses a low vocal pitch and little inflection. His speech breathing is inappropriate; he initiates phonation at high lung volumes and inevitably holds his breath after inspiration. Palpation of the abdomen during speech reveals no distention during inspiration. There is no palpable laryngeal excursion during inspiration or speech. Examination with the transnasal flexible endoscope and stroboscopy demonstrates laryngeal bracing, anteroposterior supraglottal compression, and a long closed phase during phonation. During the hyperadducting voice breaks, the true vocal folds are adducted firmly, and the ventricular folds are also active. During diagnostic voice therapy, Allen speaks with vocal fluency when he uses a "nasal chanting" mode with vowel prolongation and while phonating simultaneous with pivotal jaw movements at a rate of one jaw drop per syllable. He also responds positively to the sensations associated with coordinated voice onsets during repetitive "Hm!" productions.

As is usually the case with spasmodic dysphonia, it is difficult to confirm a neurological component is contributing to Allen's spasmodic dysphonia. We speculate that the viral illness he suffered may have effected a change in his neurological system. The psychiatrist diagnoses a mild obsessive-compulsive disorder and some chronic anxiety responses. His tendency to blame himself for his voice problem and to employ a "feedforward" mechanism to ensure muscle misuse and dysphonia on the phone are inappropriate.

The etiological platform components that are most relevant during treatment planning for Allen are psychological and technical. We discuss all relevant and available treatment options and combinations. Allen is not keen on the idea of botulinum toxin injections at this time; he is still convinced he "poisoned" himself with drugs. He is very willing to deal with maladaptive psychological responses and demonstrates some insight

that is encouraging to the psychiatrist. Allen wants to participate in a voice therapy program. An intensive program is recommended, and luckily, he is pursuing treatment with the blessing of his boss, who tells Allen to do "whatever it takes." Allen will be able to take a full month of medical leave immediately, and an intensive therapy program can be initiated.

To best take advantage of motor learning principles, a program of simple physical drills is initiated to form the foundation of Allen's vocal responses. In association with relaxation and relevant postural adjustments, Allen is coached in drills for CVO, humming at a slightly higher pitch than is typical for him, and a syllable repetition task simultaneous with jaw movements. These are selected to reprogram speech responses at three levels: voice onset, resonance awareness, and the use of articulatory movements to free the larynx from supraglottal tension. Allen agrees to practice 5 hours daily and to refrain from speaking in his spasmodic dysphonia voice for the first 2 weeks, unless absolutely necessary. Allen quickly discovers that immediately following each practice session, he can produce simple utterances: "Hey!", "Sure!", "Fine", and even his name, using the CVO response rather than his SD behavior. The humming exercise becomes a technique for extending the CVO sensations into longer voice segments, and the jaw movement exercise provides a model for articulating while maintaining the sensation of abdominal control. After 2 weeks of intensive therapy, Allen can apply these principles in the controlled therapy environment to carry on a conversation with his clinician. He agrees to continue with intensive drills daily at the fundamental level.

Transfer of Allen's new repertoire vocal behaviors is planned carefully. He creates a graph of increasingly difficult communication situations to determine the order and timing of skill transfers. On the advice of his speech-language pathologist, Allen's boss agrees he will be permitted to return to work on a modified work assignment for 1 month, with fewer phone-contact hours. Allen works through the hierarchical plan methodically to apply his consciously controlled vocal technique in progressively more difficult communication situations. This is the most challenging part of the program for him. He returns to work, his technique slips whenever he becomes distracted or anxious, but he continues to work with the psychiatrist and *speech-language pathologist to refine his skill application. He discovers that he needs to practice his vocal techniques every morning, lunch break, and evening to maintain familiarity with the sensations he is trying to achieve in his "good" speaking style. He notes that if he skips a morning warm-up, his voice is "lousy" all day. The time required for warm-up seems to shorten, however, and after 6 months, Allen is confident that he is in the "driver's seat."*

4.6.3 Voice Therapy for Gender Dysphoria (Transsexual Voice)

The challenge facing gender dysphoria patients undergoing gender reassignment and their voice management team is a complex one. It generally is agreed that the most immediate voice problem relates to inappropriate pitch. Because the male larynx is larger than the female larynx (the membranous vocal folds are longer by a factor of 1.3 to 1.6)[41,84], the congenital gender of a male-to-female transsexual determines a low natural f_0. The gender-based laryngeal size discrepancy does not pose as great a problem for the female-to-male transsexual, because increased vocal fold mass is an expected result of the administration of male hormones[20,21]. Individuals undergoing male-to-female transitions represent the majority of patients consulting the voice clinic because administration of female hormones has no demonstrated effect of raising f_0.

The effect of f_0 on pitch perception is only one of several factors differentiating male from female voices. The average adult male vocal tract is considerably larger than that of women, but the size differences are not linear. For example, in addition to having longer vocal tracts, men have proportionally larger pharyngeal cavities[43]. Both size and shape differences contribute to formant frequencies which undoubtedly affect a listener's perception of "maleness" or "femaleness". Perceptual studies of gender identification support the notion that glottal source and vocal tract

filter functions both contribute to these judgements[18,19,75,89]. Voice source and vocal tract filter functions also contribute to voice quality differences between men and women that may affect gender identification judgments[18,44,54,62,74,89]. Breathiness in women's voices, the primary acoustic effect of phonation with posterior glottal chink, and short closed phase ratios also can be seen in the vocal tract filter function. Both f_0 and glottal posture may contribute to greater harmonic-formant interaction and less distinct formant frequencies in women[19,43].

Therapeutic strategies to feminize the speech of male-to-female transsexual patients must account for both glottal source and vocal tract adjustments. In addition, male-female differences in articulatory style, suprasegmental features, vocabulary, and pragmatics must be considered to optimize results. Of course nonlinguistic gestures may also facilitate feminine perceptions; these often develop vicariously.

Therapy activities for the transsexual patient include techniques to alter pitch and sometimes register use, unless a phonosurgical approach is planned as the primary treatment to change pitch. (Phonosurgical procedures for pitch elevation are discussed in Chapter 3, Section 3.4.8.) Individuals using a speaking f_0 range at or above 160 Hz are identified more often as female, other factors held constant[75,89]. In male-to-female transsexuals, however, mean f_0 may need to be targeted closer to 200 Hz for individuals to be identified as female in all communication situations[31]. Transgender speakers may need to compensate for larger vocal tracts by speaking above the typical f_0 critical range for female identification. Computerized visual feedback devices often are useful to assist patients in establishing and maintaining a higher f_0. When the patient's natural f_0 is very low, it may be necessary for her to use a falsetto register to achieve a speaking f_0 in the female range. This obviously is not as desirable as use of high modal register phonation, because of the limitations in intensity and timbre that are imposed by falsetto register, and extra care may be necessary to avoid excessive muscle misuse.

Most patients learn a breathy voice quality by imitating the therapist or another appropriate vocal model. If it is difficult to achieve, the laryngoscope may provide visual feedback of a glottal chink posture[62]. If the use of a breathy voice quality causes discomfort or palpable tension in extrinsic muscles, it may be abandoned in favor of a clearer tone with minimal muscle misuse.

Some patients may be able to adopt an altered laryngeal posture during speech, for example, an elevated larynx to shorten the resonance tract and raise formant frequencies. This maneuver may also effectively narrow the pharyngeal cavity, which is known to be larger in men. Biofeedback may be useful to establish these changes, including tactile monitoring of larynx position, visual monitoring with a mirror, or use of more sophisticated visual feedback equipment such as spectrograms that provide information about formant frequencies. Vocal tract length and formant frequencies may be affected by facial postures, for example, slight lip retraction may compliment an elevated larynx and further decrease vocal tract length. Any such postural adjustments should be monitored closely, and they should be pursued only if the therapist can incorporate hygienic muscle use so that discomfort and vocal misuse will not develop as a result of posturing changes.

Some attention should be focused on precision of articulation, which is greater in women[15,75]. Acoustic and visual feedback devices may be necessary to monitor this speech behavior change. Anecdotal reports have suggested that male-to-female transsexuals who have been living as women for some time tend to develop slightly forward articulatory postures. This style may be accompanied by a desired elevation of the larynx.

The therapy program may include work on intonation and stress patterns, which may influence impressions of maleness and

femaleness, in particular the tendency for women to have wider ranges of intonation and upward inflection at phrase endings has been demonstrated[10,65,83,88].

Vocabulary and syntactic changes may also provide cues to the intended gender (e.g., men tend to say "maybe", whereas women say "perhaps"). Use of modal verb constructions ("can," "will," "may," "shall," etc.) may feminize speech[15]. As with nonlinguistic gestures, this characteristic often is learned vicariously as individuals undergoing gender reassignment adjust to their changing roles.

Individuals with gender dysphoria are faced with ongoing physical, psychosocial, and economic stress. These factors greatly increase their susceptibility to muscle misuse. The voice use profiles of many transsexuals may reflect this susceptibility, so specific relaxation exercises need to be incorporated at all stages of the voice rehabilitation program. The voice-care team needs to remain sensitive to the lifestyle dynamics of these patients to determine treatment priorities. A voice therapy program demands considerable time and motivation and, in some cases, a large financial commitment. It therefore is critical that this portion of an individual's rehabilitation be timed appropriately so that he or she is not further distressed by unsuccessful treatment.

4.6.4 Communication Rehabilitation Following Laryngectomy

Individuals who undergo total laryngectomy (typically to treat laryngeal cancer) require an interdisciplinary approach to rehabilitation. Ideally, the team approach is adopted prior to surgery, when a patient is still able to express emotions and request information with the speech mechanism intact. Psychological counseling is an ongoing aspect of rehabilitation and often becomes part of the speech-language pathologist's role. Speech and voice rehabilitation may be expedited if the psychologist or psychiatrist can provide expertise to facilitate a patient's psychosocial adjustment postsurgically. Peer group support systems are also invaluable during the critical period of emotional healing.

Doyle has summarized the rehabilitation goal: "Rehabilitation following laryngectomy should be guided by one primary goal: to provide the patient with the greatest opportunity for returning to as normal a life as possible."[23] It is the primary responsibility of the speech-language pathologist to ensure that each patient has an adequate means of communication to express practical and emotional needs during the adjustment period. During the immediate postoperative period, writing on paper or a "magic slate" may be the most comfortable alternative. In some acute care settings, augmentative communication devices may be available to help the laryngectomee communicate with a computer-generated voice, a visual display or a typed hard-copy of basic requests. Ultimately, the speech-language pathologist endeavors to provide each individual with information and access to the most effective long-term method of communication. Currently, three primary methods of voice rehabilitation exist: artificial larynges, esophageal voice, and tracheoesophageal voice.

4.6.4.1 Artificial Larynx

Artificial larynges (AL) may be *electronic* or *pneumatic*. *Electronic* ALs may be *of neck-contact (cervical)* or *intraoral* variety. Cervical ALs are typically placed on the neck surface, and an electronically generated tone is transmitted to the vocal tract (Figure 4–8a). Articulatory movements provide the tone modification to make AL speech intelligible. The ideal placement of the cervical AL determines maximum transmission of sound into the vocal tract and minimal extraneous buzz. Because cervical ALs require contact with the neck surface, they are not typically introduced during the immediate postoperative period. Many cervical ALs are equipped with

intraoral adaptors so they can be used as intraoral mechanisms as well. Electronic intraoral larynges transmit the battery-generated tone to the vocal tract by means of a tube that is held in the mouth (Figure 4–8b). Appropriate placement of the tube is necessary to ensure optimal sound transmission and resonance, minimal interference with articulatory movements, and maximum intelligibility. Casper and Colton advocated introduction of the intraoral AL soon after surgery to maximize communication[17].

Traditional electronic ALs tend to be simple devices with limited options for pitch and loudness adjustment. Because the power source is electronic and no connection exists between pulmonary air and the oral cavity, speakers need to find a new way to generate airflow-dependent articulatory effects of plosion and aspiration. Typically, ingressive airflow techniques can be trained. Most speakers find they need to exaggerate articulatory dynamics to ensure maximum intelligibility when using electronic ALs. Training in AL placement, intelligibility, prosody and phrasing, and other tactics to improve communication effectiveness and speech naturalness are primary goals for therapy.

Pneumatic ALs were designed to use pulmonary air as the alaryngeal power source. This is achieved by placing a cuffed cup over the tracheostoma to receive exhaled air (Figure 4–8c). The stoma cup is attached to a housing unit that contains a potential vibrator; typically a reed or a rubber disc or band (Figure 4–8d). The tone generated is transmitted to the mouth by means of a rubber or plastic tube connected to the housing unit. Placement of the tube is typically in the buccal cavity. This affords good sound transmission with minimal articulation interference. Because they use the respiratory system in a way similar to laryngeal voice, pneumatic ALs offer the greatest potential for a natural speech product. The respiratory system is used for pitch and loudness changes in much the same way that it was preoperatively.

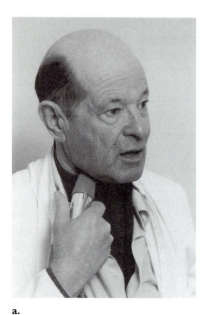

a.

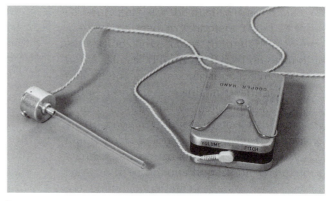

b.

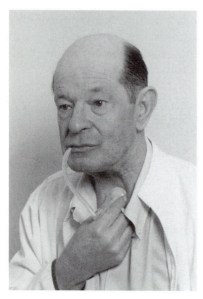

c.

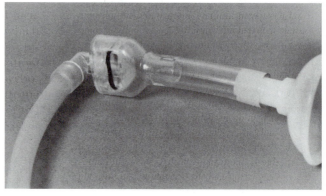

d.

Figure 4–8. Artificial larynges (AL); (**a**) cervical electronic AL, (**b**) intraoral electronic AL, (**c**) pneumatic intraoral AL, (**d**) vibrating apparatus (voice source) for pneumatic AL.

Initially, pneumatic ALs may require two-handed operation, to ensure proper placement of one end at the tracheostoma and the other end in the mouth. Because the stoma cup must be placed directly over the tracheostoma during speech, the pneumatic AL is not a viable alternative in the immediate postoperative period. Therapy goals include proper placement, appropriate phrasing, maximizing intelligibility, and effective use of suprasegmental aspects of speech that are possible with the pneumatic AL.

Regardless of the ultimate primary voice restoration method, a laryngectomy patient may benefit from introduction to and training in the use of an artificial larynx. Some individuals are willing to learn some alaryngeal speech skills preoperatively. Others become highly motivated soon after surgery and may become proficient in use of an intraoral artificial larynx within a few days. In this case, the frustration associated with inability to talk is minimized.

4.6.4.2 Esophageal Voice

Within the esophagus, the constrictor muscles of swallowing, including the cricopharyngeus muscle can provide a vibratory source for alaryngeal voice. One does not need to be a laryngectomee to have experienced the potential voice source in the esophagus; as air passes noisily from the stomach after a particularly rich meal or a carbonated drink, we are inadvertently producing esophageal voice. Systematic training to refine this vocal potential in the pharyngoesophageal (PE) segment of the aerodigestive tract has been a responsibility of the speech-language pathologist for many decades.

Traditional esophageal voice training involves identification and development of a method to reliably inject or inhale air into the esophagus, followed by release of the air to create a controlled tone that can be shaped by articulators into speech. Typically, the intraoral air pressure buildup from plosive and fricative consonant production is exploited to facilitate injection of air into the esophagus, followed by relaxation of the PE segment to create a vibratory source as the air is released upward.

The process of alaryngeal speech is a motor speech skill that requires considerable training and practice and takes up to 1 year to perfect[9,14,17,27,55]. Not all laryngectomees are successful in achieving an esophageal voice that allows for effective communication; estimates of success among laryngectomees in achieving functional esophageal voice range from 50% to 70%. Nevertheless, good esophageal speech has been achieved by many individuals under the patient and skilled direction of voice therapists and is a source of pride to the speaker and therapist. Since the development and refinement of tracheoesophageal puncture techniques for postlaryngectomy voice restoration, speech-language pathologists are called upon less frequently to direct programs in esophageal voice training.

4.6.4.3 Tracheoesophageal Voice

In the late 1970s two pioneers of laryngectomy rehabilitation introduced a method for restoring voice in laryngectomized patients[9,72]. The technique had two primary requirements:

1. a surgical procedure to create a fistula between the posterior wall of the trachea and the anterior wall of the esophagus—the *tracheoesophageal puncture* (TEP; Figure 4–9a), and

2. a small tracheoesophageal prosthesis (TEP) tube that could be placed into the fistula to keep it open, thus providing a channel for air to flow from the trachea to the potential esophageal voice source (the PE segment) while guarding against aspiration of food, fluid, and saliva from the esophagus into the trachea (Figure 4–9b).

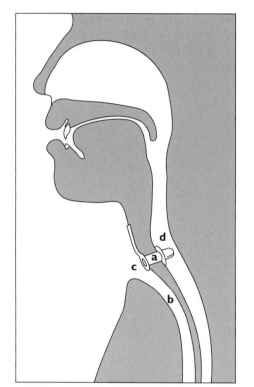

legend

a   TEP Prothesis
b   trachea
c   stoma
d   P-E segment
    (voice source)

a.

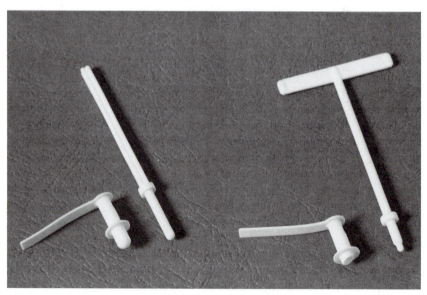

b.

Figure 4–9. Tracheoesophageal (TE) puncture and prosthesis; (**a**) sagittal section showing TE puncture site and prosthesis placement, (**b**) TE prosthesis with duckbill valve (left) and low-profile valve (right).

For many laryngectomees, the many months of traditional esophageal voice training can now be replaced by a few days of learning to refine their essentially instant tracheoesophageal voice. Tracheoesophageal voice restoration procedures and prostheses have evolved significantly since their introduction by Blom and Singer 2 decades ago, but this has become the primary vocal rehabilitation approach for laryngectomees. The majority of laryngectomees now can be offered a TEP option for voice restoration either at the time of their laryngectomy (primary TEP) or following recovery from the laryngectomy surgery (secondary TEP). For reasons related to tumor size or location or surgical complications, patients may not have the option of having a primary TEP procedure. Decisions about having a surgical procedure for secondary TEP voice restoration are based on the patient's desire, as well as certain criteria that best predict success for voice restoration. These criteria influencing patient selection for secondary TEP intervention are adapted from Blom and Singer[9,72] and Andrews et al[3]:

➤ Patient expresses motivation and mental stability to improve communication
➤ Patient demonstrates adequate self-care skills to maintain stoma and TEP hygiene: good eyesight, and manual and digital dexterity.
➤ Patient demonstrates realistic expectations regarding speech outcome
➤ Tracheostoma is not situated inferior to sternal notch and is not less than 2 cm diameter at its widest point
➤ Patient can phonate fluently during transnasal insufflation test: 8s /ɑ/; count to 10
➤ No medical contraindications to surgery or TEP method exist (eg, tracheoesophageal fistulas)
➤ No significant hypopharyngeal stenosis

The speech-language pathologist's role in voice rehabilitation with TEP includes:

➤ Determining the suitability of the patient for a TEP procedure in cooperation with the otolaryngologist, patient, and family
➤ Educating and counseling the patient and family on the nature of the procedure(s), care of the prosthesis and fistula site, and expectations and limitations for speech with TEP
➤ When TEP is a secondary procedure, administering an esophageal insufflation test to determine the prognosis for good voice (Figure 4–10); if results are equivocal

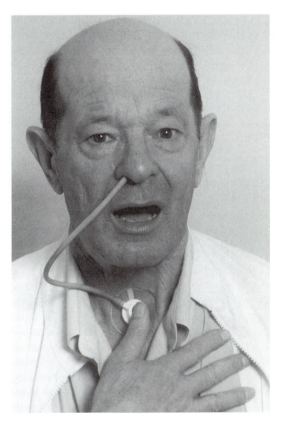

Figure 4–10. Transnasal insufflation test for preoperative evaluation of esophageal voice. The catheter is dropped to a level just below the pharyngoesophageal (PE) segment, and then air is forced into the esophagus. The PE segment should vibrate continuously as long as the driving force is sufficient. The test is used extensively before secondary TEP procedures. It also may be used to determine prognosis for traditional esophageal voice acquisition.

or negative, discussion with the surgeon may ensue to determine if further surgical procedures can be used to improve the prognosis

➤ Determining the appropriate size and type of prosthesis; fitting and placing the prosthesis

➤ Training the patient or family in replacing, cleaning, and maintaining the prosthesis and TEP site, as determined by the type of prosthesis (the role of the patient in maintenance of the prosthesis varies with prosthesis type)

➤ Assisting the patient to employ tracheostoma finger occlusion or a *tracheostoma valve* optimally to ensure expiratory air is directed through the prosthesis to allow the PE segment to vibrate (Figure 4–11)

➤ Training optimal breath control and effort to optimize phrasing, intonation, and other suprasegmental aspects of speech

➤ Monitoring changes in the TEP system: different prosthesis size and type requirements, prosthesis deterioration, troubleshooting other problems with speech, and prosthesis management

The reader is encouraged to seek detailed information about procedural aspects of voice restoration using the three primary alternatives in current literature, including references in the recommended reading at the end of this chapter. Special postgraduate training is sometimes necessary for speech-language pathologists to meet required competency levels to direct speech rehabilitation programs for laryngectomees.

4.6.4.4 Other Considerations in Laryngectomee Rehabilitation

Because the vocal intensity potential of esophageal voice and TEP voice may not meet the demands of some communication situations, full vocal rehabilitation may include acquisition and training in use of a vocal amplification system. The speech-language pathologist can help the esophageal speaker determine the need for this type of augmentative device and assist with selection and implementation of the appropriate system.

The emotional impact of a cancer diagnosis and subsequent laryngectomy is enormous. Laryngectomees will inevitably experience all the stages of grieving that are associated with loss of a loved one, a job, or a significant body function. The clinicians involved in laryngectomy rehabilitation need to be aware of these recovery characteristics to provide the appropriate support and to schedule therapy activities appropriately. A particularly poignant personal account of the emotional conflicts and adjustments required of a laryngectomee is referenced[33]. The events leading up to and following a laryngectomy procedure inevitably contribute to anxiety and depression, which

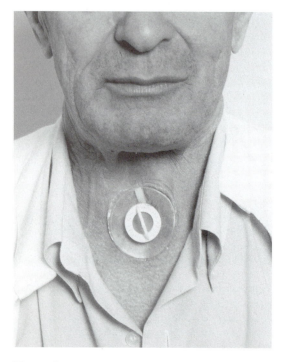

Figure 4–11. TEP speech using a tracheal stoma valve.

may translate into muscle tension. Muscle misuses may inhibit optimal development and application of alaryngeal voice, therefore initial therapy goals often are directed toward general and specific relaxation.

Whenever possible, family and friends are included in the communication rehabilitation program. This allows the team to provide support and education for the patient and family together. Communication partners are also trained to adapt to an alternative set of speech-voice-communication systems and to be effective listeners and communication facilitators.

Laryngectomees are typically middle-aged or older; the physiological changes associated with aging may need to be considered as therapy is planned. Factors such as hearing acuity, dentition, and general reduction in speech dynamics may all influence therapy goals and expectations. Other factors that should be considered when planning therapy with elderly persons are presented in Section 4.6.6.

4.6.5 Voice Therapy for Children: Special Considerations

Voice management for the pediatric population demands special consideration of the role that care-givers, educators, and peers play in influencing a child's behavior. Aspects of development, evaluation, and etiology of voice disorders in children are presented in detail in Chapter 6.

4.6.5.1 Cerebral Palsy

The child with **cerebral palsy** often is deprived of normal early-childhood cognitive and sensory experiences because of reduced mobility, and sensory deficits. In cases in which a child has a severe congenital disorder that impairs voice function, the speech language pathologist may provide counseling to parents and other caregivers

regarding the best ways to ensure that the child has access to experiences that are prerequisite to cognitive and linguistic development. If nonvocal communication is to be long term, then all appropriate augmentative and alternative methods should be explored to provide the most effective and efficient expression of the child's needs and thoughts.

A high incidence of voice problems has been documented in children with communication deficits related to disordered phonology-articulation, language, fluency, hearing, and structurally based resonance problems (eg, cleft palate)[7,14,51,69,77,78,87]. Intervention for the vocal dysfunction may be incorporated into a broader based therapy program, particularly in younger children, or may be addressed as a special aspect of the therapy program.

4.6.5.2 Hearing Impairment

Children who are **congenitally deaf** or **hard-of-hearing** are deprived of auditory input from their environment and appropriate feedback regarding their own vocalizations. In cases of severe hearing impairment, this typically results in a complex developmental communication profile. Delayed speech and language are common, and speech is typically characterized by inappropriate pitch, resonance, voice quality, and prosody, as well as abnormal phonological patterns. When hearing is augmented with cochlear implants or customized hearing aids, children have the best opportunity to monitor and modify abnormal voice features.

In Chapter 8, we describe speech-breathing differences that are commonly observed in individuals with hearing impairment. These include high levels of lung volume loss after inspiration and before onset of phonation, high lung volume expenditure during speech limbs, initiation of utterances at relatively low lung volumes, frequent termination of utterances below FRC, linguistically-inappropriate pauses for inspiration, and wide variability in lung-volume excursions across and within speaking tasks. Because speech-breathing forms the foundation for appropriate speaking patterns, preliminary therapy goals may focus on naturalizing speech-breathing patterns. Tactile and kinaesthetic feedback should be particularly useful in demonstrating inappropriate breathing tactics and providing models for more appropriate strategies. In some instances, visual feedback of airflow or flow volume levels or graphic representation of kinematic measures of speech-breathing patterns (using dedicated instrumentation as described in Chapter 8) may be useful.

Habitually high speaking pitches, low pitch variability, and exaggerated pitch variability have been reported in children with congenital hearing impairment[11,32,53,80,87]. These speech features are addressed by exposing children to other voice models, using optimal hearing augmentation, and by working directly on pitch with biofeedback instrumentation[13]. Analog or computer software instrumentation can be used to provide real-time visual feedback of f_0 and intonation contours. Tactile feedback may also be useful when the child attends to sensations of resonance associated with different pitch ranges or registers.

Another commonly reported voice characteristic in congenitally hard-of-hearing children is inappropriate resonance, sometimes termed "cul-de-sac," often in association with oral-nasal resonance imbalances (hypernasality or hyponasality)[11,52,87]. These are typically associated with a backed tongue posture, and inappropriate posturing of the velopharyngeal port during speech. Visual and kinaesthetic feedback may be useful in helping children alter tongue posture to a more forward position. If the suprahyoid muscles are hypertonic, tactile feedback may facilitate a more anterior tongue posture and relaxation.

The "tongue is a rug" image, in combination with direct visual monitoring, will provide a model for neutral tongue positioning at rest and during simple syllable repetition drills. Jaw relaxation and natural pivotal jaw movements may facilitate tongue relaxation and improve resonance. Relaxation of the base of tongue and jaw may allow for more appropriate palatal posture and more balanced oral-nasal resonance. Additionally, use of tactile feedback and of visual feedback with acoustic instrumentation that provides appropriate spectral information about nasality can assist children in adjusting resonance balance. When increased oral space and articulatory dynamics are used to treat hypernasality, palatometry may be used to provide feedback about articulatory targets and vocal tract postures (B. Bernhardt, personal communication). When hyponasality is the primary feature, humming exercises may be useful as they provide dramatic kinaesthetic feedback regarding resonance sensations in the face.

Finally, abnormal voice quality features, such as harshness, have been noted in children with hearing impairment, and these present a management challenge when auditory feedback is limited[87]. A combination of visual, kinaesthetic, and auditory feedback offer the best opportunity of altering vocal quality features. General and specific relaxation exercises also may effectively change voice quality by facilitating more appropriate vocal fold vibratory patterns.

4.6.5.3 Structural Deficits

Voice therapy may be required to assist children who use inappropriate strategies to compensate for structural deficits in the vocal tract, most commonly cleft palate[51]. When the glottis is being used as an articulator to compensate for inadequate valving at the velopharyngeal port, phonological intervention strategies may be the primary focus. In instances where compensatory muscle misuse results in dysphonia and secondary vocal fold lesions such as nodules, a comprehensive voice rehabilitation program, such as the one described earlier in this chapter and in the next case example, may be required.

Children with other **phonological-articulatory problems** may also develop compensatory strategies that cause muscle misuse in the larynx and consequent dysphonia. In some instances, the therapy activities for speech disorders may contribute to onset of a voice problem.

Case 4.6

Billy Ho is an 8-year-old second-generation Asian-Canadian, who has been referred to the voice clinic by his pediatrician under the recommendation of his parents and speech-language pathologist. Billy has been undergoing speech therapy since his early preschool years to expedite his phonological development. His parents first expressed concern to Billy's pediatrician about his "unclear" speech when he was approximately 3 years old. By that age, Billy's older brother had had "perfect" speech, but Billy seemed to his parents to be making many speech errors. They were especially aware that he used "l" or "w" for "r" and "th" for "s" when he spoke. (They had, as immigrants worked hard on their own speech to extinguish their Cantonese accents and English speech errors.) They eventually contracted a private speech-language pathologist to work with Billy, because the speech-language pathologist in the public health clinic felt his speech was within the normal range for his developmental stage and could not accommodate him on her caseload.

Billy has passed through his developmental milestones normally, according to his pediatrician, and is a healthy, exuberant young boy. He does fairly well in school, although his parents are concerned that he does not focus on academics as well as his older brother does. He loves sports and is often seen organizing a soccer game among his friends at recess. He comes across as a very "happy-go-lucky" fellow, and has a quick sense of humor. He speaks Cantonese and English with equal ease and has been enrolled in extracurricular French and Spanish classes because his family travels frequently. Recently, his teacher, speech-language pathologist, and family have noticed his voice is progressively hoarser and sometimes it "disappears" on a word or syllable. Billy has also noticed it, but says he is "not too worried"—he never liked choir anyway, and is often told to "mouthe the words;" pitch control has never been his forte. People also have noticed that Billy clears his throat frequently, even when he is not talking. His voice is hoarse in the morning. The speech-language pathologist based in Billy's school district has been continuing his articulation therapy because he still has an inconsistent "s" in speech.

During the assessment, we note a low-pitched, breathy voice with some aphonic breaks. Billy uses aggressive glottal attacks during voice onset. He is mildly hyponasal (his tonsils and adenoids are quite hypertrophic, but his nasal passages are clear). His pitch range is limited to five tones when he demonstrates a scale, but he produces a 2-octave continuous pitch range when he phonates simultaneously with a lip trill (which he thinks is hilarious). He initiates phonation at high lung volumes and uses a large portion of his vital capacity during speech limbs. His inspiratory speech-breathing pattern is characterized by no palpable abdominal distention. His jaw appears immobile during speech, and he wears a "perma-smile." His suprahyoid and thyrohyoid muscles are hypertonic at rest and during speech. His cricothyroid visor does not open during downward pitch glides. His cricopharyngeus muscle is also hypertonic, and the larynx cannot be moved laterally. On videolaryngostroboscopy, we note anteroposterior supraglottal compression, a large posterior glottal chink, and bilateral fleshy vocal fold nodules. His posterior larynx is moderately erythemic. His larynx rises during upward glissandos. A fairly consistent /θ/ ("th") for /s/ articulation pattern is noted. He demonstrates the therapy exercise he has been using over the past 2 years to make the proper /s/: "push your tongue up against that ridge behind your top teeth, smile, and blow hard" (try it yourself!). During a trial of facilitation techniques, we note Billy's vocal quality is clear during humming with "nasal buzz"; syllable repetition with loose mandibular movements (one jaw drop per syllable); coordinated voice onsets (Hm!); and lip trilling. When we ask Billy to talk about his recent summer vacation activities, he informs us about the 4-week summer camp he attended in a foreign country. Camp consisted of some outdoor activities judiciously scheduled around 5 hours daily of "speech, geology, math, and history." Asked how he felt about this type of vacation, Billy responded "I didn't really like it, but they had a good swimming pool." Billy likes using his voice to "organize" and encourage his friends during sports and finds it no problem to get a loud clear voice on the soccer field. His "soccer" voice is loud, clear, and remarkably free of muscle misuses.

A multifaceted treatment program is necessary to help Billy. His reflux is treated with typical lifestyle-modification measures, in particular skipping the bowl of cereal he has been eating before bed for the past few months, sleeping on a tilted bed, and cutting back on the cola drinks. The unrealistic expectations of Billy's parents for his academic and speech excellence need to be addressed, and this is undertaken initially by the psychiatrist, who finds Billy "remarkably well adjusted considering the pressure he is under to be the perfect child." His parents are asked to encourage Billy's diverse interests (compared with those of his academically inclined brother, who has decided at age 11 to be a corporate financial advisor) to widen his developmental and future professional potentials. The extracurricular activities focusing on "speech" (other language classes) are deferred for now.

The voice clinic speech-language pathologist confers with the clinician in Billy's school district to adjust his articulation therapy program, so that muscle misuses in his face, jaw, tongue, and abdomen are not reinforced by the "s" strategies. She admits she was not documenting much improvement in his speech and welcomes suggestions for new strategies. A technique that incorporates loose pivotal jaw movements and the "tongue is a rug" placement are explored (awsaw . . ., eesee . . ., oso . . ., oosoo . . .) and we find Billy can place his tongue appropriately more consistently when he actually thinks about relaxing it and letting his jaw do the work. During this exercise, he can also extinguish the "perma-smile" that

he wasn't even aware of wearing outside the therapy room and which contributed to jaw tension. Finally, during this exercise, Billy discovers his voice is clearer, and as he learns to apply the jaw movements to other speech sequences, he is able to maintain a clearer voice.

Despite his somewhat clearer voice, Billy continues to exhibit some postural and speech-breathing misuses that contribute to inappropriate laryngeal muscle use. Rather than expanding his speech therapy program, which he says causes him miss too much of his physical education class, the speech-language pathologist discusses a classroom-based "voice class" for Billy in his homeroom. Billy's teacher thinks this is a "grand" idea; she is willing to provide time for the clinician to direct the class twice a week; and maybe it will help her strained voice too. A series of exercises are presented, one set each class, to improve alignment; speech-breathing, and voice onset; relaxation and mobility in the articulators; resonance; intonation and phrasing. Voice class becomes a favorite subject because the students are permitted to move about, make goofy noises, and explore the effect of different voice styles on each other. From the exercises, a set of vocal warm-up exercises is selected to be used by the entire class each morning and afternoon, directed by the teacher. Billy excels in many of the exercises because he has learned about some of them during his speech therapy. By the time the class gets to "Martian-jaw speech," Billy is a pro, and his /s/ is becoming consistent enough that the daily voice warm-up sessions in class serve as his speech therapy practice. The teacher and class are all thrilled to learn how to shout without undue strain on their throats, and Billy is at the top of the class. They also learn that excessive shouting can make their throats sore and their voices hoarse; they explore alternative ways to get attention or their important points across. Billy's voice becomes clearer gradually as he gains confidence and skills, and it attracts less and less attention.

Voice therapy to remediate abusive vocal behaviors or muscle misuse voice disorders in children should involve cooperation of family, educators, peer, and friends as appropriate. In instances where vocally aggressive behavior (or conversely, reduced vocal dynamics) is an expression of a need for the child to gain control over his social or home environment, the origin of the psychosocial needs should be explored. In some cases, the community or school psychologist or psychiatrist may be included in evaluation and counseling of the child and family when a difficult psychosocial dynamic exists.

Direct therapy with children may be appropriate in cases where the family, educators, and other significant persons can attend treatment sessions to provide support and carryover. In general, for children under the age of 8 or 9 years or for the immature and dependent child, a home-based or school-based program (or both) that integrates new vocal behaviors into the child's everyday activities will be most successful. In such cases, the family (with or without the teacher) is trained to adopt the primary role as therapist. As such, the caregiver provides appropriate models for voice production, helps the child monitor his or her own behavior, participates in vocal games and exercises to reinforce good posture and vocal use, and supports the child's attempts to modify behavior. When behavior changes are required during activities with peers (such as sporting events or group discussions) the entire team may be educated and involved in appropriate voice use. In this situation, the important peer influence may become a supportive and integrated one, rather than a factor precipitating or perpetuating abusive vocal behavior. Further, peer involvement in an indirect voice therapy program relieves the stigma for the child with a voice disorder, and may provide vicarious learning of more effective communication skills for all participants.

Although anecdotal reports suggest that nodules regress spontaneously in boys after puberty, the muscle misuses that often accompany and may have been the primary cause of these lesions can persist into adulthood if not treated. Further, in some cases, the presence of a mild dysphonia may represent a variety of organic or psychosocial problems (or both), which require attention so as not to negatively affect communication development in the long term.

4.6.6 Voice Therapy for the Geriatric Population—Special Considerations

Age-related voice changes result from the expected physiological degenerative processes that are described in Chapter 8. Additional physiological or disease processes that may arise most commonly in geriatric years can complicate the picture. When a neurological, systemic, or structural disorder are dominant etiological factors contributing to a voice or speech problem, they should be addressed in the appropriate manner, while natural aging changes are also considered in therapy planning.

Therapy for voice disorders in the elderly frequently is focused on reducing the muscle misuses that accompany attempts to compensate for natural aging changes. The therapy program may be directed toward exploring the naturally higher pitch in the elderly man who is attempting to compensate for his atrophied vocal folds by pushing out a lower pitch that resembles what he has been accustomed to hearing. The postmenopausal woman may need help adapting to a naturally lower f_0 that results from mucosal thickening. Strategies to employ a more natural, if unfamiliar, pitch range may include specific relaxation exercises, optimizing speech-breathing and voice onset strategies, resonance enhancement, manual massage or manipulation techniques if laryngeal muscle misuse is inhibiting use of the appropriate pitch, and use of auditory or visual feedback devices to monitor and reproduce the target range. An important aspect of skill carryover to daily communication will be reassurance that the new voice is audible, intelligible, and socially acceptable. The therapist can facilitate development of this reassurance by inviting the patient's friends, relatives, or caregivers to therapy sessions to provide the appropriate feedback. It may also be helpful to accompany the patient to some typical communication settings to provide support and engage in troubleshooting for difficult situations.

Inadequate loudness may be a problem in elderly persons, particularly men who are experiencing glottal incompetence with senile vocal fold atrophy. Sometimes strategies that are adopted inadvertently to compensate for inadequate loudness are inappropriate and cause discomfort or more severe dysphonia. In these instances, techniques should be sought to reduce muscle misuse and optimize function. When indicated, forced glottal adduction exercises may be used in conjunction with optimizing breath support strategies, specific relaxation, and resonance enhancement to improve glottal closure. In cases of significant vocal fold atrophy, voice therapy may be an adjunct to surgical intervention to augment the vocal folds for better adduction. Vocal amplification systems can be introduced to provide the extra vocal power in elderly persons who do not improve sufficiently with surgery or therapy or who are not candidates for these treatment modalities.

Because compromised hearing acuity is often a reality in elderly persons, the speech-language pathologist may need to work closely with an audiologist to ensure that communication and therapy are optimized by providing the best auditory rehabilitation program possible. Often the communication partners of elderly persons are also elderly and hearing impaired. Whenever possible, elderly partners of voice clinic patients should be included in the therapy process so they can provide support and come to understand the role and responsibilities of the listener. Voice rehabilitation in the elderly some-

times is focused on learning strategies for effective communication, including achieving optimal hearing in a communication partner.

The aging process typically results in slower speech rates and reduced articulatory precision. Changes in the oral structures may result in poor or missing dentition and poorly fitting dentures. These factors may influence the types of therapy techniques that are employed and expectations for performance level during various stages of rehabilitation. If general physical or cognitive function is also deteriorating, therapy goals will necessarily need to be simpler, and more time may be required to reach specific goals. It is best to be honest and realistic when planning a voice program for elderly persons so they can enjoy the achievement of appropriate therapy goals without being unduly constrained by physical or cognitive limitations.

4.6.7 Principles and Voice Techniques for Treating Patients with Conversion Dysphonia/Aphonia

Conversion reaction voice disorders are relatively uncommon; however, appropriate diagnosis, timing, and selection of intervention strategies may be critical to ensure muscle misuses are not reinforced over a long period. A sample case is presented in Chapter 5 (Cases 5.1, 5.4 and 5.5). The primary approach in voice therapy for individuals suffering conversion dysphonias or aphonias may be symptomatic, particularly if symptoms are recent and precipitating psychological conflicts have resolved. The program is generally short term. In most cases, full restoration of voice is the goal for the first therapy session, followed by brief follow-up visits or telephone conversations.

If therapy is undertaken on the same day as the evaluation, supportive family members or friends who may have accompanied the patient to the clinic are encouraged to attend the therapy session in its entirety, assuming there are no obvious aspects of the relationship that would be detrimental to therapy progress (for example, and overly protective mother who has been reinforcing poor voice behavior). If therapy is scheduled for a subsequent day, the patient is requested to bring a supportive friend or family member. Following are typical goals and activities.

4.6.7.1 Education and Sound Introduction

The consulting physician and speech-language pathologist reassure the patient that no structural abnormalities or disease processes are present to account for the dysphonia. Most patients seek reassurance that no carcinoma or other life-threatening diseases are present. If an upper respiratory tract infection coincided with dysphonia onset, the patient often must be convinced that no residual signs are present to threaten voice recovery. Samples of the videolaryngostroboscopic exam are reviewed with the patient to reinforce the clinicians' reports and to demonstrate evidence of normal voice function, for example, during cough, sigh, or inhalation phonation.

The clinician describes relevant principles of normal phonation and the specific mechanisms of muscle misuse that result in the patient's dysphonia. The final common pathway, muscle misuse, is emphasized as the mechanism of dysfunction, *not* psychopathology.

The clinician describes and demonstrates mechanical adjustments that are necessary to produce normal phonation. If diagnostic therapy has not been undertaken yet to determine which techniques facilitate change most effectively, it is incorporated at this stage. The nature of the techniques selected, and explanation for their success depends on observations made during the diagnostic therapy probes. For a comprehensive list of techniques, see Section 1.9 in Chapter 1.

Examples of explanations to effect change include the following:

Problem: Vocal folds are hyperabducted (held open tightly).

Solution: Adduct (close) the vocal folds to phonate.

How? Cough, throat-clear, hum, push-pull, squeak at high pitch, use low-pitched glottal fry phonation, inhalation phonation, sigh, laugh, manipulate larynx, and so forth.

Problem: Vocal folds, ventricular folds, or both are hyperadducted.

Solution: Relax the vocal tract and vocal folds.

How? Yawn, sigh, breathy voice, inhalation phonation, alter target pitch, phonation with simultaneous head, shoulder or jaw movements, manipulate larynx, and so forth.

Problem: Vocal folds are inconsistently adducted.

Solution: Feel the sound consistently.

How? Use continuous voicing: prolong vowels, use phrases that have only voiced segments and palpate larynx during phonation to gain kinesthetic awareness of vibration and resonance.

When generalized muscle and postural misuse is present during phonation attempts, holistic and specific relaxation exercises, such as those described earlier in this chapter, may be introduced to increase success with voice restoration.

Once a facilitation exercise has been applied successfully to initiate phonation, the patient is encouraged to combine this technique with sound extension, typically on a vowel or nasal phoneme /m/. Tactile, auditory, and visual feedback devices may be used to provide information regarding phonation consistency. At this point, the clinician and support person provide reinforcement and encouragement generously. The first attempts at extending phonation may not represent the patient's normal phonation style, but he or she is reassured that a more natural style will develop, and tactics are introduced to shape the sound production.

4.6.7.2 Guidelines for Shaping Sound Extension

If the patient's dysphonic voice sounds too high pitched and squeaky, a glissando pitch change with continuous phonation may facilitate transition to a lower pitch. Alternatively, glottal fry register might be employed to experience lower pitched phonation, with maximum kinesthetic feedback from the larynx. When pitch or intensity of consistent glottal fry phonation are increased, a transition into modal register generally occurs.

If the patient's voice sounds too low pitched, phonation in falsetto register might be introduced to interrupt the misuse pattern. High-pitched phonation on /i/ *(ee)* or /u/ *(oo)* may be most successful. A siren imitation may ease the transition to a more appropriate pitch range. Also, exercises designed to increase oral resonance often facilitate a more natural pitch range. The CVO using spontaneous vocalizations (such as /hm/ or /m hm/) may provide a pitch reference that is more appropriate.

If the larynx tends to rise with phonation attempts, manual pressure or altered head position may be used to maintain an appropriate larynx posture. Tactile kinesthetic feedback is useful to help the patient gain control over phonation consistency. Light palpation on the thyroid lamina region, lips, cheeks, or nasal bone may provide the tactile feedback necessary for continuous phonation.

Once continuous relaxed phonation is achieved on a single sound in an appropriate pitch range, the clinician advises the patient that successful phonation techniques can be extended to all sound productions. Principles of articulation are discussed and simple relaxed tongue, jaw, lip, and velar movements are introduced to practice sound transitions during sustained phonation, for example,

extending a hum-to-vowel transition: /mama-mamamama/, /mimimimimimi/, /mememememe/, /momomomomomo/, /mumumu-mumumu/. Some patients will recognize the speech approximation and spontaneously apply phonation to conversational use at this point. Others may require further coaching and gradual approximations to recognizable speech. Transitional stages include multiple sound transitions on sustained phonation: /mamamimimama/, /nananunano/, /malamalama/, /namolunabe/. Voiceless phonemes may be introduced at a later stage, once consistent phonation is achieved on all voiced sequences: /mapadapala/, /nesila muta/. A few words and speech phrases may sneak into the sound sequences: /senotumi/ ("say no to me"). At this stage, distraction from the mechanics may be useful to allow for generalization of the phonation to speech. The support person may begin to recognize the speech phrases and react accordingly. Encouragement and praise again are offered generously to the patient, who is required to continue with phonation exercises until he or she is confident enough to apply them to spontaneous speech. Serial speech may be introduced as a further transitional stage (counting, reciting days of week, months of year, etc.). Responsibility to select and apply techniques is gradually transferred to the patient.

4.6.7.3 Putting the Voice to Work: Transferring Responsibility to the Patient

The patient, clinician, and support person engage in conversation to build the patient's confidence and to troubleshoot for potential problems. If inconsistency is noted, the patient is requested to select and apply a technique to facilitate a more appropriate phonation pattern and coached as required. Suggestions are made for ongoing practice, generally at the nonsense syllable or serial speech stage, to build confidence and reinforce appropriate motor patterns. The patient and support person are instructed to continue conversing at home throughout the day. The patient is reassured that the restored voice represents the most natural and efficient method of speaking, and for that reason, it will be easy to maintain. Further information is exchanged with the patient and support person at their request.

4.6.7.4 Follow-Up

A recheck phone conversation or office visit is scheduled for the following day, depending on the level of success achieved during the initial session. During follow-up phone calls, further office visits are scheduled as indicated by the patient's report and clinician's observations. The patient is encouraged to call immediately if any questions or concerns arise.

4.6.7.5 Prognostic Factors in Treatment of Psychogenic Dysphonias

The following questions need to be considered to establish treatment priorities and predict therapy outcome with voice therapy alone. In cases where negative prognostic factors are identified, voice therapy may need to be augmented with psychotherapy, pharmacotherapy, or surgical therapy (eg, botulinum toxin injections).

➤ Has the precipitating stressor or conflict been resolved? *(yes = positive prognosis)*
➤ How long has the dysphonia persisted? *(long duration = negative prognosis)*
➤ How consistent are the symptoms? *(consistent may or may not = negative prognosis)*
➤ Has the patient experienced unsuccessful treatment consultations before this one? *(yes = negative prognosis)*
➤ Was the patient prescribed voice rest for the current problem? *(yes = negative prognosis)*
➤ Is the patient self-assured that persistent somatic symptoms (muscle pain, globus pharyngeus, dysphonia) do not represent a serious or life-threatening medical problem such as cancer? *(yes = positive prognosis)*
➤ Is the patient receiving attention or reinforcement as a result of the dysphonia (secondary gain)? *(yes = negative prognosis)*
➤ Does the patient have confidence that you can help restore his or her voice today? *(yes = positive prognosis)*

4.6.7.6 Indications for Psychiatric Referral

During a voice evaluation or treatment program, several factors may indicate that psychiatric consultation or intervention is necessary to improve prognosis for voice therapy. These are outlined below.

During the Initial Evaluation
➤ Evidence in patient's history of psychiatric disorder
➤ Predisposing personality factors: narcissistic preoccupation with voice or perfect performance, inhibition of expression of assertiveness, inability to permit vocal crying, hypochondriacal traits, or a tendency to somatize psychological conflicts
➤ Coincidence of psychological stressors or 'event' and onset of dysphonia, when the conflict is not clearly resolved
➤ Psychological distress concomitant with physical illness that commonly affects the voice (e.g., flu)
➤ Patient consistently experiences anticipatory anxiety about voice production
➤ Cause and effect relationships are unclear (Figure 4–12)
➤ Patient requests a psychiatric referral

During the Voice Therapy Program
➤ Reduced patient motivation
➤ Inappropriate patient response to a demonstrated voice improvement
➤ Recurrence of dysphonia following an initial recovery

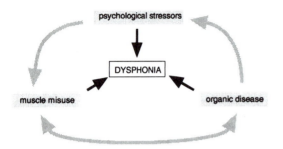

Figure 4–12. Interacting etiological factors in dysphonia symptom formation.

➤ Persistent signs of anxiety, depression, or psychological conflict
➤ Patient requests a psychiatry referral

4.6.8 Therapy for Adductor Breathing Disorders: Vocal Cord Dysfunction

The speech-language pathologist often is called upon to participate in treatment of individuals with respiratory vocal cord dysfunction (VCD). This disorder is characterized by adduction of the true vocal folds during inspiration, causing dyspnea (shortness of breath and associated symptoms). Muscle misuse voice disorders often accompany VCD. Choice of therapy techniques depends on aspects of the etiological profile that are known, other relevant treatments, and results of diagnostic therapy. Because psychological factors, reflux, and irritable larynx syndrome often are present, an interdisciplinary approach may be necessary.

In some cases, VCD is treated primarily with botox injections to weaken the vocal folds (see Chapter 3, Section 3.5.2). When this primary treatment is ongoing, the speech-language pathologist may focus treatment on optimizing vocal function in the presence of an induced laryngeal myasthenia. Techniques

that increase vocal intensity, clarity, and minimize air wastage during speech may predominate. A vocal amplification system may be necessary to augment voice use in difficult acoustic environments.

When behavioral therapy is the primary treatment modality, strategies are developed for general relaxation; specific relaxation of articulators, larynx, and pharynx; and positioning to minimize symptoms during a VCD attack. Frequent "sniffing" drills may be prescribed to maximize vocal fold abduction. Von Berg et al described a 4-step program that includes patient education, upper-body relaxation, oral-cavity breathing focus, and identification and reduction of precipitators[86]. Some individuals find the transnasal flexible endoscope useful to provide visual feedback regarding vocal fold positioning and associated kinaesthetic sensations. Because many individuals with VCD have developed inappropriate compensatory muscle misuses during speech and breathing (such as jaw jutting, abdominal clenching, and tongue retraction), they may benefit from a more comprehensive vocal rehabilitation program.

4.6.9 Therapy for Vocal Performers: Special Considerations

Professional singers, actors, comedians, broadcasters, and other vocal performers rely on their voices to earn income. Beyond the economic dependence on their voices, the identity of professional voice users often is heavily invested in their voices: "I'm a coloratura;" "I'm the voice of Mickey Mouse." The combined economic and emotional significance of the voice may contribute to a high incidence of hypochondriacal and narcissistic behaviors among professional voice users. The professional voice user typically must use his or her voice in extraordinary ways that are more physically demanding than speech and, if performed improperly, more harmful to the vocal system. Some vocal performers have had extensive training to prepare them for their voice use in performance venues, whereas others have had no formal training. Some may experience problems related primarily to performance voice use, others may have more generalized vocal misuse and abuse issues. Most professional voice users seeking treatment admit that, although they may apply learned techniques to performance voice use, they do not attend to technical issues during daily social or occupational talking.

A multidisciplinary approach to treatment of the professional voice user often is required, and may include the laryngologist, speech-language pathologist, psychiatrist, and a singing teacher or voice coach.

In the vocal performer, careful assessment at all four etiological platform levels is critical. When preventive or rehabilitative voice therapy is indicated, the program should address not only performance voice issues, but also the amount, type, and techniques of daily conversational voice use. Vocal performers often have other jobs that require talking; they tend to be socially exuberant individuals, and other psychological and lifestyle factors may lead them to overuse and abuse their bodies and their voices (Figure 4–13). A comprehensive vocal rehabilitation program as described earlier in this chapter is appropriate for all professional voice users. Group therapy offers the best arena for support, brainstorming, and motivation. When techniques for vocal performance are to be included in the voice therapy program, the clinician needs to be familiar with the performance style and conditions and have appropriate training in the particular pedagogical field. Most often the technical aspects of vocal performance are managed primarily by the singing or acting-voice teacher. Specific aspects of technique for vocal performance are provided in Chapter 7.

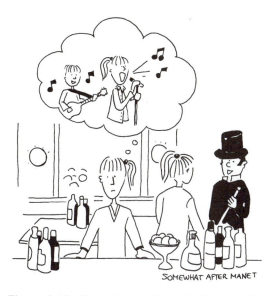

Figure 4–13. The aspiring professional voice user often is an occupational voice user. From *Vocalizing with Ease: A Self-Improvement Guide* (p. 28), by L. A. Rammage, 1996, Vancouver: Pacific Voice Clinic. Copyright 1996, by L. A. Rammage and M. Haijtink.

4.7 Monitoring Change In Voice Therapy Programs

Documentation of changes, anticipated or otherwise, is a critical part of the voice therapy program. The requirement by employing agencies, primary and secondary insurance programs, and professional certification programs for outcome measures is only one reason to document change. Patient and clinician can both benefit from the continuous monitoring of change in behaviors, symptoms, and instrumental measures. Regular documentation of perceptual-acoustic, acoustic, aerodynamic, stroboscopic, or other diagnostic data can guide the clinician in decisions about accelerating, decelerating, or modifying therapy activities and goals. Ongoing access to outcome measures can provide the patient with objective proof of progress and increase motivation. The legal benefit of outcome measurement cannot be understated. When a patient, employer, insurance company, or other interested party requires "proof" of therapy success (or lack thereof) a carefully-documented series of measures supports the clinician's professional opinion.

At the completion of therapy programs a comprehensive reevaluation of the voice is recommended. All the voice care professionals who participated in the pretreatment assessment should be included, and all relevant phonatory function measures should be repeated. Care should be taken to control for important confounding variables in each outcome measure that is to be compared with pretherapy data, for example, controlling for intensity and f_0 while making phonatory flow-rate measures. For phonatory function measures, formal data collection forms such as the Treatment Efficacy Response Form (TERF) are useful for documenting baseline and treatment response data. This can be compared against normative data over time by overlaying the appropriate graph on the patient's TERF chart (Figure 4–14)[45].

It is important to provide outcome measures that are patient based. Self-evaluation forms such as the Vocal Handicap Index (VHI) allow the patient to document changes in physical, functional and emotional impact of the voice disorder over time (see Appendix 1–1).

Unfortunately only a few well-designed therapy effectiveness studies are available to date to guide the speech-language pathologist in selecting and planning treatment. Clinicians are in the best position to provide relevant outcome measures to document effectiveness of specific therapy protocols for the voice-disordered population. The responsible clinician treats each patient with two intentions: to assist the individual in achieving the best voice function possible and to use each therapy experience to contribute to our understanding of the most efficient and effective means to reach this end.

4.8 Summary

Voice therapy programs are designed to improve, stabilize, or "normalize" voice function in individuals with a wide diversity of voice problems. Techniques employed may be symptomatic or holistic or may be incorporated into a comprehensive vocal rehabilitation program. In some instances, the etiological factors creating a voice problem may determine the type of therapy program and prognostic indicators. In other instances, therapy goals may be designed to address maladaptive compensatory behaviors, in particular, muscle misuses.

Because phonation is only one link in the speech chain, and voice problems often are associated with other speech, language, perceptual, or physical problems, many voice therapy programs may be incorporated into more global communication rehabilitation programs. In any case, the clinician planning a voice therapy program should consider the role of the voice in speech and language development and production, as well as its importance as an occupational or vocal performance tool and as a physical mechanism for the expression of emotions. In the next chapter, we will explore the relationships between voice and the psyche further and discuss principles for psychological treatment of voice disorders.

TREATMENT EFFICACY RESPONSE FORM

PATIENT: _____

DIAGNOSIS: _____

POST BASELINE TREATMENT: _____

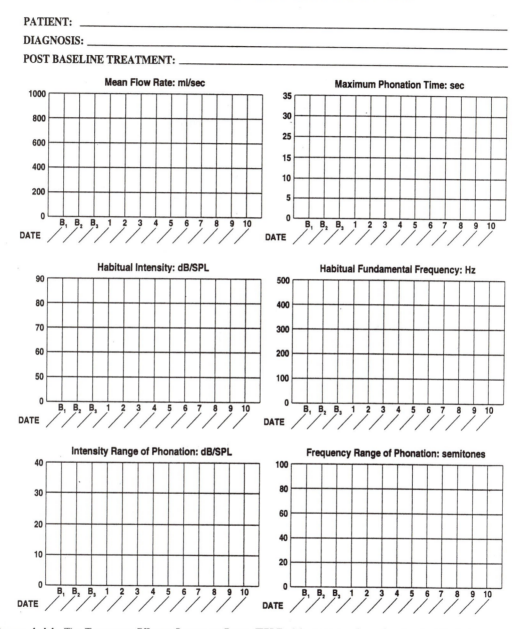

Figure 4–14. The Treatment Efficacy Response Form (TERF); (**a**) response form for six physiological measures of voice function, (**b**) normative chart for women, for comparison with TERF measures, (**c**) normative chart for men, for comparison with TERF measures, (**d**) normative chart for children, for comparison with TERF measures. From *Voice Care in the Medical Setting* (pp. 174–177), by D. L. Koschkee and L. A. Rammage, 1997, San Diego: Singular Publishing Group, Inc. Copyright 1997, by Singular Publishing Group, Inc. Reprinted with permission.

(continued)

Typical Values for Adult Females

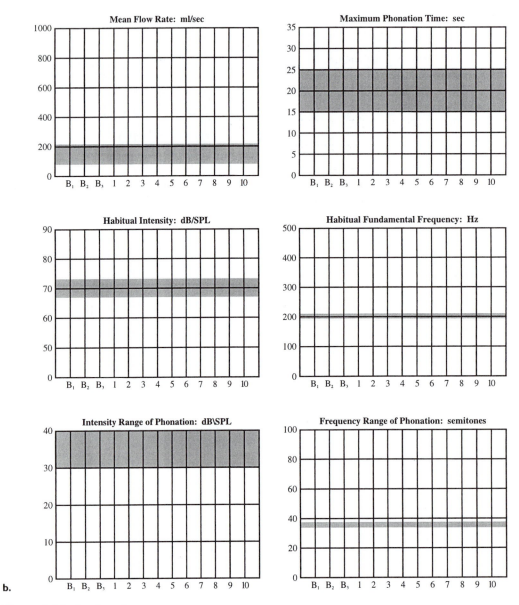

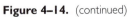

Figure 4–14. (continued)

Typical Values for Adult Males

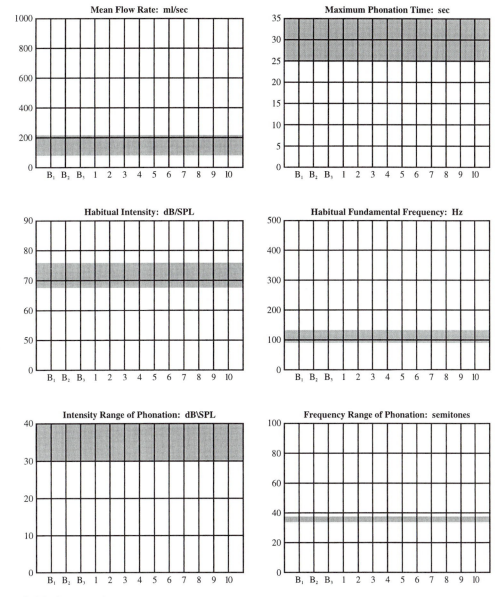

c.

Figure 4–14. (continued)

Typical Values for Children
(8-10 years)

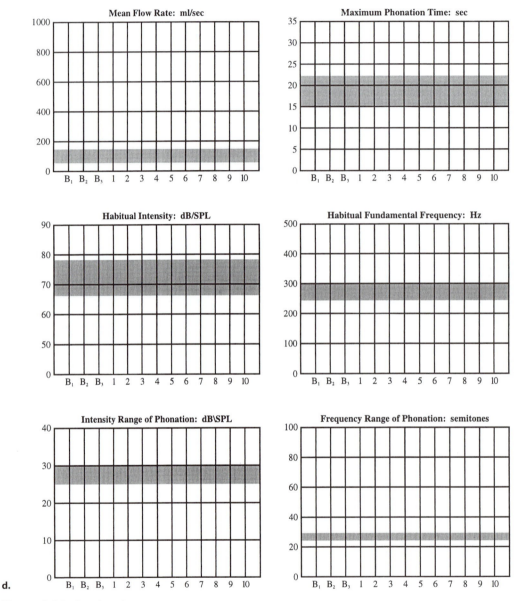

d.

Figure 4–14. (continued)

References

1. Adams, J. A. (1971). A closed-loop theory of motor learning. *Journal of Motor Behavior, 3*(2), 111–149.

2. Adams, J. A. (1987). Use of the model's knowledge of results to increase the observer's performance. *Journal of Human Movement Studies, 12,* 89–98.

3. Andrews, J. C., Mickel, R. A., Hanson, D. G., Monahan, G. P., & Ward, P. H. (1987). Major complications following tracheo-esophageal puncture for voice rehabilitation. *Laryngoscope, 97,* 562–567.

4. Aronson, A. E. (1985). *Clinical Voice Disorders An Interdisciplinary Approach,* (2nd ed.). New York: Thieme.

5. Barkmeier, J., & Verdolini-Marston, K. (1992, July). *Behavioral treatment for adductory spasmodic dysphonia.* Handout distributed at the Second Biennial Phonosurgery Symposium, Madison, WI.

6. Barlow, W. (1973). *The Alexander Technique.* New York: Warner Books.

7. Baumgartner, J. M., Ramig, L. A., & Kuehn, D. P. (1986). Voice disorders and stuttering in children. In T. J. Balkany, & N. R. T. Dashley (Eds.), *Clinical Pediatric Otolaryngology.* St. Louis: CV Mosby.

8. Belau, M., Machado, L., Guides, Z., Pontes, P. & Pontes, A. (1998). Using vocal fry to treat nasality problems. *Phonoscope, 1*(1), 4.

9. Blom, E. D., & Singer M. I. (1979). Surgical-prosthetic approaches for postlaryngectomy voice rehabilitation. In R. L. Keith, & F. C. Darley (Eds.), *Laryngectomee Rehabilitation.* Houston: College-Hill Press.

10. Boone, D. R. (1997). *Is Your Voice Telling on You?* (2nd Edition). San Diego: Singular Publishing Group, Inc.

11. Boone, D. R. (1966). Modification of the voices of deaf children. *Volta Review, 68,* 686–692.

12. Boone, D. R. (1993). *The Boone Voice Program for Children* (2nd Edition). Austin: Pro-Ed.

13. Boone, D. R., & McFarlane, S. C. (2000). *The Voice and Voice Therapy* (6th Edition). Boston: Allyn and Bacon.

14. Carlson, K. A. (1992, July). *Recognition of voice disorders in children.* Paper presented at the Phonosurgery Symposium, Madison, WI.

15. Case, J. (1996). *Clinical Management of Voice Disorders* (3rd Edition). Austin: Pro-Ed.

16. Casper, J. (1999). Voice therapy in the treatment of vocal fold stiffness and scar: A roundtable. *Phonoscope, 2*(3), 139–144.

17. Casper, J. K., & Colton, R. H. (1992). *Clinical Manual for Laryngectomy and Head and Neck Cancer Rehabilitation.* San Diego: Singular Publishing Group, Inc.

18. Coleman, R. O. (1976). A comparison of the contributions of two voice quality characteristics to the perception of maleness and femaleness in the voice. *Journal of Speech and Hearing Research, 19,* 168–180.

19. Coleman, R. O. (1971). Male and female voice quality and its relationship to vowel formant frequencies. *Journal of Speech and Hearing Research, 14,* 565–577.

20. Colton, R. H., & Casper, J. K. (1990). *Understanding Voice Problems: A Physiological Perspective for Diagnosis and Treatment.* Baltimore: Williams & Wilkins.

21. Colton, R. H., & Casper, J. K. (1996). *Understanding Voice Problems: A Physiological Perspective for Diagnosis and Treatment* (2nd Edition). Baltimore: Williams & Wilkins.

22. Dagenais, P. A., Southwood, M. H., & Lee, T. L. (1998). Rate reduction methods for improving speech intelligibility of dysarthric speakers with Parkinson's Disease. *Journal of Medical Speech-Language Pathology, 6*(3), 143–157.

23. Doyle, P. C. (1999). Postlaryngectomy speech rehabilitation: Contemporary considerations in clinical care. *Journal of Speech-Language Pathology and Audiology, 23*(3), 109–116.

24. Duffy, J. R. (1995). *Motor Speech Disorders—Substrates, Differential Diagnosis and Management.* St. Louis: Mosby.

25. Dworkin, J. P., & Culatta, R. A. (1996). *Dworkin-Culatta Oral Mechanism Examination and Treatment System (D-COME-T).* Nicholasville, KY: Edgewood Press, Inc.

26. Dworkin, J. P., & Meleca, R. J. (1999). Behavioral therapy for organic voice tremor. *Phonoscope, 2*(2), 113–119.

27. Edels, Y. (1983). *Laryngectomy: Diagnosis to Rehabilitation.* Rockville, MD: Aspens Systems.

28. Feldenkrais, M. (1949). *Body and Mature Behaviour.* New York: International University.

29. Froeschels, E. (1952). Chewing method as therapy. *Archives of Otolaryngology, LVI,* 427–434.

30. Froeschels, E. (1932). Uber eine neue Behandlingsmethode der stimmstorungen bei einseitiger Rekurrens lahmung. *Monatschr Ohrenhiekd, 66,* 1316–1320.

31. Gelfer Pausewang, M. (1999). Voice treatment for the Male-to-Female Transgendered Client. *American Journal of Speech-Language Pathology, 8,* 201–208.

32. Gilbert, H. R., & Campbell, M. I. (1980). Speaking fundamental frequency in three groups of hearing-impaired individuals. *Journal of Communication Disorders, 13,* 195–205.

33. Gunderson, S. (1999). Please listen to me. *Journal of Speech-Language Pathology and Audiology, 23*(3), 106–108.

34. Harris, T., Harris, S., Rubin, J. S., & Howard, D. M. (1998). *The Voice Clinic Handbook.* London: Whurr Publishers Ltd.

35. Hixon, T. J. et al. (1987). *Respiratory Function in Speech and Song.* Boston: College-Hill Press.

36. Howie, P., & Andrews, G. (1984). Treatment of adults stuttering: Managing fluency. In R. F. Curlee, & W. H. Perkins (Eds.), *Nature and Treatment of Stuttering: New Directions* (pp. 423–445). San Diego: College-Hill Press.

37. Iwarsson, J., & Sundberg, J. (1998). Effects of lung volume on vertical larynx position during phonation. *Journal of Voice, 12*(2), 159–165.

38. Iwarsson, J., Thomasson, M., & Sundberg, J. (1998). Effects of lung volume on the glottal voice source. *Journal of Voice, 12*(4), 424–433.

39. Izdebski, K., Ward, R. R., & Dedo, H. H. (1999). Voice therapy following surgical (or chemical) treatment for adductor spasmodic dysphonia. *Phonoscope, 2*(3), 149–158.

40. Jacobson, E. (1938). *Progressive Relaxation* (2nd Edition). Chicago: University of Chicago.

41. Kahane, J. C. (1983). Postnatal development and aging of the human larynx. *Seminars in Speech and Language, 4*(3), 189–203.

42. Keith R. L., & Darley F. L. (1979). *Laryngectomee Rehabilitation.* Houston: College-Hill Press.

43. Kent, R. D., & Read, C. (1992). *The Acoustic Analysis of Speech.* San Diego: Singular Publishing Group, Inc.

44. Klatt, D. H., & Klatt L. C. (1990). Analysis, synthesis and perception of voice quality variations among female and male talkers. *Journal of the Acoustical Society of America, 87*(2) 820–857.

45. Koschkee, D. L., & Rammage, L. (1997). *Voice Care in the Medical Setting.* San Diego: Singular Publishing Group, Inc.

46. Kotby, M. N., El-Sady, S. R., Basiouny, S. E., Abou-Rass, Y. A., & Hegazi, M. A. (1991). Efficacy of the accent method of voice therapy. *Journal of Voice, 5*(4), 316–320.

47. Lessac, A. (1973) *The Use and Training of the Human Voice.* New York: Drama Book Specialists.

48. Linklater, K. (1976). *Freeing the Natural Voice.* New York: Drama Book Specialists.

49. McFarlane, S. C., Holt-Romeo, T. L., Lavorato, A. S., & Warner, L. (1991). Unilateral vocal fold paralysis: Perceived vocal quality following three methods of treatment. *American Journal of Speech-Language Pathology, 1,* 45–48.

50. McFarlane, S. C., Watterson, T. L., Lewis, K., & Boone, D. R. (1998). Effect of voice therapy facilitation techniques on airflow in unilateral paralysis patients. *Phonoscope, 1*(3), 187–191.

51. McWilliams, B. J. (1969). Diagnostic implications of vocal fold nodules in children with cleft palate. *Laryngoscope, 79,* 2072–2080.

52. Monsen, R. B. (1976). Second formant transitions in speech of deaf and normal-hearing children. *Journal of Speech and Hearing Research, 19,* 279–289.

53. Monsen, R. B., Engebretson, A. M., & Vernula, N. R. (1979). Some effects of degrees on the generalization of voice. *Journal of the Acoustical Society of America, 66,* 1680–1690.

54. Nittrouer, S., McGowan, R. S., Milenkovic, P. H., & Beehler, D. (1990). Acoustic measurements of men's and women's voices: A study of context effects and covariation. *Journal of Speech and Hearing Research, 33* 761–765.

55. Prater, R. J., & Swift, R. W. (1984). *Manual of Voice Therapy.* Boston: Little Brown.

56. Ramig, L. O. (1995). Voice therapy for neurological disease. *Current Science,* ISSN 1068–9508.

57. Ramig, L. O. (1997). *Voice Treatment for Parkinson Disease and Other Neurological Disorders LSVT(SM)* . Rockville, MD: American Speech-Language Hearing Association.

58. Ramig, L. O., Bonitati, C. M., Lemke, J. H., & Horii, Y. (1994). Voice treatment for patients with Parkinson disease: Preliminary efficacy data. *Journal of Medical Speech-Language Pathology, 2*(3), 191–209.

59. Ramig, L. O., Countryman, S., Thompson, L. L., & Horii, Y. (1995). Comparison of two forms of intensive speech treatment for Parkinson disease. *Journal of Speech and Hearing Research, 38,* 1232–1251.

60. Ramig, L. O., Horii, Y., & Bonitati, C. (1991). The efficacy of voice therapy for patients with Parkinson's disease (pp. 61–86). *National Center for Voice and Speech Status Progress Report,* Iowa City: National Center for Voice and Speech.

61. Ramig, L. O., & Scherer, R. C. (1992). Speech therapy for neurologic disorders of the larynx. In A. Blitzer, M. F. Brin, & C. T. Sasaki, et al. (Eds.), *Neurologic Disorders of the Larynx* (pp.163–181). New York: Thieme Medical Publishers, Inc.

62. Rammage, L. A. (1992). *Acoustic, aerodynamic and vibratory characteristics of phonation with variable posterior glottis postures.* Doctoral dissertation, University of Wisconsin, Madison.

63. Rammage, L. A. (1996). *Vocalizing with Ease: A Self-Improvement Guide.* Vancouver: Pacific Voice Clinic.

64. Rammage, L. A., Morrison, M. D., & Nichol, H. (1986). *Muscular Tension Dysphonia* (videotape). New York: Voice Foundation.

65. Richards, D.M. (1975). *A comparative study of the intonation characteristics of young adult males and females.* Doctoral dissertation, Case Western Reserve University, Cleveland.

66. Schmidt, R. A. (1975). A schema theory of discrete motor skill learning. *Psychological Review, 82*(4), 225–260.

67. Schmidt, R. A. (1988). *Motor Control and Learning.* Champaign, IL: Human Kinetic Publishers.

68. Schneider, C. M., Dennehy, C. A., & Saxon, K. G. (1997). Exercise physiology principles applied to vocal performance: The improvement of postural alignment. *Journal of Voice, 11*(3), 332–337.

69. Shriberg, L. D., Kwiatkowski, J., Best, S., Hengst, J., & Terselic-Weber, B. (1986). Characteristics of children with phonological disorders of unknown origin. *Journal of Speech and Hearing Disorders, 51*(2), 140–160.

70. Shulman, S. (1989). *Spasmodic Dysphonia: Techniques and Approaches in Successful Voice Therapy.* Rockville, MD: American Speech-Language-Hearing Association.

71. Silverman, F. H. (1992). *Stuttering and Other Fluency Disorders.* Englewood Cliffs, NJ: Prentice-Hall.

72. Singer, M. I., & Blom, E. D. (1980). An endoscopic technique for restoration of voice after laryngectomy. *Annals of Otology, Rhinology and Laryngology, 89,* 529.

73. Smith, S., & Thyme, K. (1976). Statistic research on changes in speech due to pedagogic treatment (The Accent Method). *Folia Phoniatrica, 28,* 98–103.

74. Sodersten, M., & Lindestad, P-A. (1990). Glottal closure and perceived breathiness during phonation in normally speaking subjects. *Journal of Speech and Hearing Research, 33*(3), 601–611.

75. Spencer, L. E. (1988). Speech characteristics of male-to-female transsexuals: A perceptual and acoustic study. *Folia Phoniatrica, 40,* 31–42.

76. Spielberger, C. D., Gorsuch, R. L., Lushene, R., Vagg, P. R., & Jacobs, G. A. (1983). *The State-Trait Anxiety Inventory.* Palo Alto, CA: Consulting Psychologists Press, Inc.

77. St. Louis, K. I., Hansen, G., Buch, J., & Oliver, J. L. (1992). Voice deviations and coexisting communication disorders. *Language, Speech and Hearing Services in the Schools, 23*(1), 82–87.

78. St. Louis, K. I., & Hinzman, A. R. (1988). A descriptive study of speech, language and hearing characteristics of school-aged stutterers. *Journal of Fluency Disorders, 40,* 211–215

79. Stemple, J. C., Glaze, L. E., & Gerdeman, B. K. (1996). *Clinical Voice Pathology: Theory and Management.* San Diego: Singular Publishing Group, Inc.

80. Subtelny, J., Whitehead, R., & Klueck, E. (1989). Therapy to improve pitch in young adults with profound hearing loss. *Volta Review, 91,* 261–268.

81. Sundberg, J. (1999, May). *Breathing and phonation.* Presentation at the 4th International Care of the Professional and Occupational Voice Symposium, Canadian Voice Care Foundation, Banff, Alberta.

82. Sundberg, J., Leanderson, R., von Euler, C., & Knutsson, E. (1991). Influence of body posture and lung volume on subglottal pressure control during singing. *Journal of Voice, 5*(4), 283–291.

83. Terango, L. (1966). Pitch and duration characteristics of the oral reading of males on a masculinity-femininity dimension. *Journal of Speech and Hearing Research, 9*, 590–595.

84. Titze, I. R. (1989). Physiologic and acoustic differences between male and female voices. *Journal of the Acoustic Society of America, 85*, 1699–1707.

85. Titze, I. R. (1994). *Principles of Voice Production.* Englewood Cliffs, NJ: Prentice-Hall, Inc.

86. Von Berg, S., Watterson, T. L., & Fudge, L. A. (1999). Behavioural management of paradoxical vocal fold movement. *Phonoscope, 2*(3), 145–147.

87. Wirz, S. (1992). The voice of the deaf. In M. Fawcus (Ed.), *Voice Disorders and Their Management* (2nd Edition, pp. 283–303). San Diego: Singular Publishing Group, Inc.

88. Wolfe, V. I., Ratusnik, D. L., Smith, F. H., & Northrup, G. (1990). Intonation and fundamental frequency in male-to-female transsexuals. *Journal of Speech and Hearing Disorders, 55*, 43–50.

89. Wollitzer, L. (1994). *Acoustic and perceptual cues to gender identification: A study of transsexual voice and speech characteristics.* Master's Thesis, University of British Columbia, Vancouver, British Columbia, Canada.

Recommended Reading

Andrews, M. L. (1991). *Voice Therapy for Children: The Elementary School Years.* San Diego: Singular Publishing Group, Inc.

Andrews, M. L. (1991). *Voice Therapy for Adolescents.* San Diego: Singular Publishing Group, Inc.

Blom, E. D., Singer, M. I., & Hamaker, R. C. (1998). *Tracheoesophageal Voice Restoration Following Total Laryngectomy.* San Diego: Singular Publishing Group, Inc.

Boone, D. R. (1993). *The Boone Voice Program for Children* (2nd Edition). Austin: Pro-Ed.

Boone, D. R., & McFarlane, S. C. (2000). *The Voice and Voice Therapy* (6th Edition). Boston: Allyn and Bacon.

Casper, J. K., & Colton, R. H. (1992). *Clinical Manual for Laryngectomy and Head and Neck Cancer Rehabilitation.* San Diego: Singular Publishing Group, Inc.

Doyle, P. C. (1994). *Foundations of Voice and Speech Rehabilitation Following Laryngeal Cancer.* San Diego: Singular Publishing Group, Inc.

Duffy, J. R. (1995). *Motor Speech Disorders—Substrates, Differential Diagnosis and Management.* St. Louis: Mosby.

Dworkin, J. P., & Culatta, R. A. (1996). *Dworkin-Culatta Oral Mechanism Examination and Treatment System (D-COME-T).* Nicholasville, KY: Edgewood Press, Inc.

Edels, Y. (1983). *Laryngectomy: Diagnosis to Rehabilitation.* Rockville, MD: Aspens Systems.

Fawcus, M. (1992). *Voice Disorders and their Management.* San Diego: Singular Publishing Group, Inc.

Gunderson, S. (1999). Please listen to me. *Journal of Speech-Language Pathology and Audiology, 23*(3), 106–108.

Harris, D. (1998). Singing and therapy. In T. Harris, S. Harris, J. S. Rubin, & D. M. Howard (eds.), *The Voice Clinic Handbook* (pp. 207–245). London: Whurr Publishers Ltd.

Harris, S. (1998). Speech therapy for dysphonia. In T. Harris, S. Harris, J. S. Rubin, & D. M. Howard (eds.), *The Voice Clinic Handbook* (pp. 139–206). London: Whurr Publishers Ltd.

Journal of Voice (1987 -). San Diego: Singular Publishing Group, Inc.

Koschkee, D. L., & Rammage, L. (1997). *Voice Care in the Medical Setting.* San Diego: Singular Publishing Group, Inc.

Lieberman, J. (1998). Principles and techniques of manual therapy: Applications in the management of dysphonia. In T. Harris, S. Harris, J. S. Rubin, & D. M. Howard (eds.), *The Voice Clinic Handbook* (pp. 91–138). London: Whurr Publishers.

Ramig, L. O. (1997). *Voice Treatment for Parkinson Disease and Other Neurological Disorders LSVT*$_{(SM)}$ Rockville, MD: American Speech-Language Hearing Association.

Rammage, L. A. (1996). *Vocalizing with Ease: A Self-Improvement Guide.* Vancouver: Pacific Voice Clinic.

CHAPTER

5

Psychological Managment of the Patient with a Voice Disorder

5.1 Introduction

The function of voice is principally to communicate with other people. It thus is seen to have a major social component that serves to disperse feelings of psychological isolation. To speak, one requires an organic apparatus capable of producing sound, a psychological intent to communicate, and a social context in which one feels the desire to talk (because most people do not talk much to themselves; they think instead). Voice production, therefore, clearly rests on the outcome of the interaction of factors that can be conceptualized as being at organic, psychological, and social levels. These assertions are obvious and hardly warrant mention. What does require emphasis is the principle underlying all our work in the voice clinic. Namely, that human beings are complex unitary organisms constituted so that their functioning is the outcome of the constant interplay of thoughts, emotions, and actions, the last being mediated by the voluntary musculature.

An individual's voice is a sensitive indicator of emotions, attitudes, and role assumptions. It therefore is not surprising that impairments of voice function are not uncommon accompaniments of psychological conflicts. Nonetheless,

the factors producing a dysphonic voice are a complex mixture of organic and psychological features occurring in a social context. A relatively minor organic problem may trigger muscle misuse and a voice problem that is primarily of psychological origin. This is particularly likely to happen if another organic predisposing condition exists, such as reflux esophagitis and acid laryngitis. Similarly, psychologically and socially induced vocal misuse may lead to a secondary laryngeal organic problem, such as polypoidal degeneration. For example, the hoarseness associated with an early cancer of the vocal fold may be due as much to the anxiety engendered ventricular band dysphonia as to the malignancy itself. Interestingly, when the carcinoma is resolved after radiation, the dysphonia of psychological origin that was causing most of the hoarseness may also be improved; however, this dysphonia may persist and lead to continuing concern about the tumor still being present. A conscious individual cannot fail to have a psychological response to a real or suspected organic illness. The frequently expressed apprehension of anxious dysphonic patients that their hoarseness arises from cancer illustrates this all too clearly. In cases such as this, it is easy to see that the assessment and management of patients with voice disorders has confronted clinicians with their limitations. Both the absence of more objective and standardized assessment tools and procedures and the failure of professionals to use uniform diagnostic terminology have complicated our understanding of the problem as well as its treatment.

A thought that engenders an emotion of joy, anxiety, sadness or anger induces an impulse to action, which requires the use of voluntary musculature. If an individual perceives the social context to be one that permits expression of the emotionally charged idea without negative consequences, then that ends the matter; the activity is performed. If, however, the individual feels obliged to inhibit overt expression of the emotionally charged idea, then the tonus of those muscles that would have been used to express it is typically increased, with normal tonus and posture being restored over time. Should the individual experience repeated episodes of inhibition of the impulse to cry or to speak angrily, which are the emotional expressions most commonly deemed to be unacceptable, then the muscles of phonation and respiration will have been primed for the advent of dysphonia. Thus, we are confronted with the obligation to disentangle the organic, psychological, and social factors occasioning a dysphonia.

5.2 Brief Review of the Literature

Let us go back in time to Shakespeare to consider Hamlet's assertion: "Tears in his eyes, distraction in's aspect, a broken voice". Even in Shakespeare's time we see recognition of a connection between emotionally laden ideas and voice disorders. For more than a century, aphonia and dysphonia have long been associated with the psychiatric disorder of hysteria[22].

Although voice disorders commonly are seen in general medical practice[24], there are few epidemiologic data on their incidence and prevalence. Dysphonias afflict individuals of all ages, women more often than men[10,19]. Although no predominant predisposing personality types have been found to be linked to the general symptom of dysphonia, earlier literature tended to emphasize the association with hysterical personality[5], whereas more recent studies have described a number of patients with voice disorders as introverted[15].

There is widespread belief in the close association between personality traits and voice characteristics. Experimental confirmation has been found that the voice conveys correct information concerning characteristics of personality[3]. The same study showed, however, that there is not uniformity in the expression of personality through voice; rather, many features of many personalities can be determined from voice characteristics. The personality trait of dominance and the voice characteristics of loudness, resonance, and lowered pitch were found to be associated; submission, by contrast, was not[31]. This study supported the hypothesis that certain personality traits and certain voice characteristics may have developed together as reactions to situations involving social communication. One thinks of the modeling that parents provide for their children—not only vocal but also emotional and postural. The association of personal characteristics and emotion with the suprasegmental properties of speech (including pitch, loudness, and temporal features) has been demonstrated[11,20,27,32,33]. The complexity of the effect of emotion on voice is easily recognized when one accepts that the human voice simultaneously conveys semantic content, momentary emotional states, and the more enduring characteristics of the speaker, all modified by the social context in which the communication is taking place[14]. It has long been recognized that certain disorders are adversely affected by the repression of certain conflicting ideas and their accompanying affects[1].

Theories of emotion abound, but this publication is not the place for a detailed review of them. It is worth noting, however, that in a major publication on human emotions[23], there is no mention of the voice as a transmitter of emotion, whereas a substantial emphasis is given to facial expression as the supreme center of sending and receiving social signals. Each emotion is deemed to have an inherently adaptive function based on a specific and innately determined neural substrate, a characteristic facial expression, or neuromuscular expressive pattern, and a distinct subjective quality.

What is true for the face as an organ of emotional and social expression is also true for the voice. Just as an individual's attitudes are entrenched in characteristic facial expressions and generalized body posture, as Alexander long ago made clear[2,8,9,16], so will the muscles of phonation be programmed either to express emotions or to suppress them if giving vent to them would be too anxiety provoking. This last point introduces the usefulness of the concept of **state dependent memory, learning, and behavior**. This is a state in which specific muscle misuses become entrenched by significant psychological events that arouse emotions and an impulse to action, but the action is inhibited by anxiety. The state later can be reactivated by the individual perceiving any feature of the earlier event, often outside the individual's full awareness[42,43]. To avoid awareness of such anxiety-provoking stimuli, whether from the environment or from within, individuals heighten their recognition threshold, thereby defending themselves from the perception, which is then kept out of conscious awareness[12]. We see what it is safe to see and feel what we can permit ourselves to feel without distress.

The role of the voluntary muscle system is of particular interest to those seeking to help patients with voice disorders, yet most of the psychiatric literature makes no mention of the role played by musculature in controlling unacceptable thoughts and emotions[18] and those who do have made no reference to voice disorders[30,40]. In the treatment of voice disorders, however, particular emphasis has been

given to manipulation of the muscles of phonation[29]. Clinicians and many patients acknowledge motor and sensory manifestations of inappropriate levels of muscular effort during speech. For example, awareness of the somatic sensations of effortless breathing is of vital importance to an individual's well-being[6]. This is especially true for patients with muscle misuse voice disorders, who may be well aware that the level of effort in their speech-breathing muscles is inappropriate.

Suppression of awareness of emotionally charged cues has been recognized in patients who have difficulty distinguishing between emotions, giving verbal expression to them, and recognizing that some physical sensations are indeed manifestations of emotions. In addition, they have a limited fantasy life, tending to direct their attention to external reality, such as their physical ailments, with little reference to their inner emotional experience. These individuals are deemed to have **alexithymia** and frequently are burdened with psychosomatic disorders[25,26,28,47,48]. Given that the voice is a principal means of conveying emotion in a social context, it is no surprise that a number of dysthymic (chronically depressed) patients who are resistant to the idea that their voice problems have psychological and emotional components also display alexithymic features. This makes the treatment of their voice disorders much more difficult to conduct[36].

Dysphonia may, and often does, present in individuals who are free of clinical psychiatric disorder[17]. A study confirming our own findings of this showed that two-thirds of patients evaluated for dysphonia of psychogenic origin did not receive a formal psychiatric diagnosis[19]. A common finding is that dysphonic patients have a minor psychiatric disturbance[49] and the suggestion of traitlike vulnerability[44]. Where psychiatric disorders are recognized, they include major depression and dysthymic disorders, adjustment disorders with depression or anxiety, generalized anxiety disorder, conversion and phobic disorders, posttraumatic stress disorder, and personality-trait difficulties. Only occasionally is dysphonia due to a schizophrenic disorder.

5.3 Indications for Referral for Psychiatric Consultation

The recognition by the voice clinic team that a patient has a psychiatric disorder should prompt referral when the patient is not already seeing a psychiatrist. In a number of incidences, evidence of formal psychiatric disorder is not forthcoming. Rather, personality factors that may predispose the patient to dysphonia are evident. These vary considerably and include a narcissistic preoccupation with voice, preoccupation with perfect performance, and a tendency to somatize psychological conflicts[45]. In addition, a number of patients show a marked inhibition in the expression of emotions: assertiveness, let alone the overt expression of anger, may be restrained; whereas other patients reveal an inability to permit themselves to cry. A hypochondriacal trait should not go unrecognized.

In taking the history from the patient, it is important to note any psychological stressors that were impinging on the individual at the time of the onset of the disorder. This is particularly relevant when psychological distress in the patient occurred concomitantly with a physical illness affecting the voice. Once a dysphonia has been present for a while, a carefully taken history often will reveal that the patient experiences anticipatory anxiety about voice production, typified in such statements as: "When the phone rings, I just know my voice will be bad." In each of these cases, the patient's attitude can lead to perpetuation of the dysphonia, which may require assistance of a psychiatrist for its resolution (Figure 5–1).

During the course of voice therapy, it may become evident to the speech-language pathologist that expected outcomes are not being realized. When there are no structural or neuro-

logic explanations for a lack of progress in therapy, psychological factors should be considered. Indications for psychiatric referral during the course of voice therapy are discussed in Chapter 4 and represented in case examples below.

The approach to the evaluation and treatment of the patient with a voice disorder advocated in this text clearly requires the close collaboration of the otolaryngologist, speech-language pathologist, and psychiatrist. The context in which we work has made this possible for our patients. In Canada, universal medical care has eliminated all financial barriers to access to treatment. Impediments remain, however, to the implementation of a satisfactory treatment plan. Speech-language pathologists and psychiatrists familiar with the management of voice disorders are in short supply, and their distribution is such that many patients from smaller communities do not have ready access to them. Another factor often encountered is the attitude of a number of patients. Having been relieved of the fear that they may have cancer, a substantial proportion of them show little motivation to carry out the exercises prescribed by the speech-language pathologist or to clarify and resolve the psychological factors sustaining their dysphonia.

5.4 Types of Pathogenesis Observed in Dysphonia of Psychological Origin

Tensional symptoms arise from overactivity of the autonomic and voluntary nervous systems in individuals who are unduly aroused and anxious. This leads to voluntary muscle misuse, usually with generalized muscle hypertonicity. Specifically, hypertonicity of the intrinsic and extrinsic muscles of the larynx cause muscle misuse voice problems; at times these are associated with psychiatric disorders such as adjustment disor-

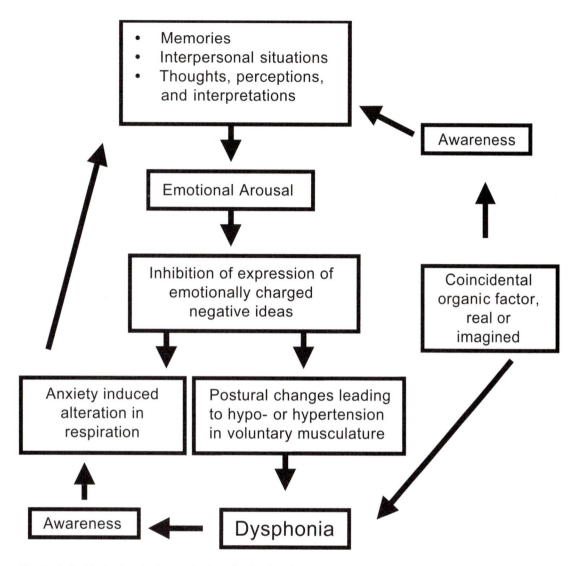

Figure 5–1. Mechanisms in the production of voice disorders.

ders and anxiety disorders or with personality trait disturbances.

Symbolic symptoms occur when a somatic symptom involving the sensory or voluntary motor nervous system is unconsciously substituted for a psychological conflict. This is the conversion disorder referred to so frequently in the psychiatric literature. It gives rise to aphonia or dysphonia when the muscles involved are those of phonation. Some recent work suggests the involvement of conscious mechanisms in the production of conversion symptoms[21]. This should come as no surprise to voice clinicians who have seen a substantial improvement in voice when the patient with conversion dysphonia is distracted, only to have a deterioration occur when the patient is again focused on the voice problem.

Increasingly, practitioners are recognizing that the concept of psychological conflicts and pathologic effects as a model of pathogenesis is not valid in patients with psychosomatic disorders[38]. Rather, many of these individuals burdened with **alexithymic features** have substantial difficulty in recognizing, describing, and expressing their feelings. This apparent intellectual deficit, coupled with an inability to relate thought, feeling, and the impulse to action leads them to present puzzling physical symptoms[26], one of which is dysphonia.

Hypochondriacal symptoms, or the self-fulfilling anticipation of poor voice production, occur in those who are unduly aware of, or responsive to, sensations arising from a particular portion of their anatomy—in the case of those with dysphonias, usually their mouth, throat, and respiratory system. The associated psychiatric diagnoses often are personality-trait disturbances involving obsessive-compulsive and dependent features, as well as hypochondriacal ones.

Depressive equivalent symptoms may arise in those individuals who are not complaining overtly of depressive symptomatology but are suppressing the impulse to cry or to express anger verbally. Adjustment, dysthymic, and affective disorders of the depressive type are the psychiatric diagnoses found in these cases.

A single patient may show symptoms of several categories, such as those of symbolic, tensional, or hypochondriacal origin, at any particular time[34]. One type of pathogenesis may reinforce another; for example, there may be a hypochondriacal exaggeration of a tensional symptom. It is relevant to note these differing types of pathogenesis because the treatment of the individual symptoms may need to be different. Finally, organic and psychogenic processes frequently are combined and obviously require differing therapeutic approaches[46].

The factors producing a dysphonic voice often are a complex mixture of organic, psychological, and social features, any one of which may be predisposing, precipitating, or perpetuating agents. Several case examples of this are provided at various points in this text.

5.5 Function of Psychogenic Dysphonia

The function of the symptom of psychogenic dysphonia may vary substantially from patient to patient, and these differences must be understood to direct therapy appropriately. The term **primary gain** refers to the reduction of anxiety, tension, and conflict that is provided by the production of a symptom of psychogenic origin, such as a dysphonia, through the employment of various defense mechanisms such as regression, repression, denial, reaction formation, and isolation of affect. Psychogenic dysphonia, although unpleasant in itself, constitutes for the patient a lesser evil than the personal problems from which it arose. This is exemplified in the following case.

Case 5.1

Delores, a middle-aged woman, had a respiratory tract infection that produced dysphonia while she was awaiting triple-bypass cardiac surgery. Delores was very apprehensive about the upcoming surgery. The infection resolved, but her dysphonia persisted even after her operation, which she did not believe had been as successful as her cardiologist asserted. Her husband kept saying to her: "It is better to have a hoarse voice to worry about, rather than a bad heart," thereby helping to perpetuate the symptoms. At the clinic, Delores was seen jointly by the otolaryngologist, the speech-language pathologist, and the psychiatrist. In the presence of all three professionals the otolaryngologist showed and discussed with her the videotape of her structurally normal larynx. A sample of her voice was audiotaped, after which she was interviewed by the psychiatrist, during which her doubts about her heart operation, as well as her reluctance to stand up to her domineering husband, were recognized. "As I get older, it bothers me more that he is the decision maker. I'd like to have my voice back, but it would only lead to more arguments." Delores was encouraged to retrieve her voice and to take the risk. The psychiatrist met with the speech-language pathologist to pass on his findings before voice therapy was started. The husband was advised to change his behavior.

Secondary gain is the benefit derived by the individual from the external environment when others perceive his or her evident distress; this may take the form of monetary compensation, increased attention or sympathy, and the satisfaction of dependency needs. These secondary gains may serve to reinforce the patient's disorder and perpetuate its persistence.

Sociologists have emphasized that an individual's assumption of the **sick role** and display of **invalid behavior** may convey many valuable privileges. Invalids may not only be exempted from normal social obligations, they also may be freed from their responsibilities. Society requires individuals to seek appropriate treatment for their disability so that they exercise the privileges of the sick role for as brief a time as possible. Failure to do this is perceived correctly as the employment of the symptom for secondary gain. The next two cases provide examples of secondary gain derived from a voice disorder.

Case 5.2

Kenneth was a schoolteacher with an obsessively perfectionist personality trait, coupled with a paranoid attitude. He was having problems in his marriage. During this difficult time, he was confronted by an extremely defiant group of young adolescents whom he described as "that class of destroyers trying to get me." He would lose his

voice for 5 to15 minutes when he raised it to try to restore order in the classroom; his failure to succeed in doing so increased feelings of depression. Before attending the clinic, Kenneth had been placed on long-term disability leave, which would support him on full salary until he reached retirement age. He was reluctant to accept speech therapy, to take medication, or to engage in psychotherapy.

In appraising our patients and their response to treatment, it is necessary to differentiate the extent to which the symptom of dysphonia has primary or secondary gain attributes because this will influence the manner in which treatment needs to be directed. It is often necessary to alter the behavior of those in the patient's immediate social network to diminish the rewards conferred by the assumption of the sick role; this frequently is not easy to do.

Case 5.3

Bobby, a 14-year-old high school student, was referred to the voice clinic because of episodes of aphonia, which had led to his refusal to go to school; his mother had accepted this behavior. It emerged that he was his mother's only child and had never known his father. He had been brought up in the house of his maternal grandparents with his grandmother as his principal caregiver; she had been extremely indulgent of his every wish so that the description of him as a spoiled child was accurate. When his mother moved several hundred miles away with her son to be the housekeeper for a relative, the indulgent atmosphere to which Bobby had been accustomed was lost in a household where other children also received consideration. On examination, it became evident that Bobby was deliberately producing the dysphonia. At times, he would refuse to respond at all, merely glaring at members of the voice clinic team. Nothing in the history obtained from the mother or in the examination of Bobby suggested the presence of a formal psychiatric disorder. He made it clear that his voice would undoubtedly return the moment he went back to live with his grandmother, which his mother adamantly opposed. The grandparents were convinced that Bobby was physically ill and would not drive him and his mother several miles to the clinic for his speech therapy and psychiatric follow-up interview. The mother said she could not bring herself to take the bus to bring Bobby to the clinic. He returned to his distant small town to the care of his family physician, who had neither a speech-language pathologist nor a psychiatrist to assist him in the resolution of Bobby's condition.

In many patients referred to a voice clinic, the dysphonia has been present for a long time. This often leads to difficulty in determining the precise etiologic factors in dysphonias of psychological origin. Not only do patients tend to forget some of the important anxiety-laden events surrounding the onset of their dysphonia, but the natural psychological adaptive mechanisms lead to the resolution of these conflicts with the passage of time. The voice clinicians are faced with the difficult situation of being unable to elicit the hard facts indicative of psychological conflicts, which would enable them to make a positive psychiatric diagnosis. At the time of the consultation, the patient will seem relatively free of psychological conflict while still burdened with the dysphonia, the latter being the residue of the muscle misuse which arose during the earlier time of acute psychological conflicts.

The habitual pattern of muscle misuse, irrespective of pathogenesis of the symptom, often persists in situations where the psychological conflicts seemed to have receded[13]. This situation strongly suggests that voice disorders should be evaluated as soon as possible after their onset for one to be able to identify the psychological etiologic factors. Providing therapy is also much more effective at this earlier time. It cannot be emphasised too strongly that, in the absence of organic structural change in the organs of phonation, the muscles of phonation are the final common path of all dysphonias of psychogenic origin, and the voice problem will certainly persist if the misuse is not remedied.

As mentioned in Chapters 1 and 2, facial expressions give clues to underlying emotional states (Figure 1–22). Long-standing failure to give expression to feelings of sadness or anger result in postural changes which, in some individuals, serve to perpetuate dysphonia. Conversely, it is not surprising that the abreaction of the suppressed emotion results in a return of normal muscle tonus because the previous hypertonicity or hypotonicity no longer are needed to restrain overt expression of the feeling; marked improvement in voice often is noted subsequently. The next two cases illustrate this.

Case 5.4

William was a 55-year-old accountant. His weak, hoarse voice had responded quite well during voice therapy sessions, but the improvement was not sustained. He was a reserved man who had spoken little about himself in the initial assessment by the otolaryngologist and the speech-language pathologist. William demonstrated many postural misuses that could be altered during therapy, but he could not sustain the improvements. He was referred to the psychiatrist because of the lack of progress in his voice therapy. During the psychiatric interview, it emerged that William had been obliged to leave the small country town where he had lived because of the behavior of his ex-wife, which could only be described as paranoid. Besides telephoning his employers, she had portrayed him to his three children in such terms that they had refused to speak to him. He thought that he dared not express directly to her any of the considerable anger he felt for fear of the inevitable repercussions. In addition, he had reluctantly accepted his children's rejection of him without defending himself, as he felt their mother needed whatever support they were willing to give her. On reviewing these topics in subsequent sessions, the quality of William's voice fluctuated considerably. He was encouraged to write what he would like to have said to his ex-wife but dared not. In the privacy of his car parked on remote beaches, he was encouraged to say angrily, even to shout, his views. This he did conscientiously. There was steady improvement in the strength and quality of his voice. The gains he subsequently made in voice therapy carried over into everyday use. Finally, he agreed to write and telephone his children to reestablish contact; his pent up feelings were further relieved when two of the three responded favorably.

When medical and laryngeal examination have established the absence of organic pathology affecting the vocal folds and the patient has received appropriate voice therapy, failure to improve should lead to a consultation between the otolaryngologist and the speech-language pathologist, the outcome of which might be reexamination by the former or consultation with an interested psychiatrist. A further illustration is provided in the next case.

Case 5.5

Lance, a 50-year-old man who had developed baker's asthma necessitating the sale of his business, was referred to the psychiatrist by the speech-language pathologist. She was treating him to reduce his persistent falsetto phonation; no improvement had resulted despite their diligent efforts. The psychiatrist was involved in the review by the otolaryngologist and speech-language pathologist and then interviewed Lance. With great reluctance and over lengthy interviews, this stalwart individual added to the sparse history he had been willing to provide earlier. Not only was he being bankrupted by the failure of the purchaser of his bakery to pay him, but also the Workers' Compensation Board refused to recognize that his asthma was work related. While he and his wife were contemplating the sale of their hard-won home, the middle of his three teenaged daughters had run away from school and home with a drug pusher. Lance had not told his wife of his apprehension that his chest pains were due to heart disease. At this point the "stiff Scottish upper lip" and determined smile gave way to muffled sobs; he was thoroughly ashamed of this unmanly behavior. Further questioning established the presence of a masked depressive disor-

der, the treatment of which led to the resolution of the dysphonia. The return of his daughter, the improvement of his financial affairs, and the absence of heart disease all played their part.

A patient's negative reaction to detectable improvement in voice or detection of undue anxiety in a patient during voice therapy are further indications for a psychiatric referral, revealing as they do conflicting attitudes in the patient. Consider the following case:

Case 5.6

One such case was that of Sally, 27-year-old school teacher who had dysphonia of the spasmodic disorder type. During voice therapy sessions, there would be substantial improvement in her voice, to which she responded by complaining that her throat hurt and she was not being helped at all. Paradoxically, she was most reluctant to end the sessions. With some difficulty, she was persuaded to accept psychiatric consultation. During the interview Sally was most defensive, denying any psychological disability and emphasizing that her family could not accept the idea of her seeing a psychiatrist. It emerged that she was an extremely dependent young woman, whose dysphonia had been precipitated by the principal of her school mocking her ethnic background and failing to praise her work despite the many opportunities she gave him to do so. She proved to be an extremely difficult case to manage psychiatrically. Consultations between the otolaryngologist, the speech-language pathologist, and the psychiatrist were gloomy affairs. Sally dismissed the psychiatrist on several occasions, neglected do her voice therapy exercises, and demanded that the otolaryngologist find some organic explanation for her disability. Although she did become more independent and less demanding in her general functioning and there was some improvement in her voice, it was only when she was given botulinum toxin injections that substantial improvement occurred.

In adults free of dysphonia, the production of the spoken word has become an automatic activity. The brain has been programmed to produce appropriate speech without the individual having to give specific thought as to how muscles are used to accomplish it. Similarly, a person skilled in riding a bicycle does not particularly think about what he or she is doing, but simply rides. Once an individual becomes aware of having a dysphonic voice, whether of organic or psychogenic etiology, the stage is set for him or her to interfere with the previously automated voice production. The likely consequence of this awareness is a perpetuation of the voice problem when speech is involved, but not during singing or spontaneous vocalizations in many cases[21]. The following exercise has helped patients understand their reactions and persuaded them to stop listening anxiously to the way in which they are speaking, so as to reduce their anticipatory anxiety and improve voice function.

The following instructions are given: *Run up carpeted stairs as quickly as possible; then come down and repeat the operation. On the second trial, think carefully about placing each foot as precisely and quickly as possible on each tread of the stairs.* Patients will discover that this is difficult to do, that their speed of ascent is slowed and that they might even stumble forward (hence the injunction to do the activity up carpeted stairs!). Those patients who are willing to learn from the exercise feel somewhat liberated from the bonds of dysphonia and are more readily able to diminish their anticipatory anxiety about speaking, thereby reducing inappropriate muscle and postural misuse. Voice production is improved when they are able to distract their attention from the voice while speaking.

5.6 Preparation of the Patient for Psychiatric Referral

As we are all only too aware, a number of patients regard the referral to a psychiatrist as tantamount to being offered an insult. That

being the case, it is important that the otolaryngologist or speech-language pathologist should prepare the patient carefully for the referral. He or she should portray the psychiatrist as a colleague interested in voice disorders and should refer to a close working relationship between them. A psychiatrist can be portrayed as more skilled in evaluating whether or not psychological factors are contributing to the voice disorder. Where appropriate, the patient can be assured that he or she is not seen as having a definitive psychiatric disorder. It is worthwhile to explain to the patient the role of precipitating psychological factors, muscle tension, and anticipatory anxiety in the production of dysphonia. The interaction and additive effects of organic and psychological factors also should be reviewed as a part of the preparation.

5.7 The Psychiatric Consultant

The dysphonic patient is more likely to be helped if the attributes and interests of the consulting psychiatrist include some, if not all, of the following:[39]

There should be a willingness to engage in active dialogue with the patient to establish a therapeutic alliance, rather than the maintenance of a rather silent and distant interviewing style. The psychoanalytical approach exemplified in the latter is particularly disconcerting to patients with voice disorders, who usually have more than enough embarrassment about their speech for it to be emphasized by silence. Several patients whom we have seen at the voice clinic left previous psychiatric treatment for this reason.

Willingness to become familiar with the physical findings on laryngoscopy, which requires a close working relationship with the otolaryngologist, is highly desirable. This is frequently helpful in diminishing any reluctance the patient has to communicate freely with the psychiatrist. This reluctance also is lessened if the psychiatrist works closely with the speech-language pathologist providing treatment[4,7]. In taking the history, it is particularly important for the psychiatrist to focus on each episode of voice dysfunction that the patient has experienced and the context in which it occurred; this is important in itself but it also facilitates rapport.

Competence in the use of hypnotic suggestion is also of value in a number of cases of dysphonias[35,37,41]. A proper understanding of the misuse of voluntary musculature in patients with psychological conflicts enables the psychiatrist to collaborate more readily with both the speech-language pathologist and the otolaryngologist[2,8,9,13]. Regrettably, psychiatrists with these attributes are relatively rare.

It is reasonable to expect that the psychiatrist will understand the terminology used by the laryngologist and the speech-language pathologist, with both of whom he or she will collaborate closely. Further, the psychiatrist should provide relevant consultation findings and focus his or her work with the patient seeking to improve the voice disorder. Many of those psychiatrists who have psychoanalysis as their theoretical basis hold to the belief that removal of a symptom such as aphonia or dysphonia will inevitably lead to the manifestation of another symptom unless major work in conflict resolution is undertaken. This has not been our experience, nor has it been found by those who work with behavior therapy. Where ongoing psychoactive medication or psychotherapy is required, it is to be expected that the voice clinic psychiatrist will provide this in addition to the initial consultation.

5.8 Summary

Human beings are unitary organisms in whom thought, feeling, the impulse to action, and the action itself are bound together. We are all of a piece, not separate minds and bodies. The final common path of all the variables that impinge on voice production is the voluntary musculature. Addressing voice disorders with this frame of reference has been found to help substantially in diminishing the tendency of some patients to dismiss the significance of psychological factors. This is particularly so when the frame of reference for muscle misuse is explicitly declared to patients and when they are made aware that the psychiatrist is familiar with the physical status of their larynx. In addition, it serves to enhance their cooperation in both psychotherapy and voice therapy.

References

1. Alexander, F. (1950). *Psychosomatic Medicine.* New York: Norton & Co., Inc.
2. Alexander, F. M. (1932). *The Use of the Self.* London: Methuen & Co., Ltd.
3. Allport, G. W., & Cantril, H. (1934). Judging personality from voice. *Journal of Social Psychology, 5,* 37–55.
4. Andersson, K., & Schalen, L. (1998). Etiology and treatment of psychogenic voice disorder: Results of a follow-up study of thirty patients. *Journal of Voice, 12,* 96–106.
5. Aronson, A. E., Peterson, H.W., & Litin, E. M. (1966). Psychiatric symptomatology in functional dysphonia and aphonia. *Journal of Speech and Hearing Disorders, 31,* 115–127.
6. Bakal, R. (1999). *Minding the Body. Clinical Uses of Somatic Awareness* (p.188). London: The Guilford Press.
7. Baker, J. (1998). Psychogenic dysphonia: Peeling back the layers. *Journal of Voice, 12,* 527–535.
8. Barlow, W. (1973). *The Alexander Principle.* London: Victor Gollancz.
9. Barlow, W. (1978). Anxiety and muscle tension. In W. Barlow (Ed.), *More Talk of Alexander* (pp. 109–126). London: Victor Gollancz.
10. Bridger, M. W. M., & Epstein, R. (1983). Functional voice disorders. A series of 109 patients. *Journal of Laryngology and Otology, 97,* 1145–1148.

11. Costanzo, F. S., Markel, N. N., & Costanzo, P. R. (1969). Voice quality profile and perceived emotion. *Journal of Counselling and Psychology, 16,* 267–270.

12. Eriksen, C. W. (1965). Perceptual defence. In *Psychopathology of Perception, Proceedings of the 53rd Annual Meeting of the American Psychopathological Association.* New York: Grune and Stratton.

13. Feldenkrais, M. (1949). *Body and Mature Behaviour.* New York: International University.

14. Friedhoff, A. J., Alpert, M., & Kurtzberg, R. L. (1962). An effect of emotion on voice. *Nature, 193,* 357–358.

15. Gerritsma, E. J. (1991). An investigation into some personality characteristics of patients with psychogenic aphonia and dysphonia. *Folia Phoniatrica, 43,* 13–20.

16. Gray, J. (1991). *Your Guide to the Alexander Technique.* London: Victor Gollancz.

17. Guze, S. B., & Brown, D. L. (1962). Psychiatric disease and functional dysphonia and aphonia. *Archives of Otolaryngology, 76,* 96–99.

18. House, A., & Andrews, H. B. (1987). The psychiatric and sound characteristics of patients with functional dysphonia. *Journal of Psychosomatic Research, 31,* 483–490.

19. Horowitz, T. (1979). *States of Mind* (p. 76). New York: Plenum Medical Book Company.

20. Hunt, R. G., & Lin, T. K. (1967). Accuracy of judgements of personal attributes from speech. *Journal of Personal and Social Psychology, 6,* 450–453.

21. Hurwitz, T. A. (1989). Ideogenic neurological deficits. Conscious mechanisms in conversion symptoms. *Neuropsychiatry, Neuropsychology and Behavioral Neurology, 1,* 301–308.

22. Ingals, E. F. (1890). Hysterical aphonia. *Journal of the American Medical Association, XV,* 92–95.

23. Izard, C. E. (1977). *Human Emotions.* New York: Plenum Press.

24. Johnson, A. F., Jacobson, B. H., & Benninger, M. S. (1990). Management of voice disorders. *Henry Ford Hospital Medical Journal, 38,* 44–47.

25. Kinzl, J., Bierl, W., & Rauchegger, H. (1988). Functional aphonia. A conversion symptom as a defensive mechanism against anxiety. *Psychotherapy and Psychosomatics, 49,* 31–36.

26. Kooiman, C. G. (1998). The status of alexithymia as a risk factor in medically unexplained physical symptoms. *Comprehensive Psychiatry, 39,* 152–159.

27. Kramer, E. (1963). Judgement of personal characteristics and emotions from nonverbal properties of speech. *Psychology Bulletin, 60,* 408–420.

28. Lane, R. D., Sechrest, L., Reidel, R., Weldon, V., Kaszniah, A., & Schwartz, G. E. (1996). Impaired verbal and nonverbal emotion recognition in alexithymia. *Psychosomatic Medicine, 58,* 203–210.

29. Lieberman, J. (1998). Principles and techniques of manual therapy: Applications in the management of dysphonia. In T. Harris, S. Harris, J. S. Ruben, & D. M. Howard (Eds.), *The Voice Clinic Handbook* (pp. 91–138). London: Whurr Publishers Ltd.

30. Lowen, A. (1967). *The Betrayal of the Body.* London: The Macmillan Company.

31. Mallory, E. B., & Miller, V. R. (1958). A possible basis for the association of voice characteristics and personality traits. *Speech Monographs, XXV,* 255–260.

32. Marxel, N. N., Meisels, M., & Houck, J. E. (1964). Judging personality from voice quality. *Journal of Abnormal and Social Psychology, 69,* 458–463.

33. Markel, N. N. (1969). Relationship between voice-quality profiles and MMPI profiles in psychiatric patients. *Journal of Abnormal Psychology, 74,* 61–66.

34. Matas, M. (1991). Psychogenic voice disorders: Literature review and case report. *Canadian Journal of Psychiatry, 36,* 363–365.

35. McCue, E. C., & McCue, P. A. (1988). Hypnosis in the elucidation of hysterical aphonia: A case report. *American Journal of Clinical Hypnosis, 30,* 178–182.

36. McHugh-Munier, C., Scherer, K. R., Lehmann, W., & Scherer, U. (1997). Coping strategies, personality and voice quality in patients with vocal fold nodules and polyps. *Journal of Voice, 11,* 452–461.

37. Morsley, I. A. (1982). Hypnosis and self-hypnosis in the treatment of psychogenic dysphonia: A case report. *American Journal of Clinical Hypnosis, 24,* 277–283.

38. Nemiah, J. C. (1996). Alexithymia; Present, Past—and Future? *Psychosomatic Medicine, 58,* 217–218.

39. Nichol, H., Morrison, M. D., & Rammage, L. A. (1993). Interdisciplinary approach to functional voice disorders: The psychiatrist's role. *Otolaryngology-Head and Neck Surgery, 108,* 643–647.

40. Reich, W. (1949). *Character Analysis, Edition 3.* New York: Orgone Institute Press.

41. Rosen, D. C., & Sataloff, R. T. (1997). *Psychology of Voice Disorders* (p.151). San Diego: Singular Publishing Group, Inc.

42. Rossi, E. L. (1986). *The Psychobiology of Mind-body Healing.* New York: Norton.

43. Rossi, E. L., & Cheek, D. B. (1988). *Mind-body Therapy.* New York: Norton.

44. Roy, N., McGrory, J.J., Tasko, S. M., Bless, D. M., Heisey, D., & Ford, C. H. (1997). Psychological correlates of functional dysphonia: An investigation using the Minnesota Multiphasic Personality Inventory. *Journal of Voice, 11,* 443–451.

45. Salkovskis, P. M. (1989). Somatic problems. In K. Hawton, P. M. Salkovskis, J. Kirk, & D. M. Clark (Eds.), *Cognitive Behaviour Therapy for Psychiatric Patients: A Practical Guide,* (pp. 235–276). Oxford: Oxford University Press.

46. Sapir, S., & Aronson, A. E. (1987). Coexisting psychogenic and neurogenic dysphonia: A source of diagnostic confusion. *British Journal of Direct Communication, 22,* 73–80.

47. Sifneos, P. (1973). The prevalence of alexithymic characteristics in psychosomatic patients. *Psychotherapeutics and Psychosomatics, 22,* 255–262.

48. Sifneos, P. E. (1996). Alexithymia: Past and present. *American Journal of Psychiatry, 153*(7) (Festschrift Supplement) 137–142.

49. White, A., Deary, I. J., & Wilson, J. A. (1997). Psychiatric disturbance and personality traits. *European Journal of Disorders of Communication, 32,* 307–314.

CHAPTER

Pediatric Voice Disorders: Special Considerations

6.1 Descriptions, Definitions, And Epidemiology

The multifactorial platform model of dysphonia presented in Chapters 1 and 2 can be applied to individuals of all ages. Nonetheless, voice disorders in children differ from those in adults in several respects.

➤ Anatomically, the larynx is not only smaller, but also is structurally and functionally different.
➤ The types of disorders included in the differential diagnosis include consideration of a wide range of congenital and genetic disorders.
➤ Voice pathology may occur in association with disorders of speech, language, and other developmental disorders. The mechanical inability to communicate may occur with, or be a manifestation of, disorders of communication at the cognitive level.
➤ In the prelingual child, the clinician must be aware of the relationship of voice to respiratory and feeding function, as a localizing and diagnostic symptom in aerodigestive tract disorders.

➤ The limited cooperative ability of young children dictates that the clinician take special care to select and administer evaluation and treatment techniques in the least invasive and frightening manner.
➤ The clinician must include the parents, family, caregivers, and educators as therapists.

The overlap of language, speech, and voice disorders is frequent, and many patients with developmental disabilities have difficulties in all areas. In the mildest cases, a disordered voice in a child may be an indication of a focal laryngeal defect that may have minimal influence on overall health or communication. In other cases, the abnormal voice may be a clue to a systemic disorder of congenital or acquired nature, and recognition of the voice symptoms may play a critical role in localizing a potentially life-threatening condition.

It is unlikely that the clinician seeing children with abnormal voices will be considering underlying malignant diseases, but potentially fatal lesions such as foreign body ingestion, acute inflammatory conditions, or histologically benign lesions (such as mucoceles or papilloma) may all have serious airway complications.

Case 6.1

Sara, an 18-month-old girl who previously has been healthy, suddenly vomits and becomes agitated and short of breath while playing at home. At the local hospital, a diagnosis of "sudden severe croup" is made. Sara is unresponsive to inhaled racemic epinephrine (adrenaline) and systemic steroids. Urgent transfer to the regional pediatric hospital is arranged. Further interview with her parents reveals that Sara has been unable to speak or cry since the sudden onset of symptoms. Direct laryngoscopy under general anesthesia reveals a spiral-shaped fragment of plastic wedged in her larynx. Severe associated swelling of the vocal folds is noted, as well as minor lacerations and contusion. A minor chink at the anterior glottis remains patent. Following removal of the foreign body, Sara is intubated to allow for resolution of the laryngeal edema. Antibiotic and steroid therapy is given. Her parents recognize the foreign body as a component of one of Sara's toys.

Regrettably, training of general pediatricians frequently does not emphasize abnormalities of voice as an important diagnostic symptom or localizing sign in the manner that auscultation (evaluation by listening) of cardiac sounds or focal neurological abnormalities might be evaluated.

Voice is regarded as a function of the larynx that has arisen as a late evolutionary process for communicative purposes. The primal function of the larynx is to provide an airway to the lungs and a sphincteric valve to protect the lower respiratory tract. These functions are vital to the health and functioning of the individual. Nonetheless, it is the secondary function of voiced language that provides a unique role in societal organization.

In Chapters 1 and 8, perceptual-acoustic features of voice are described along several perceptual dimensions including pitch, loudness, and quality. Wilson noted that a normal voice should have a pleasing quality, proper balance of oral and nasal resonance; appropriate loudness; habitual pitch level suitable for the age, size, and gender of an individual;

and appropriate voice inflections[35]. Additionally, timing characteristics of voice should be appropriate to contribute to speech fluency. Voice characteristics convey information not only related to the individual's laryngeal status, but also to social origins, emotional state, physique, age, and gender.

A voice disorder is noted to occur when these parameters are deviant. Wilson summarizes this impression by stating that if a voice is distracting or unpleasant or if it interferes with the content of the communication, a disorder is present. The disturbed voice quality may occur from laryngeal dysfunction and result in perceptual descriptions such as the following:

➤ hoarse, harsh, or breathy glottal source features
➤ abnormal loudness
➤ inappropriate pitch for age, size, or gender
➤ inappropriate stress or intonation patterns

Laryngeal dysfunction frequently is associated with disturbances of balance between oral and nasal coupling, resulting from lesions affecting the velopharyngeal sphincter, obstruction in the nasopharynx, or glosso/pharyngeal hypertonicity. In this case, hypernasal or hyponasal resonance may contribute to voice-quality perception.

The study of voice disorders in the pediatric population often is overshadowed by concerns related to language development and speech disorders. It is important that the clinician has a working understanding of the nonphonatory aspects of speech and language disorders to be able to distinguish between the voice disorder and other unrelated or interacting aspects of communication disorders. A brief review of these disorders serves to place pediatric voice disorders in the context of communication.

Language refers to a system of symbolic designations for objects, relationships, and activities that are shared and learned. Language symbols serve to classify experiences for the purpose of communication. Oral language is transmitted vocally and received aurally, whereas writing, sign language, and other non-vocal language systems are transmitted manually and received visually or through tactile sensation. Each language, whether oral or manual, has a grammar or **syntax**, a system of rules by which words or meaningful units are organized to make phrases and sentences. In oral languages, voice contributes to **suprasegmental** aspects of speech, in particular stress and intonation, which can change the meaning or structure of a sentence. Consider the sentence, "You are going," for example. If the voice rises in pitch at the end of the sentence, it conveys a question; if the pitch drops, it becomes a statement of fact or a command.

Speech refers to the oral expression of language. **Articulation** is the motor function by which internal language is converted into series of **phonemes** or sound segments by movements of the lips, tongue, palate, pharynx, larynx, and respiratory system[4], for example: rounding of the lips for /u/, closure-release of the lips for /p/, or lowering of the velum for nasals /m/; /n/; /ŋ/. **Phonology** is the pattern or system of rules by which the sounds are organized.

Disorders in the development of speech and language have been studied extensively[5,11,33]. These problems account for the major caseload for speech-language pathologists working with verbal communication problems in children and are usually the major source of parental concern when evaluation and intervention are sought. Developmental language disorders frequently are associated with other disorders of development and intellectual function. Parameters of language skill form major components of test batteries used to assess intellectual function.

Speech development is a maturational learned process that occurs in stages over a 4-to-6 year period. The majority of speech disorders are articulation or phonological problems. Disordered or delayed articulation may be associated with organic disorders such as **cerebral palsy**, **cleft palate**, **orofacial abnormalities**, **dental problems**, or **neuromuscular disorders**.

Stuttering represents a dysfluent speech pattern in which rhythm is interrupted by stoppage, prolongation, or repetition of sounds, words, or phrases. The etiology may be neurological, but stress and learned factors can also contribute. Many children demonstrate a brief period of developmental dysfluency as they are struggling with the application of new vocabulary, syntax, and phonological rules.

Autism may be characterized by failure to develop appropriate language and social responsiveness, as well as deficiency or distortion of speech. Stereotyped behaviors or echolalia may also occur in autistic children.

The incidence of speech, language, and voice disorders is higher in individuals with **mental retardation**. Behavioral disorders are associated with higher incidence of speech and language disorders. Restless behaviors, attention deficit, or hyperactivity may occur in these patients.

Facial movements, throat clearing, sniffing, and coughing may occur along with abnormal vocalizations known as tics in patients with *Gilles de la Tourette's syndrome*, a neurological syndrome of uncertain etiology[23].

Reliable estimates of the prevalence of voice disorders in children are not available, but estimates range from 5% to 25% in the school-aged population[25,35]. Only approximately 1% of the children in the caseload of pediatric otolaryngologists is referred for voice problems, however[30].

6.2 Natural History Of Voice And Vocal Tract Development

The pediatric larynx differs from the adult larynx in several respects that have important clinical implications. According to two studies, the average length of vocal folds in adults is approximately 21 mm for women and 29 mm for men[20,21]. The new-born vocal folds may range from less than 4 mm to 8 mm in length[22]. In newborns, the vocal processes of the arytenoids form a greater relative proportion of the glottis such that the membranous and cartilaginous parts of the vocal folds are approximately equal. The relatively larger area of the respiratory (posterior) glottis structures in infants serves important functions for deglutition and respiration; it is designed to alternately valve rapidly and effectively to protect the airway during swallowing and open rapidly for inspiration between swallows. Dejonckere reported that at birth, the lower border of the cricoid is located at level C3 to C4 but descends to the level of C5 at 2 years, mid-C6 at 5 years, and the level of C6 to C7 at 15 years (see Figure 8–22).[13] At birth, the thyroid and hyoid structures are contiguous then separate craniocaudally. The alae of the thyroid cartilage form an angle of 110° at birth in the male and 120° in the female. The angle remains stable in the female with growth, but narrows to 90° in the male at puberty. The hyoid is cartilaginous at birth and then begins to ossify at 2 years. The remaining cartilages ossify during adulthood. The narrowest diameter of the pediatric airway is at the subglottal (cricoid) level[31].

In more than 50% of individuals, the infant epiglottis is omega-shaped in cross section, rather than a gentle curve as it appears in the adult. The infant's softer cartilages and lax supporting ligaments tend to collapse on inspiration. The subepithelial tissues are less dense and more vascular and are therefore more subject to inflammatory or posttraumatic edema.

The functional correlates of these differences are that the infant larynx appears more anterior and higher in the neck and is more difficult to intubate. The posterior subglottis bears the brunt of intubation injuries. The point of maximal vocal fold vibration occurs more anteriorly and may influence the site of nodule formation.

Minor changes in laryngeal soft tissue edema in the infant result in marked changes in the airflow resistance at the laryngeal level. Airflow resistance is proportional to the inverse of the radius to the power four[10] (for example, a 1 mm edematous swelling at the laryngeal level increases work of breathing by approximately 40%).

The histological development of the larynx is described in Chapter 8. The vocal fold structure is simpler in infancy. The mucosal layers are thick, and there is no vocal ligament (see Figure 8–23b). The infant larynx has fewer of the type I muscle fibres which are responsible for slow, prolonged contraction. In contrast, a larger proportion of type II fibres may serve the infant's need for rapid glottic movement to allow rapid inspiration without aspiration during feeding.

The change in fibre populations with growth is thought to be correlated with increased refinement and variety of vocalization and the potential for training in later life. Corresponding increases in tongue strength and coordination occur to facilitate speech development. The vocal ligament differentiates in the preschool years and the vocal fold becomes two-layered at puberty. Throughout childhood the larynx grows in a relatively linear fashion provided that bodily growth follows normal patterns. In specific growth disorders such as achondroplasia, laryngeal size correlates better with individual weight than individual age.

The functional characteristics of laryngeal growth include a decrease in fundamental frequency as the larynx increases in size and decrease in formant frequencies as the pharyngobuccal tube elongates. At birth the cry averages 500 Hz and then declines to an average of 286.5 Hz at 7 years, and 275.8 Hz at 8 years[13]. Average pitch range at 1 to 2 years is 5 semitones, then 14 to 19 semitones in 12-year-old boys and 16 to 22 semitones in 12-year-old girls. During adolescence a rapid descent of fundamental frequency (up to an octave) typically occurs within the course of several months in boys until it reaches an average speaking f_0 of 100 Hz. The female voice declines an average of 2.4 semitones over the course of several years into early adulthood when an average speaking f_0 of approximately 200 Hz is reached. In addition to the laryngeal changes noted, the vocal tract grows and changes shape dramatically from infancy to adulthood. The growth patterns of the vocal tract during puberty are different for boys and girls. The pharyngeal region increases proportionally more in boys than in girls, compared with growth in the oral cavity. These structural developments alter the resonance characteristics in complicated ways. The frequency of vocal tract formants drops as the vocal tract grows larger, but shape changes also determine the frequency of individual vocal tract formants. These developmental and gender differences are discussed in greater detail in Chapter 8.

Emotive or communicative intent in the voice is recognized early in infancy. Specific cues for hunger, pain, comfort, pleasure, or discomfort are recognized, particularly by the infant's mother or other experienced caregivers. Loss of communicative variation in infant vocalization is recognized in infants deprived of social stimulation (P. Rodenberg, personal communication, May, 1993). There is a characteristic harsh, incessant, high-pitched, inconsolable quality to crying in newborns in withdrawal with neonatal abstinence syndrome after exposure in utero to opiate drugs.

6.3 Causes Of Voice Disorders in Children

The four etiological platform components of voice disorders (technique-skill level, lifestyle, psychological factors, and gastroesophageal reflux) can be applied to children within the context of relevant developmental stages. The most common etiologies of voice disorders in children arise from the technical, lifestyle, and psychological platform components and are typically referred to as **vocal abuse** and **muscle misuse**. Within this clinical

group, vocal nodules predominate as the most likely secondary organic component associated with dysphonia. The classification scheme for muscle misuse voice disorders outlined in Chapter 2 can be applied to describe the nature of muscle misuse voice disorders associated with secondary organic lesions, as well as those that are not associated with structural changes.

In describing the nature of organic problems associated with voice dysfunction in children, it is valuable to differentiate *primary* and *secondary* organic disorders. The most common pediatric laryngeal lesions are reviewed below.

6.3.1 Primary Organic Disorders

Many of the potential organic causes of voice disorders in children are very rare and are beyond the scope of this text. The reader is referred to Maddern, Campbell, and Stool[25] and Dejonckere[13] for detailed listings of etiologic lesions. These comprehensive analyses cluster causes accordingly to pathologic etiology and include conditions such as disorders of resonance and disorders in which involuntary (noncommunicative) sound (such as stridor) emanates from the vocal tract.

The rarer causes of voice disorders frequently provide the most challenge to investigate and treat, particularly when the voice is a clue to a systemic disorder or represents an indication that a threat to airway or vital functioning is present. The association of stridor and airway obstruction with dysphonia implies a serious obstructive lesion in the glottis. Delayed diagnosis and intervention may place the child at severe risk.

Case 6.2

Mickey, a 2-year-old boy, is noted to have progressive hoarseness over the course of 1 year. Medical attention is not sought until shortness of breath is noted. Prescribed antibiotic treatment produces no benefit. Direct laryngoscopy at a regional hospital is attempted. Mickey becomes cyanotic at induction of general anesthesia, and the procedure is abandoned without visualization of the glottis. Mickey is transferred by air ambulance to the regional pediatric hospital. On arrival, he is noted to be aphonic with biphasic stridor and moderate costocervical indrawing. Slow induction of general anesthesia by inhalation agents is undertaken by an experienced pediatric anesthesiologist.

Direct laryngoscopy reveals severe laryngeal papillomatosis such that 80% of the glottis is obstructed. Inspiratory-expiratory movement of partially pedunculated clusters of papilloma is noted. After biopsy and rapid debulking with cupped forceps the remaining papillomata are vaporized using a carbon dioxide laser. Postoperatively, Mickey's voice quality improves dramatically, and the airway obstruction resolves. Subsequently he requires repeated laser treatments at 6-month intervals for modest papilloma regrowth. Good voice function is maintained.

Recurrent respiratory **papillomatosis** is a relatively common disorder in which benign wartlike growths repeatedly grow in the larynx. The etiology is viral, and acquisition from maternal genital papillomata is presumed to occur. The pediatric form of the condition recurs more aggressively and diffusely than in adults. The lesions may spread to the distal tracheobronchial tree and can be associated with a fatal outcome. The condition has been refractory to a wide range of treatments including surgical removal, fulgurization (heat destruction), cryotherapy (destruction by freezing), antiviral agents, radiation, and locally applied toxins. Currently, the best method of control to maintain airway patency is repeated treatments with a CO_2 laser. Surgery should conserve the underlying laryngeal tissues especially at the posterior and anterior glottis. Tracheotomy is associated with distal dissemination of disease and is to be avoided. Current research includes evaluation of immune system adjuncts, such as interferon, phototherapy (light therapy), cidofovir,® and isotretinon[1]. Spontaneous regression occurs with age in

many cases. This condition forms a significant and frequently worrisome caseload for pediatric laryngologists. Voice therapy has little role in treating this disorder but may assist the child to optimize communication strategies when significant persistent hoarseness occurs following medical-surgical management.

Congenital malformations of the larynx include **webs** and **aplasias**. Aplastic conditions may be associated with malformations and fistulae involving the gastroesophageal tract. The condition can be fatal at birth unless prompt recognition and airway bypass is undertaken. Laryngeal webs vary in thickness and extent. Tracheotomy is frequently required when surgery to divide the web is undertaken[7,8]. Residual voice function is usually adequate for most speech communication situations but may be enhanced by voice therapy to reduce inappropriate compensatory strategies and optimize and augment vocal loudness, pitch, and quality once the child is old enough to cooperate in a rehabilitation program. An example of a laryngeal web is presented in Chapter 2, Figure 2–12.

Laryngomalacia is the most common congenital laryngeal disorder. The condition is associated with nonvoluntary, noncommunicative respiratory noise known as stridor. It may be evident shortly after birth and persist for up 18 months. The noise represents a loud inspiratory crowing related to airflow turbulence because the supraglottal structures (epiglottis, aryepiglottic folds, and arytenoids) tend to collapse with the inspired breath. The condition is a result of immaturity of cartilaginous development and is most evident in omega-shaped larynges. The majority of cases require no therapy other than diagnosis of the condition and exclusion of other lesions. In a few cases, the cartilaginous collapse may impair the airway and secondarily affect growth and feeding. Surgical resection of the collapsing tissue by epiglottopexy or laser vaporization may be needed.

Other laryngeal lesions such as **subglottal stenosis** or **subglottal hemangioma** have been of concern primarily for effects on respiration. Choice of therapy including endoscopic or open surgery may affect the ultimate outcome for voice function.

Vocal fold paralysis represents the second most common diagnosis of congenital laryngeal disorders. Grundfast reviewed this condition extensively and described the association with myelodysplasia and Arnold-Chiari malformation, which is characterized by caudal displacement of the cerebellum and brainstem into the cervical canal[18]. It is believed that stretching of nerve rootlets occurs, resulting in neurogenic laryngeal paralysis in patients with spina bifida and meningomyelocele.

In cases in which speech and language development may be threatened by impairment of vocal pitch, loudness, or quality, ongoing input from the speech-language pathologist is recommended. Surgery to restore anatomic competence to the vocal tract frequently is required before direct speech and voice therapy can be effective. In the interim, the speech-language pathologist may need to provide augmentative communication options to ensure that the child is maintaining motivation to communicate and receiving adequate feedback during verbal discourse.

Case 6.3

Tanya, a 9-year-old girl who was born with left unilateral cleft lip and cleft palate is reviewed by a multispecialty cleft disorders team. Past history includes extreme prematurity, hydrocephaly, and ventriculoperitoneal shunting. Left vocal cord paralysis (neurogenic) has been diagnosed previously. Mild hearing loss, velopharyngeal incompetence, bucconasal fistula, malocclusion, and a weak, breathy voice quality are noted. Management recommendations include alveolar bone grafting, teflon injection to the paralysed vocal fold and subsequent speech therapy.

Surgical intervention to attempt to reposition or reinnervate paretic vocal cords should not be undertaken until the possibility of spontaneous recovery has passed. The choice of procedure needs to be safe to permit laryngeal growth through to adulthood. Intracordal injection of teflon has now been discontinued because of inflammatory reactions. Fat and gelfoam tend to dissipate. Research for other suitable materials is ongoing.

Other congenital lesions associated with vocal fold paralysis include spastic and neuromuscular disorders (eg, cerebral damage may result in any combination of the cerebral palsy dysarthrias) and specific thoracic abnormalities including cardiac defects. Acquired causes of vocal fold paralysis include nerve injury during birth or related to cardiac, thoracic, or neck surgery.

Gastroesophageal reflux disease (GERD) increasingly has been recognized as a common cause of voice disorders in adult patients. In infants, there is mounting evidence that success in the management of subglottal stenosis, choanal atresia, laryngomalacia, and intubation related laryngeal edema is improved if associated GERD is controlled. Reflux should also be considered as a dysphonia platform component in preschool and older children, particularly those who exhibit the typical signs and symptoms of GERD: frequent throat clearing, nocturnal coughing and choking, hoarse voice or throat clearing in the morning, globus pharyngeus, postnasal drip, water brash, acid taste, or heartburn[16]. The lifestyle and diet measures outlined in Appendix 3–1 often are sufficient to manage GERD in children.

6.3.2 Secondary Organic Disorders

The most common voice disorders in children arise from vocal misuse and abuse. Vocal fold **nodules** represent the majority of associated secondary lesions and are identified in more than 50% of children examined with voice disorders. The nodules are typically bilateral and occur at the usual point of maximum vocal fold vibration at the junction of the anterior and middle thirds of the membranous cords. Histologically, the lesions represent local fibrotic thickening of the vocal folds.

The etiology and management of nodules is discussed extensively in this text. Typically, bilateral vocal fold nodules in children represent an effect of muscle misuse voice disorders, and a laryngeal isometric laryngeal posture often is identified during laryngoscopy. Common observations include an exaggerated posterior glottal chink, extralaryngeal muscle misuses, and postural misuses typical of the features seen in adults who develop bilateral nodules. Precursor stages include local edema and then an organized inflammatory reaction before mature fibrosis develops[24]. Children with this symptom complex may be observed to shout loudly during play and may be participating in sporting or other activities where shouting and excessive voice use occurs. Throat clearing, coughing, and abrupt glottal attacks may occur. The condition is more common in boys. Psychobehavioral characteristics that often are identified in children with vocal nodules include extroversion, aggression, frustration, immaturity, poor coping or problem-solving skills, argumentativeness, disobedience, and use of voice as a method of asserting a role in the family or peer structure[17,28,32,36]. In Chapter 4, a case example is presented (Case 4.6) demonstrating the multifactorial etiology that may contribute to voice problems in children with secondary vocal fold nodules.

Von Leden presented a comprehensive review of management of nodules in children[34]. He stated that "all current authorities concur that treatment of vocal nodules in children should be conservative" and that surgical ablation is unnecessary and potentially harmful as vocal fold injury may occur. He reported a favorable outcome with voice therapy and noted a spontaneous tendency toward symptom regression at puberty. If the causal factors persist, the nodules tend to recur. Voice improvement and partial or full resolution of nodules with behavioral management have been reported in a number of other studies[9,12,26,29]. Some guidelines for developing vocal rehabilitation programs for children with muscle misuse voice problems are presented in Chapter 4.

Benjamin and Croxson advocated surgical removal in specific conditions refractory to previous therapy in children older than 8 years[3]. The preconditions for surgery include long-standing symptoms with social or educational compromise. They advocate forceps and scissor removal, preserving the underlying vocal ligament and vocalis muscle, rather than laser ablation. Hirschberg and colleagues also suggested reserving surgery for the most severely affected cases[19].

Cases of previously diagnosed vocal nodules, which have been refractory to treatment by voice therapy, require reevaluation. Mistaken diagnosis can occur when initial laryngeal examination has been difficult to attain.

6.3.3 Disorders of Muscle Misuse

The most common muscle misuse voice disorder in children has been discussed in the previous section: the laryngeal isometric pattern associated with generalized muscle misuse in the head, neck and larynx, often associated with vocal abuse and secondary bilateral vocal fold nodules. Other muscle misuse voice disorders can occur in the pediatric population as a result of factors operating at technical, psychological, and GERD platform levels, sometimes in combination with adjustments made to compensate for developmental changes.

Case 6.4

Tim, a 14-year-old-boy, is referred for voice evaluation because of teasing about a high-pitched, feminine voice quality. Peer comments include references to possible homosexuality. Pediatric endocrinological evaluation indicates normal pubertal growth with no evidence of hypogonadism. Laryngological examination shows evidence of normal male growth. Mild prognathism and high laryngeal position are noted. Vocal pitch range that fluctuates between approximately 140 Hz and 290 Hz (typical for adolescent male transitional stage) is recorded, but a fronted resonance and articulation pattern is noted to convey an effeminate mannerism. Voice therapy and psychiatric evaluation are initiated and reveal no significant psychopathology. The voice clinic team determine that this is represents a form of adolescent transitional voice disorder. Tim demonstrates good motivation to effect changes to his voice. Therapy is directed toward encouraging a consistent speaking pitch below 160 Hz and adjusting his tongue carriage and resonance quality.

Children may exhibit muscle misuse voice disorders in the absence of primary or secondary organic lesions. Psychopathological processes may play a role in symptom formation, including psychological states such as anxiety and personality traits such as obsessional behaviors. In adolescence, **adolescent transitional voice disorders**, such as the one represented above and in Chapter 4 (Case 4.1), may occur in boys, and **conversion reaction dysphonias**, such as the one represented below, are seen more frequently in girls. A coping style that includes repression of the overt vocal expression of negative emotions may also play a role, as is depicted in the following case. An interdisciplinary approach to assessment and management of individuals with these disorders has obvious advantages.

Case 6.5

Megan, an 11-year-old girl, is seen in the voice clinic with aphonia. She has been whispering for 5 months. Her previously normal voice had changed overnight with a "mild cold." She had no accompanying complaints of pain, stridor, dysphagia, or shortness of breath. During the voice evaluation, a normal cough is elicited. Flex-

ible endoscopic laryngoscopy shows complete adduction of the vocal folds with voluntary coughing but failure of adduction with attempted voicing. Glottal fry register cannot be elicited. Inhalation phonation does occur with modeling and encouragement. An interview with Megan's mother reveals that her sibling had died of leukemia before the onset of dysphonia. Grief counseling is currently underway with a family counsellor. A diagnosis of conversion dysphonia is made. Partial recovery of voice occurs after one joint session with the voice clinic psychiatrist during which the grieving girl allows herself to cry audibly. Subsequently, she regains her voice fully after 2 voice therapy sessions, in which she learns to extend and shape phonation using an inhalation-exhalation technique.

Detailed descriptions of voice therapy approaches are provided in Chapter 4. In addition to the many possible psychosocial influences on muscle function, muscle misuses may represent compensation for anatomical defects (e.g., cleft palate), linguistic incompetence (e.g., language encoding difficulties), or second-language learning. In many cases, the voice disorder may not be treated directly in children with primary structural, phonological, or language disorders. Initial focus may be placed on rehabilitation of general speech and language functions. Muscle hypertonicity in the larynx is a common manifestation of stuttering and strategies for vocal relaxation and fluency can be incorporated into a speech management program[2].

6.4 Application of Technological Advances to the Management of Pediatric Voice Disorders

The development of technological devices that allow for examination of children's vocal tracts without general anesthesia represents a great advance in the management of these patients. In the past, the clinician was faced with the inevitable decision to recommend direct laryngoscopy under general anesthesia when indirect (mirror) laryngoscopy failed because of a child's age or limited cooperation. In selected cases in high-risk neonates, direct examination with physical restraint with or without topical anesthesia may have been advocated.

The development of fine-caliber (2 mm or less) flexible fiber-optic endoscopes has permitted minimally invasive examination of a wide range of patients with only topical anesthesia or no anesthesia at all. The use of video recording has enhanced documentation for purposes of comparison with subsequent examination, parent and colleague education, medical and legal records, and visual feedback for patients during therapy.

Visualization of the child's larynx during vocalization gives better diagnostic information about function than can be obtained by observation during spontaneous respiration, but no phonation, under general anesthesia. This is particularly important in vocal fold paralysis, which requires judgement and experience to assess[18].

The techniques for flexible fiber-optic nasopharyngolaryngoscopy are demonstrated in Figures 6–1 to 6–3. For infants, the traditional positioning places the child supine and requires one assistant or parent to immobilize the head and another to immobilize the body (Figure 6–1). Suctioning of pharyngeal secretions may be required via a catheter passed into the nares opposite the endoscope.

Some parents of young infants prefer not to witness the examination, becoming anxious, tearful, or faint at the prospect. In this circumstance, an alternative positioning is recommended using one trained assistant with the parents waiting elsewhere. Stabilizing the infant in an upright position with trunk and head support allows good visualization with less pharyngeal stimulation and less reflux or retention of secretions (Figure 6–2).

Occasionally, airway, cardiovascular, or

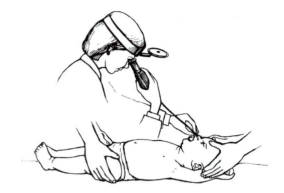

Figure 6–1. Technique for supine positioning of infants for nasopharyngolaryngoscopy.

other conditions may compromise the safe conduct of the examination[18]. Significant airway compromise, cardiac anomaly, or arrhythmia history suggests that monitoring equipment, intravenous access, and resuscitation equipment should be available. Such cases may be best evaluated in the operating room with an anesthesiologist, rigid endoscopes, and endotracheal tubes on standby.

In healthy children, the examination can be well tolerated in cooperative patients as young as 4 or 5 years. The toddler to early preschool child remains the most difficult patient to evaluate because safe restraint is difficult to maintain and cooperative maturity is not yet attained. These children (and older patients with mental or behavioral disorders) may still require general anesthesia for evaluation.

Chait and Lotz described the examination technique in detail in older children[6]. These techniques are applicable for both velopharyngeal and laryngeal examination.

Whereas the flexible endoscopic examination in the adult may be undertaken by one clinician, it is helpful in younger children to have a second trained team member working in cooperation with the endoscopist, particularly when video equipment is to be operated

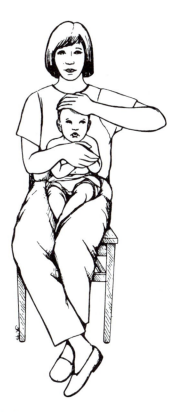

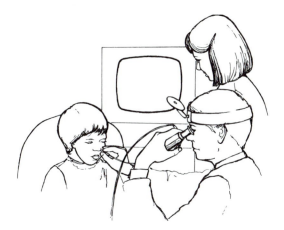

Figure 6–3. Positioning for endoscopist and trained assistant during nasopharyngolaryngoscopy.

Figure 6–2. Sitting position of infants for naso-pharyngolaryngoscopy.

during the examination (Figure 6–3). It may be useful to maintain direct contact between the child's face and the practitioner's hand that is used to advance the endoscope into the nose. This helps anticipate and discourage the child's movement during examination. Effort should be made to create a pleasant environment with a comfortable lounge-style chair, and the absence of frightening medical equipment and "white coat" clothing. The child can be encouraged by the prospect of "being on television" and allowed to examine the endoscope and camera. During the preparation and examination, the child may be distracted by being offered a choice from a selection of small toys or to work with a pegboard

or puzzle activity during the procedure. Most examiners find that the effort to introduce topical anesthesia into the nose is rewarded by better cooperation for the examination. The least invasive techniques are best tolerated. Local anesthetic solution with or without vasoconstrictor solution is better applied by hand-held, low-pressure atomizer or dropper followed by sniffing, rather than high-pressure or machine-generated aerosols. Similarly, the introduction of anesthetic solution on cotton-tipped applicators may be better tolerated than placing cotton pledgets with bayonet forceps or metal probes. Anaesthesia should include the middle meatus region for the purpose of velopharyngeal examination because advancement of the endoscope along the nasal floor results in movement of the scope tip with velar elevation, which distorts viewing of the velopharyngeal port area.

The use of stroboscopy in pediatric patients previously was limited when the requirements of illumination necessitated the use of the optically superior, rigid fiber-optic telescopes. The introduction of stroboscopy coupled with flexible fiber-optic endoscopes has opened up new possibilities for the examination of children with vocal fold lesions. The widespread commercialisation of video games for children has familiarized young patients to seeing animated characters or other objects on computer screens that are responsive to their input. The use of specially designed software for computer programs for visual display feedback regarding pitch and loudness parameters can be readily understood, even by preschool children.

6.5 Voice Disorders in Specific Populations

6.5.1 Hearing Impairment

As we discussed in Chapter 4, children with hearing impairment may have abnormal speech and voice characteristics because their ability to monitor and alter speech production by auditory feedback is impaired.

It is traditional to regard children with congenital hearing loss or hearing loss acquired before 2 years of age as prelingual and those acquiring impairment at an older age as postlingual. The former group has the most difficulty with control of pitch, volume, and loudness, resulting in inappropriate pitch that is usually higher than that for individuals with normal hearing. Inappropriate loudness (usually too loud) and minimal or inappropriate intonation, rhythm, and stress patterns are noted. In addition, abnormal tongue posturing may result in perception of a "backed" oral resonance characteristic, which is also associated with articulatory-phonological distortions. Wirz discussed specific phonological changes and specific voice disorders[37]. These changes are greatest in children with the most severe and earliest hearing losses.

Voice quality labels such as high-pitched, tense, flat, breathy, harsh, monotone, or lacking rhythm have been applied to describe the voices of children with hearing impairment. Possible functional correlates include abnormal breathing patterns, increased laryngeal and supralaryngeal tension, restricted pitch range, and generation of high-frequency turbulent noise in the larynx and vocal tract. Hypernasality also is reported in deaf children; however, this likely reflects a perceptual problem rather than actual velopharyngeal incompetence. Deaf children may appear to use excessive effort in speech known as over fortis. This may reflect a compensation for poor pitch control, stress, and rhythm. Reduced tongue, jaw, and lip movements during speech; reduced pitch and loudness range and variability; and generally increased pharyngeal and laryngeal tension may be noted in children with hearing impairment. Acquired laryngeal pathology including nodules, edema, and polyps may arise secondary to the misuse patterns of vocalization.

Teachers of children with hearing impairment are increasingly using visual display (biofeedback) techniques to enhance training by providing information about the level and consistency of pitch, intensity and quality of voice, and the placement of articulators during speech. Dedicated software programs may be used to provide real-time feedback of the acoustic signal, recorded from a microphone, or in conjunction with palatometry (B. Bernhardt, personal communication, March, 2000). In addition, enhanced levels of acoustic amplification and tactile input (eg, touching the larynx, feeling respiration or lip position) may improve proprioception and articulatory accuracy.

In otolaryngology clinics, the parental complaint of poor speech development or loud voice is a frequent trigger for the request for hearing evaluation. Children with fluctuating mild hearing loss related to intermittent serous otitis media are noted to have periodic deterioration in acquisition of language and articulatory accuracy, as well as loud speech.

Case 6.6

Bonita, a 4-year-old girl, has required prolonged hospitalization for severe asthma and chronic respiratory disease that is steroid dependent. She has suspected immune incompetence and has heptatocellular disease and ascites. Depressed affect is noted. Adenotonsillectomy had been performed for upper airway obstruction. She has a past history of recurrent otitis media and has mild mixed bilateral hearing loss for which hearing aids have been prescribed. Bonita has had chronic hoarseness with a breathy low-pitched voice and cushingoid facies. Previous laryngoscopy suggested edematous changes consistent with steroid use. Biphasic stridor of sudden and progressive onset occurs. White fungating material is seen in the larynx and intubation is required. Subsequent culture grows candida. Following extubation, C0$_2$ laser therapy is used to vaporize residual inflammatory swelling and intubation granuloma in the larynx. Hoarseness persists postoperatively. Voice pathology consultation is requested to improve communication skills. Psychology counselling is provided.

In Bonita's case multiple factors contribute to laryngeal pathology. Drug use, unusual infection and intubation all contribute to changes in her laryngeal tissues. Hearing loss and abnormal respiratory function contribute to her abnormal mechanisms of voice use. Multiple speciality cooperation is required for optimal management.

6.5.2 Prematurity

The increasing survival of very premature infants (of less than 28 weeks gestation or under 1500 grams or both) is associated with a population of children with special developmental needs. Whitfield reported major handicaps in up to 10% of these patients including mental retardation, specific learning disabilities, seizures, visual disorders, hearing loss, neuromuscular disorders, and respiratory disorders (M. Whitfield, personal communication, January, 1993). In addition to the cognitive language and articulatory disorders that may result from the neuromuscular

and central processing problems, these children are at risk for laryngeal disorders related to prolonged ventilation. Extremely premature babies with bronchopulmonary dysplasia (delayed and inadequate lung development) may require weeks or months of ventilator support with chronic intubation.

The effects of red rubber endotracheal tubes in inducing glottal, subglottal, and even tracheal damage have been much reduced by the advance to smaller polyvinyl chloride tubes. Tissue edema with diminished mucosal perfusion, ulceration, then perichondritis and chondritis (cartilage inflammation) does still occur, particularly at the subglottal level where the posterior mucosa receives the major compressive and frictional effects. The induction of subglottal stenosis typically will occur in 1 to 2% of very premature babies in North American intensive care nurseries. These effects are aggravated when factors such as infection, poor tissue oxygenation, movement from seizures, or excessive mechanical movement by ventilator equipment are present.

The primary thrust of treatment for subglottal stenosis relates to the correction of the narrowed subglottal calibre and to removal of a tracheotomy cannula that is frequently required for airway management. During the past 3 decades, the development of cricoid-split techniques and a range of laryngotracheoplasty procedures in which the stenotic cricoid cartilage is divided and then augmented by the patient's own cartilage have offered increasingly reliable hope of adequate reestablishment of the airway. Cricoid resection may be required in the most severe cases.

In the past, relatively little emphasis on subsequent voice function was given in comparison with the ultimate goal of airway patency. Increasing quality of photodocumentation does reveal gross and subtle changes relating to intubation including observation of glottal tongues of granulation tissue and subsequent furrows of tissue loss, as noted by Benjamin (personal communication, November, 1992). It is speculated that premature babies will be found to have perceptual and stroboscopic abnormalities when subsequent evaluation is applied. Vocal fold damage, diminished mobility by arytenoid fixation, and potential recurrent nerve paralysis may also occur secondary to the corrective surgery.

6.5.3 The Young Patient After Tracheostomy

In previous decades, the placement of a tracheostomy cannula (by the surgical procedure of tracheotomy) was usually a short-term intervention to bypass an inflammatory upper airway obstruction. The tube was removed when the condition resolved. With developments in respiratory and ventilatory technology, temporary intubation rather than tracheotomy has become the usual treatment for short-term inflammatory conditions such as epiglottitis and croup. Long-term tracheostomy is available for many patients with chronic respiratory failure who previously did not survive. These trends result in fewer patients with tracheotomy, but those who do require the procedure usually have complex long-term special needs.

The development of expressive speech appears to be related to the ability to vocalize communication concepts and inability to use vocal communication may impair development of cognitive aspects of speech and language in some children. Thus, it is important that the voice-care team facilitate oral communication if possible for long-term tracheotomized children. Vocalization options include temporary occlusion of the tube during expiration by finger or flexion of the neck. Externally applied devices such as Passy-Muir valves have been well tolerated by children with good lung function. Electrolaryngeal speech has been accepted by some

patients and has prompted creative strategies for its introduction, such as mimicking the child's father using his electric razor vibrating against the neck for shaving. Esophageal speech may be taught to certain older children with long-term tracheostomy. Total laryngectomy for laryngeal obstruction is seldom required in pediatric patients. In the rare instances of laryngectomy, however, the child may have access to the same methods of voice rehabilitation outlined in Chapter 4 for the adult laryngectomee population. Tracheoesophageal puncture for voice restoration would not be considered until an individual has reached adult stature, as the stable positioning of the fistula is critical to long-term success of the procedure. When oral communication is not possible in the child who has had a tracheostomy, manual communication methods including signing, picture boards, or other electronic computer-assisted devices may be used[14].

6.6 Disorders Of Nasal Resonance

Nasal resonance may be regarded as a parameter of voice quality. Disorders of the velopharyngeal valving mechanism not only affect intelligibility by producing abnormal resonance quality, but also by inducing secondary changes in the function of the larynx for voice production and other compensations of speech production.

The nose is coupled to the respiratory system for the function of smell and for reasons of warming, filtering, and humidifying the inspired air. Involvement of the nose in modifying the quality of voiced communication is regarded as a relatively late function in evolutionary terms. Velopharyngeal closure serves to close off the nasal cavity during swallowing. Complex muscular interactions open the eustachian tube for middle ear ventilation. Closure is a sphincteric or valve action and comprises a component of velar elevation and a component of pharyngeal wall constriction.

6.6.1 Hypernasal Speech

In spoken English, only the nasal phonemes /n/, /m/, /ŋ/ are spoken with the velopharyngeal (VP) valve open fairly wide. Inadequate closure of the VP valve for other sounds results in hypernasal resonance on vowel and vowel-like sounds and nasal air escape ("emission") on consonant sounds with plosive-aspirate or fricative features. Associated features may include inappropriate muscle activity in the vocal tract, phoneme substitutions, dysphonia, and nasal or facial grimacing.

The disorder may range from "assimilative" nasality (only sounds preceding or following nasal phonemes are hypernasal), to no ability to prevent direction of the air stream nasally. The overall effect can vary from a slightly abnormal resonance balance, often mistaken for a regional dialectal feature, to severely impaired speech intelligibility. In the most severe cases of velopharyngeal incompetence, individuals may also experience regurgitation (or reflux) of food and fluids into the nasal cavity. Examination of the velopharyngeal port with flexible fiber-optic nasopharyngolaryngoscopy can provide specific information regarding the nature of VP incompetence leading to hypernasal speech. The VP port is examined at rest, during vegetative activities such as swallowing, and during speech. Sound sequences with a high proportion of plosive-aspirate and fricative sounds tend to reveal the poor closure-coordination most dramatically because they require tight VP closure to achieve high intra-oral pressure. Examples of test sounds and phrases used frequently include: /ɑsɑsɑ . . . /, /ɑpɑpɑ . . . /, Suzy at the sea, and Pat the puppy.

Hypernasality is readily confirmed diagnostically by the examiner alternately occluding and releasing the nares with the thumb and forefinger while the patient speaks. In the case of mild or assimilative nasality, this test may be performed while the patient is repeating sentences or exercises with a high proportion of nasal phonemes /m/, /n/, /ŋ/; during sustained high vowels /i/, /u/ (which are associated with small oral opening and thus are more readily perceived as hypernasal with VP incompetence); and sentences with a large proportion of high vowels. A cold mirror held under the nares during speech can be used to detect the presence of high levels of nasal airflow. Nasal flow during speech can be quantified with the same hardware and software used to measure phonatory airflow rates and volumes, with a specially designed nasal cone or a divided face mask, as described in Chapter 1, Section 1.5. If a divided mask is used, oral and nasal flow rates may be measured simultaneously on separate channels to allow for a flow ratio to be derived. Otherwise the same speech task (same sentence, effort level, pitch, etc.) is recorded with the full mask the nasal cone and then the oral flow determined by subtracting the nasal from overall flow rates to derive an oral-nasal flow ratio. Some acoustic software programs provide algorithms to determine the degree of "nasalance" or nasal resonance.

Velopharyngeal incompetence in children is usually associated with cleft palate. Extensive discussion of the embryogenic disorder and subsequent variation in palatal clefting are beyond the scope of this text. Notwithstanding minor interracial variations in occurrence, approximately 1 child in 750 is born with cleft palate. Clefting may involve the secondary palate (soft palate and posterior portion of hard palate) and the primary palate (premaxillary portion) to varying degrees. When clefting of the alveolus occurs, there will be associated abnormalities of dentition; when lip clefting occurs, there may be associated distortion of bilabial and labiodental sounds and abnormal structure of the anterior nose.

Other reasons for velopharyngeal incompetence include congenitally short palate, velar paralysis associated with neurological defects of cranial nerve function, cerebral palsy (particularly spastic), or posttraumatic scarring. An incomplete form of cleft palate may occur as a submucous cleft palate in which the typical findings include bifid uvula, a bony notch in the hard palate, and a submucosal defect in muscular development of the soft palate. The mass of adenoidal tissue present in the nasopharynx serves to assist with closure of the VP valve. If adenoidectomy, which is specifically contraindicated in this condition, is inadvertently undertaken, the predisposition to velopharyngeal incompetence becomes evident. Persistent hypernasality may occur following adenoidectomy in approximately 1 in 1500 children, even when no previously detected defect in palatal function was present. These cases may represent an occult form of submucous cleft that may be evident only as a muscular inadequacy. Nasendoscopy may reveal a shallow depression on the nasal surface of the velum. Advances in genetic science have identified a specific karyotype (chromosomal pattern) abnormality in Shprintzen syndome (velocardiofacial syndrome).[15]

Case 6.7

Carrie, 10-year-old girl, presents with severe hypernasality following adenoidectomy performed by another surgeon. She has a known unilateral anacusis and an unrepaired ventriculoseptal defect. Ear grommets had been inserted previously. Further evaluation reveals a history of learning difficulties. A long expressionless face is noted. The palate is long and intact but appears poorly mobile. Genetic evaluation confirms a diagnosis of velocardiofacial syndrome, and 22q11 deletion is confirmed on chromosomal testing. A trial of speech therapy is undertaken to determine prognosis for improvement with increased oral opening and exaggerated articulation. Little improvement is measured after 2 months of therapy, and pharyngoplasty surgery is planned.

Transient hypernasality may occur in many patients following tonsillectomy with or without adenoidectomy that will be self-correcting within 3 to 6 months of the procedure.

McWilliams reported a high incidence (84%) of vocal abnormalities in children with cleft palate[27]. Most common were vocal nodules. Other lesions included vocal fold hypertrophy, edema, posterior glottal chinks, and improper vocal fold approximation patterns. Because these changes are deemed to be secondary to the velopharyngeal disorder, many practitioners feel that primary therapy to improve voice quality will not be successful until the velopharyngeal disorder is corrected.

Milder cases of velopharyngeal incompetence may require speech therapy as the only treatment. The speech-language pathologist may embark on a program to help the patient improve VP valving strength with speech and nonspeech exercises. They should help the child increase the ratio of oral to nasal opening during speech; increase non-nasal articulatory dynamics; improve coordination between respiratory, phonatory, and articulatory activities; alter speech rate and prosody; and reduce compensatory articulatory strategies such as the substitution of a glottal stop for oral stop articulation.

More severe cases may require primary palatoplasty or a form of pharyngoplasty surgery that may either introduce a flap of pharyngeal tissue to span the defect or attempt to create a sphincteric muscular valve. The selection of the type of surgery is greatly assisted by radiological and nasendoscopy examination that defines the specific aspect of closure failure that is occurring. Other treatment modalities include augmenting the posterior pharyngeal wall with tissue such as cartilage or by the use of a prosthetic speech bulb, particularly in neurogenic disorders.

6.6.2 Hyponasal Speech

Hyponasal speech occurs when there is a reduction or absence of nasal airflow during the production of the phonemes /m/, /n/, /ŋ/. It usually results from structural abnormalities causing anterior or posterior nasal airflow obstruction. To the untrained listener, this resonance abnormality may be occasionally confused with hypernasality, but simple occlusion of the nares during speech will not change the speech quality in this condition. Occasionally, complex combinations of hyponasal and hypernasal resonance occur if palatal fistulae are present or if an individual with a cleft palate has anterior nasal obstruction.

Transient hyponasality occurs with upper respiratory infections or discrete episodes of allergic exposure. Chronic obstruction occurs with stenosis by bone (e.g., choanal atresia), cartilage (e.g., septal deviation), mucosal swelling (e.g., allergic rhinitis or rhinosinusitis), or neoplasms. The most common persistent cause in children is adenoidal hypertrophy that is typically evident in the preschool and early school-aged period.

Direct examination of the nose anteriorly and posteriorly (by mirror or endoscope) usually reveals the cause. Lateral soft tissue radiographs will show soft tissue masses in the nasopharynx. Rhinometry and nasometric evaluation of resonance on reading standard passages assists with diagnosis. Speech therapy does not usually have much of a role in managing these resonance disorders. Treatment is usually medical or surgical, but nonintervention frequently is advised when regression of lymphoid tissue is anticipated.

6.7 The Young Performer

The child or youth participating in dramatic or vocal performance requires special consideration. These individuals are comparable to young athletes performing to a high level of neuromuscular training. Traditional pedagogy has recommended that formal singing training not be commenced until the voice is mature for fear of damaging the vocal mechanism. Other teachers, however, maintain that training may commence at any stage during maturation provided techniques of good vocal hygiene and appropriate repertoire are applied.

Young performers may experience acute muscle misuse voice disorders when the requirements of a cluster of performances rapidly raise the frequency and intensity of voice use to a degree well beyond their usual amount. These young vocalists frequently do not have the reserves of experience to perceive when strain is occurring or to modify their technique to compensate for it.

Case 6.8

Mari, a 15-year-old girl who participates in choral singing and group singing lessons at school, develops transient dysphonia after a singing workshop of several days' duration. Her hoarseness returns during preparation for the school musical production. She complains of loss of her upper pitch range and hoarseness. She is transferred from the soprano to the contralto section of the choir.

Mari's past history includes attacks of hyperventilation associated with light-headedness and panic. A diagnosis of possible juvenile rheumatoid arthritis has been considered after complaints of pain and weakness in the hands and wrists. Antiinflammatory drugs have been used. Addi-

tionally, she has been treated with nasal steroid spray and antihistamine for allergic rhinitis.

Examination shows incomplete adduction of the posterior glottis and fullness in the anterior vocal folds. Increased suprahyoid muscle tension and high laryngeal position are noted. No inflammatory changes are seen to suggest allergy, reflux, or cricoarytenoid fixation.

The voice clinic team describes Mari's dysphonia as a muscle misuse voice disorder with laryngeal isometric posturing and vocal overuse. There is no evidence that her possible history of arthritis or rhinitis play a role in her dysphonia, although her previous "panic attacks" suggest a possible psychological predisposition to anxiety reactions and associated muscle misuse. She is provided information on voice care, and personalized singing coaching is recommended. A singing repertoire suitable for Mari's light delicate voice is carefully selected. Psychological intervention is held in reserve because she has not experienced any recent symptoms suggesting anxiety disorder.

Frequently the young performer is under great pressure to please parents and directors for monetary or social reasons and is conscious of competition and the need for early career enhancement. Changes in sleep patterns, diet, and travel and adverse environments with respect to humidity, smoke, or other pollutants may compound these pressures. Maturational changes in the voice may conflict with the performance role, such as the former boy soprano who is encouraged to maintain his previous pitch range or quality after his larynx has begun to mature. Teenage girls may be cast in musical roles that require them to produce a rich or powerful vocal sound that is not compatible with their developing vocal structure. Attempts to produce the intensity and resonance that is characterized by the voices of mature Broadway or opera singers may result in muscle misuse and mucosal lesions in younger singers. In some circumstances, the dramatic effects required for performance, such as screaming or whispering, may demand vocally abusive behavior.

6.8 Summary

Management of voice disorders in the pediatric population requires consideration of a number of factors that may influence identification and treatment of dysphonia. The voice disorder must be considered in the context of the current physical, cognitive, and emotional developmental stages of a child. Voice plays a critical role in communication development and is normally the first component of the speech system to be used by a child to communicate needs and desires. A myriad of congenital and childhood diseases and disorders can influence the development of physical, cognitive, and communicative functions including speech and voice production. Any structural deficits that impair a child's ability to express his or her needs vocally or to monitor vocal productions will contribute to delayed or disordered communication development. Identification of the underlying causes is critical to ensure appropriate management. Because voice disorders can arise at any or all of the four basic etiological platform levels, optimal management of children with voice disorders may require an interdisciplinary approach.

References

1. Avidano, M. A., & Singleton, G. T. (1995). Adjuvant drug strategies in the treatment of recurrent respiratory papillomatosis. *Otolaryngology Head Neck Surgery, 112*(2), 197–202.
2. Baumgartner, J. M., Ramig, L. A., & Kuehn, D. P. (1986). Voice disorders and stuttering in children. In T. J. Balkany, & N. R. T. Dashley (Eds.), *Clinical Pediatric Otolaryngology* (pp. 200–210). St. Louis: CV Mosby.
3. Benjamin, B., & Croxson, G. (1987). Vocal nodules in children. *Annals of Otology, Rhinology and Laryngology, 96*, 530–533.
4. Brain, W. R. (1965). *Speech Disorders: Aphasia, Apraxia and Agnosia* (2nd ed.). London: Butterworth Heinemann.
5. Casper, J. K. (1985) Disorders of speech and voice. *Pediatric Annals, 14*, 220–229.

6. Chait, D. H., & Lotz, W. K. (1991). Successful pediatric examinations using nasendoscopy. *Laryngoscope, 101,*1016–1018.

7. Cohen, S. R. (1985). Congenital glottic webs in children. *Annals of Otology, Rhinology and Laryngology,* (Supp. 121), 2–10.

8. Cohen, S. R., Thompson, J. W., Geller, K. A., & Bims, J. W. (1983). Voice change in the pediatric patient. *Annals of Otology, Rhinology and Laryngology, 92,* 437–443.

9. Cook, J. F., Palaski, D. J., & Hanson, W. R. (1979). A vocal hygiene program for school-age children. *Language, Speech, and Hearing Services in Schools, 10*(1), 21–26.

10. Crone, R. K., & O'Rourke, P. P. (1986). Pediatric and neonatal intensive care. In R. D. Miller (Ed.). *Anaesthesia* (Vol. 3, 2nd Ed., pp. 2325–2414). New York: Churchill Livingstone.

11. Curlee, R. F., & Shelton, R. L. (1983). Disorders of articulation, voice and fluency. In C. D. Bluestone, & S. E. Stool (Eds.). *Pediatric Otolaryngology* (Vol. 2, pp. 1493–1507). Philadelphia: W. B. Saunders.

12. Deal, R. E., McClain, B., & Sudderth, J. F. (1976). Identification, evaluation, therapy and follow-up for children with vocal nodules in a public school setting. *Journal of Speech and Hearing Disorders, 41,* 390–397.

13. Dejonckere, P. H. (1984). Pathogenesis of voice disorders in childhood. *Acta Otorhinolaryngologica (Belgica), 38,* 307–314.

14. Fowler, S. M., Simon, B. M., & Handier, S. D. (1985). Communication development in children. In E. N. Myers, S. E. Stool, & J. T. Johnson (Eds.), *Tracheotomy* (pp. 271–285). New York: Churchill Livingstone.

15. Goldberg, R., Motzkin, B., Marion, R., Scambler, P. J., & Shprintzen, R. J. (1993). velo-cardio-facial syndrome: A review of 120 patients. *American Journal of Medical Genetics, 45,* 313–319.

16. Gray, S. D., Smith, M. E., & Schneider, H. (1996). Voice Disorders in Children. In G. Isaacson (Ed.), *Pediatric Clinics of North America* (pp. 1357–1384). Philadelphia: WB Saunders.

17. Green, G. (1989). Psychobehavioural characteristics of children with vocal nodules: WPBIC Ratings. *Journal of Speech and Hearing Disorder, 54,* 306–312.

18. Grundfast, K. M., & Harley, E. (1989). Vocal fold paralysis. *Otolaryngological Clinics of North America, 22,* 569–597.

19. Hischberg, J., Dejonckere, P. H., Hirano, M. et al (1995). Voice disorders in children. *International Journal Pediatric Otolaryngology* (Supplement 32 - S10925).

20. Kahane, J. C. (1982). Growth of the human pre-pubertal and pubertal larynx. *Journal of Speech and Hearing Research, 25,* 446–455.

21. Kazarian, A. G., Sarkissian, L. S., & Isaakian, D. G. (1987). Length of the human vocal cords by age. (Russian). *Zhurnal Eksperimentalnoi I Klinicheskoi Meditsiny, 18,* 105–109.

22. Kent, R. D., & Vorperian, H. K. (1995). Development of the craniofacial-oral-laryngeal anatomy: A review. *Journal of Medical Speech-Language Pathology, 3*(3), 145–190.

23. Kozak, F. K., Freeman, R. D., Connolly, J. E., & Riding, K. H. (1989). Tourette syndrome and Otolaryngology. *Journal of Otolaryngology, 18,* 279–282.

24. Lancer, J. M. (1988). Vocal fold nodules: A review. *Clinical Otolaryngology, 13,* 43–51.

25. Maddern, B. R., Campbell, T. F., & Stool, S. (1991). Pediatric voice disorders. *Otolaryngologic Clinics of North America, 24,* 1125–1140.

26. McFarlane, S. C., & Watterson, T. L. (1990). Vocal nodules: Endoscopic study of their variations and treatment. *Seminars in Speech and Language, 11*(1), 47–59.

27. McWilliams, B. (1969). Diagnostic implications of vocal fold nodules in children with cleft palate. *Laryngoscope, 79,* 2072–2080.

28. Nemec, J. (1961). The motivation background of hyperkinetic dysphonia in children: A contribution to psychologic research in phoniatry. *Logos, 4,* 28–31.

29. Pizzuto, M., Emami, A. J., Simon, D. & Brodsky, L. (In press). Management of voice disorders in children.

30. Reilly, J. S. (1997). The "singing-acting" child: The laryngologist's perspective. *Journal of Voice, 11*(2), 126–129.

31. Steward, D. J. (1995). *Manual of Pediatric Anaesthesia,* (4th ed., pp. 223–247). New York: Churchill Livingstone.

32. Toohill, R. J. (1975). The psychosomatic aspects of children with nodules. *Archives of Otolaryngology, 101,* 591–595.

33. Van Dyke, D. C. (1984). Speech and language disorders in children. *Annals of Family Practice, 29,* 257–268.

34. Von Leden, H. (1985). Vocal nodules in children. *Ear, Nose and Throat Journal, 64,* 29–41.

35. Wilson, D. K. (1987). *Voice Problems in Children.* Baltimore: Williams & Wilkins.

36. Wilson, F. B., & Lamb, M. M. (1973). Comparison of personality characteristics of children with and without vocal nodules on Rorschach protocol interpretation. *Acta Symbolica, 5,* 43–55.

37. Wirz, S. (1992). The voice of the deaf. In M. Fawcus (Ed.) *Voice Disorders and their Management* (2nd ed.). San Diego: Singular Publishing Group, Inc.

Recommended Reading:

Andrews, M. L. (1991). *Voice Therapy for Children.* San Diego: Singular Publishing Group, Inc.

Dejonckere, P. H. (1984). Pathogenesis of voice disorders in childhood. *Acta Otorhinolaryngologica (Belgica), 38,* 307–314.

Fawcus, M. (1992). *Voice Disorders and their Management,* (2nd ed.) San Diego: Singular Publishing Group, Inc.

Maddern, B. R., Campbell, T. F., & Stool, S. (1991). Pediatric voice disorders. *Otolaryngologic Clinics of North America, 24,* 1125–1140.

CHAPTER

Issues in Vocal Pedagogy

7.1 Introduction: The Voice Teacher in the Voice Clinic

The voice teacher is a valuable member of the voice care team and, when interacting in a patient evaluation with the laryngologist and speech-language pathologist, and the psychiatrist, can provide extremely useful insights, particularly with the detection of errors in vocal production. The voice teacher may also provide guidance toward finding techniques that reduce vocal misuse and work directly with the singer to rebuild the voice.

7.2 Detecting Technical Errors in Vocal Production

7.2.1 Visual Observation

The first and in some ways the most reliable method of detecting errors in a singer's or actor's vocal production is observation. What should a voice teacher look for in a vocal performer with a voice-disorder? In addition to postural misuses described in Chapters 1 and 2 that may be associated with speech, specific attention should be paid to certain areas during vocal performance.

7.2.1.1 Head and Neck

The posture of the head and neck is a critical factor in body alignment, and any misalignment not only provides a visual clue to faulty technique but also is often the cause of it. The head often is held stiffly on a neck that is either hyperflexed or hyperextended. The chin can either be tucked in with the head pulled down or thrust forward with the head tilted upward. Sometimes the head is held at an angle to the left or right side or it may be observed to shake (often in time to a forced vibrato). Hypertonicity can cause the muscles and even the blood vessels in the neck to stand out in relief.

7.2.1.2 Spine, Knees, and Body Balance

The body often is seen to be held rigidly with braced knees and a "sway back" posture. Balance may be poor because of unnatural weight distribution that is either too far forward or backward in the stance. The body begins to sway halfway through a phrase so the weight distribution is constantly changing.

7.2.1.3 Shoulders and Chest

The shoulders may be held tensely so the chest is constricted, particularly on longer phrases. As the chest collapses during a sung phrase, the shoulders may fall forward. The opposite action also can be observed where shoulders are pulled back behind a firmly raised chest in a military "at attention."

7.2.1.4 Arms and Hands

The arms may be held rigidly with the elbows out and away from the body, assisting in depressing the chest and tensing the shoulders. The arm tension often leads to tense involuntary hand gestures during a phrase or song, or to the hands being rigidly clasped in front of or behind the body.

7.2.1.5 Face and Lips

The face often will give telltale signs of inappropriate tensions, such as the brow furrowing or frowning; the eyebrows twitching or lifting suddenly as a singer approaches certain pitches; or the expression of the eyes showing apprehension, fright, or even terror. These tensions, in addition to revealing the vocal performer's state of mind, often accompany postural faults of the neck and upper back. The lips can form exaggerated shapes and will sometimes quiver. They may seem to be harshly or aggressively set so the face adopts a fixed and often dramatically inappropriate expression. They can also be pulled strongly away from the teeth in a "snarl" or held very firmly over the teeth. These actions, which can be the product of some exaggerated concept of resonance or articulation, also seem to be a byproduct of neck and jaw misuse.

7.2.1.6 Tongue

Commonly, the tongue may retract by bunching up and withdrawing the tip away from the lower teeth or with the tip tilting up toward the roof of the mouth. This latter action often is observed on the higher notes. In more extreme cases, the tongue may withdraw into the mouth so that it is never visible, even on the most open vowels.

7.2.1.7 Larynx and Jaw

The larynx position can be a sign of vocal strain if it appears to be forced down when the chin is depressed or pulled up when the jaw is thrust forward. Some singers use an exaggerated depression of the larynx to produce a darker, more dramatic tonal quality. The musculature beneath the chin (the suprahyoid muscles) may be hypertonic in association with inappropriate larynx and jaw positions.

7.2.1.8 Breathing Patterns

Breathing patterns provide auditory and visual cues to vocal disorders. Noisy inhalation with a change in body balance and weight distribution will indicate an accumulation of tensions from the previous vocal phrase and often point to technical problems much more far-reaching than just the act of breathing. Inhalation accompanied by sudden changes in facial expression could herald similar problems, especially with respect to head, neck, and jaw usage. Inhalation accompanied by a sudden upward jerk of the head or raising of the shoulders may indicate breathing patterns that are focused too high in the torso and do not emphasize the essential lower rib, upper abdominal action.

7.2.2 Auditory Observation

Although a wide variety of tonal and articulatory demands are reflected in different vocal styles, some general guidelines can be given for identifying poor vocal production based on the quality of the vocal sound.

7.2.2.1 Diction

Words may be distorted and unclear in midrange singing. Factors leading to indistinct articulation include vowel shapes that are very different from those used in speech; different pronunciations of the same vowel within the same phrase or sequence of phrases; little or no movement of the jaw and lips during singing; inconsistent vowel quality (some appear to be very bright and abrasive, others dark and indistinct); and very exaggerated, unnatural movements of the lips and jaw during vocal performance.

7.2.2.2 Tone Quality

The tone may be breathy and lack clarity. Some vowels may be breathier than others. Additionally, the tone may be very different in quality from the top to the bottom of a 1 octave scale. Resonance of the voice may sound hollow or booming, or forced and constricted. Voice quality may be harsh and strident, rather than vibrant and warm.

7.2.2.3 Range

High notes may seem resonant only when they are very loud. The pitch range may be limited. The chest voice register is sometimes forced too high and sounds coarse and ugly. Sometimes a man's voice cannot find any falsetto register, or a woman's voice only functions in chest register.

7.2.2.4 Pitch

The pitch sometimes becomes sharp with increased or decreased volume, or it flattens with increased or decreased volume. Lower notes may be sharp and higher notes flat (in the female voice the reverse of this often can be the case).

7.2.2.5 Vibrato

The tone may be shrill and very straight. The voice may have a fast, nervous-sounding flutter (**tremolo**) or may waver over a wide space in a slow, exaggerated vibrato. The head may shake with vibrato, or the chest or abdomen may shake in time with the vibrato. Sometimes vibrato appears only at the end of a note. A young singer often will use a breathy and straight tone at first. This is a symptom of inexperience and lack of coordination, rather than a vocal problem.

7.2.2.6 Summary of Audible Errors in Vocal Production

➤ Although ugliness of tone is a subjective judgement and often related to the style of vocal performance, many singers with serious errors in vocal production do make an "ugly" sound. (Actors and hard rock or heavy metal singers may be called upon to make a harsh or ugly sound, and must ensure they produce it without undue strain on the vocal mechanism).

➤ Good singing should never betray great strain. Much romantic opera involves very demanding singing, but the object of technique is to make it appear controlled and easy rather than strained, shouted, or squeezed out under great pressure. Certainly there should be no evidence of great tension and strain in basic middle range scales and exercises.

➤ The resonance of the voice should be consistent throughout the range, in spite of the necessary shift in tonal quality that a voice must experience as it travels from the bottom to the top of its range.

➤ Singers should have no difficulty singing quietly and should not have to vocalize with great exertion to produce a loud tone.

➤ The words should always be clear in a comfortable midrange.

➤ The vibrato should sound natural and appropriate to the volume, range, and style of the singing.

7.3 Correcting Errors in Vocal Production

For a vocal performer, it is relatively useless to be told what not to do unless such an edict is accompanied by clear directives about what should be done. Such directives as: "Don't force," "Don't tighten your neck," "Don't breathe so high," "Don't let your posture sag," "You don't support enough," and so forth—although no doubt well meant—often do not lead to successful changes in activity because they only address what is not to be done and give no clear indications of what precisely should be happening. Only when vocal performers can make their own comparisons between one form of usage and another can a successful basis for change be established. The task of the voice trainer, therefore, is to lead the vocal performer to the experience of efficient and desirable usage of the vocal instrument. Herein lies the skill and the art of a good voice teacher, but unfortunately also the grounds for much pedagogical dispute. For example, there is a considerable body of thought that suggests it is not a good training strategy to make a singer aware of the activity of specific muscle groups during the act of singing. The argument is based on the belief that this strategy will cause the singer to tense the particular group more than it is already. The opposite side of this debate asks how can singers change the behavior of a muscle group if they have no idea what it is doing in the first place?

In the pedagogy of the former philosophy, one finds many techniques that are used to distract the singer away from the physical actions of singing. The hope is that, when distracted, singers will release some of the inhibitory behaviors that are causing inappropriate muscle use. The opposing philoso-phy may result in use of a more direct approach: giving specific directions as to what to do with the breathing apparatus, the tongue, the laryngeal position, the vowel form, the posture, and so forth.

If one can examine this situation objectively, there appears to be a point where both these approaches arrive at the same place. Regardless of whether vocal performers have traveled the distraction or the specific direction route, there is a need, when they arrive at a correct usage, to establish a clear sensory awareness of the new set of behaviors that they have established. This feedback mechanism is integral to the motor learning principles discussed in Chapter 4 and is what vocal performers must be able to apply each time they sing. If an intellectual understanding of what is going on can reinforce sensory awareness, so much the better, but this will always remain a matter of individual choice. It must be added, as a heartfelt opinion, that for any vocal performers who wish to go on to be teachers at some time in their careers, the intellectual understanding of precisely what is going on is not just a good idea, but an absolute necessity.

Once one becomes aware that there are necessary meeting points in vocal pedagogies, then many of the pedagogic disputes will be recognized as either differences in style or in the route taken toward the same goal. Students' first and perhaps most important task is to choose the style and the route that is most compatible with their needs and personality. In this text, we have chosen to offer suggestions that hail from both sides of the pedagogical argument.

7.4 Singing Pedagogy

Every culture uses the singing voice and, although the mechanism is similar (as far as we know), the cultural traditions of voice production are as different as the faces, languages, and ceremonies of the peoples of the world. In the Western tradition of classical music, there are some broadly accepted norms of what makes good and bad singing and what is healthy and unhealthy vocal behavior. Even within this tiny part of Western culture, there is enormous disagreement about the details of vocal production, and singing teachers have the reputation of being unable to agree with each other unless they belong to the same school of pedagogy. Before stating what is unequivocally "right" in singing technique and how a voice teacher should go about achieving it, it is important to establish clear terms of reference.

It is important for any voice teacher to decide whether the primary objective of voice training is to produce a singer who is maximizing the potential of the voice while gaining understanding of the process or one who is producing a series of slightly imperfect clones of the teacher's own voice. The teacher's aim should be to become redundant. The voice teacher is not dealing with a verifiable scientific experiment; there is no control subject because voices will develop in size and quality with increasing age and experience even if nothing happens to interfere with the natural process. Most important, the teacher is rarely in the position to deal with what one might delicately call a "vocal virgin." Singers always have sung before having lessons and have picked up along the way a complex amalgam of influences including those from parental singing, live and media performances, and participation in choirs and other ensembles. These all contribute to the development of a vocal personality and a singing technique. Genetic, linguistic, and cultural factors also play an important part in establishing a pattern of vocal behavior.

In training the singing voice, some general rules can be applied:

➤ Singing should be perceived by the audience as a free and natural activity. Despite its mechanical and energy requirements, singers must never display to their audience overt signs of the effort involved in the production and sustaining of vocal tone.

➤ Singing must be practiced in the same way that other musical instruments are practiced, and singers must know what and why they are practicing. Motor skills take time and perseverance to develop fully. From the investment of time and energy, singers should emerge with a solid vocal technique that will give them knowledgeable control over the mechanics and expressiveness of their voices.

➤ Vocal technique must never be an end in itself, however fascinating and engrossing the subject becomes. Singers are athletes, not bodybuilders. Most of us have had the experience of sitting through hours of technically well-schooled vocal production from a singer with no glimmer of musical intelligence or understanding. We have also been bowled over by a singer with some vocal problems, but great intensity and deep musical understanding. Singing, after all, developed in humans as a musical expression of emotions.

➤ Singing teachers should never try to make silk purses out of sows' ears. Natural talent is the most important factor in determining the ultimate potential of a voice. All voices have their individual natural limitations and a teacher's primary goal should be to help singers to reach their own potential.

The world of vocal pedagogy contains numerous conflicting ideas of how the singing voice works and how it should be trained. In the context of this book, it is not possible or appropriate to attempt to lay out a complete method of voice production. Despite the diversity of opinion, we believe that it is possible to set some basic principles with which most teachers would agree and that form the basis of esthetically pleasing and healthy voice production.

7.4.1 Posture

Good posture is of central importance to good singing, yet it often is either neglected or curiously distorted. How we organize our bodies in space and how we habitually use them in daily life is in accordance with usage patterns that have evolved over the course of our lives. These patterns that have developed since early childhood usually have grown not from a careful consideration of the most efficient and effective way to carry out a specific physical task, but from a process that evolves as each task is accomplished. It is only when we decide to pursue athletic or artistic activities that require high levels of skill, dexterity, and stamina that a qualitative evaluation of the physical organization and usage patterns becomes necessary.

7.4.1.1 Posture and Singing Performance

Public performance is filled with stress and physical fatigue, further complicated by the need to create credible characterizations and emotional body language that often is quite different from the performer's own nature. It is clear that to comply with the physical needs of transforming the body into a sophisticated musical instrument and of maintaining that instrument through the rigorous demands of a performing life, postural organization must not be left to the devices of habitual patterns that could lead to misuse.

One's posture is something that can be consciously organized and controlled, and would-be singers must assume responsibility for their correct posture if they hope to be successful. A thorough understanding of existing habit patterns and a knowledge of what must be readjusted in the best interest of singing is

required. There is in singing, as in dance and in most athletic activities, a position of "at the ready," of preparedness, the place from which something muscular and coordinated can happen. This is not a fixed position, but one of poise and balance from which easy movement can take place. The question is, how do we get there? The general principles of natural alignment presented in Chapters 1 and 4 apply equally to vocal performance.

7.4.1.2 Checklist of Good Posture for Singing

The following points (after Alexander[1] and Barlow[3]) will ensure good posture for singing (see Figure 1–15a, Chapter 1):

➤ the head is balanced comfortably at the top of the spine
➤ the back of the neck is lengthened, and the front of the neck is loose
➤ the jaw is relaxed, and the chin is level
➤ the spine feels long
➤ the back is "open" with maximum space between the shoulder blades
➤ the shoulders are released down and at maximum width
➤ the chest is comfortably raised and expanded
➤ the upper abdomen is loose with the lower abdomen moving gently in and up to maintain the position of the pelvis (the pelvis should not be in an exaggerated tucked position)
➤ the knees are not locked
➤ the body weight is distributed evenly on both the soles and heels of the feet
➤ the body weight is balanced from front to back and from side to side

From this poised, balanced position, the singer is ready to begin the cycle of activities that is responsible for creating and sustaining the singing voice. That cycle begins with the breath.

7.4.2 Breathing

In the world of singing pedagogy, breathing and breath management are subjects of much dispute, and a great deal of creative imagination has gone into methods proposed by various pedagogical schools. There is more than one way that breath can be generated by the respiratory system to create and sustain a given pitch[8]. A detailed presentation of the functions of the respiratory system is provided in Chapter 8.

7.4.2.1 Breathing for Vocal Performance

When one moves from speech-breathing to breathing for vocal performance, differing physical and acoustic requirements must be met. The first of these concerns the implications of the larger lung volumes that are necessary to sustain steady musical phrases. To understand this, we must first review some of the facts relating to normal respiration and then compare them with the requirements of singing.

If a normal man took in a full inhalation, he would have in his lungs a total volume of between 6 and 7 liters. If he then exhaled as much air as he could, between 1.5 and 2 liters would still remain in his lungs. This difference of approximately 5 liters between the total lung capacity (TLC) of 7 liters and the residual volume (RV) of 2 liters is referred to as the vital capacity (VC).

We see in Chapter 8 that the full range of VC is not often called into use; in fact the "tidal volume" used in quiet respiration is quite small, approximately .5 liters (Figure 7–1). We breathe by means of a balanced mechanical system that contains both inspiratory and expiratory forces acting as natural antagonists to each other. Inhalation during rest breathing is a result of active muscle contractions expanding the lung volume, while exhalation is relatively passive, principally

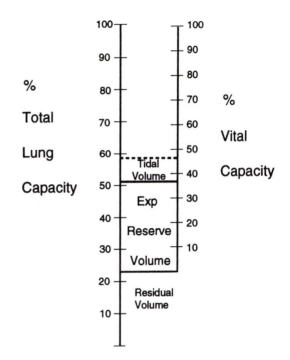

Figure 7–1. Diagram of lung capacities. Adapted from Proctor[10] with permission.

relying on the elastic recoil in the ribs and lungs and the relaxation of the diaphragm to return to the functional residual capacity.

The mechanical patterns for speech-breathing described in Chapter 8 are much more complex than those of tidal rest breathing. We note that both passive and active forces contribute to normal speech-breathing efforts. Speech at normal loudness and effort levels usually starts around 55% VC level and terminates around 35% VC level, thus using about 20% of the VC, or approximately 1 liter.

In singing and theatrical speech, lung volume requirements are often much greater, sometimes close to 100% VC in long phrases or very loud vocal productions. Control of pressure and airflow rates over this volume range is more difficult because the positive and negative elastic recoil forces of the lung tissue, thorax, and abdomen have much greater values, and these forces influence the patterns of active forces applied to the respiratory system.

Proctor has shown that after a maximum inhalation to TLC, the passive elastic expiratory force of the lungs is approximately 20 cm H_2O and that of the rib cage is 10 cm H_2O[10]. This means that if uncontrolled, these two elastic forces alone can deliver a pressure of 30 cm H_2O at the onset of the expiratory cycle. This becomes of major technical significance to the singer when it is realized that only very loud singing requires this pressure. Most singing requires pressures in the range 5 to 20 cm H_2O, and so it is clear that without control, the system is applying excess pressure against the closed vocal folds (Figure 7–2). Whatever techniques singers choose to adopt, to be safe and effective they must control this elastic recoil and its attendant pressure levels, and present air to the larynx at a pressure appropriate for the desired pitch and loudness (dynamic) level.

The solid line in Figure 7–2 represents the summation of the passive recoil forces gener-

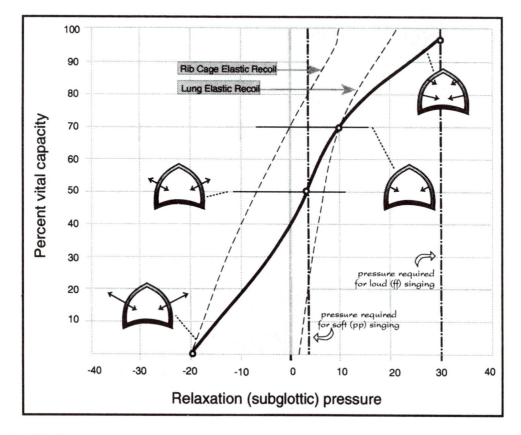

Figure 7–2. Pressures against closed vocal folds owing to elastic recoil. Adapted from Sundberg[12] and Zemlin[15] with permission.

ated by the rib cage and lungs. If the singer were to begin a vocal tone at a pianissimo dynamic after a full breath, he or she would, at this moment of onset, have to cope with an overpressure of approximately 25 cm H_2O, and this overpressure would continue to need controlling until the lung capacity was reduced to 55% VC. After this point, a continuing tone would need expiratory effort to supply an adequate air pressure to the larynx. If, however, the starting dynamic had been mezzo forte, requiring a 20 cm H_2O pressure level to sustain it, the overpressure would only exist down to approximately 86% VC, after which the expiratory forces would need to assist.

With the constant changes of pitch and dynamic and the ever-varying lung capacities that exist while the singer is in action, it can be seen clearly that the method of respiratory control that the singer adopts must be one of great flexibility and that any kind of system rigidity would render the necessary subtle actions impossible.

There is a common tendency among singers to give a deliberate inward kick with the abdominal musculature either at the onset of tone or as an aid to upward pitch change. The effect of this action is to drive the diaphragm upward against the base of the lungs and so significantly increase the pressure of the contained air. If not carefully controlled, this action will destroy the essential balance between the desired subglottal pressure and pitch, as well as the vocal fold adduction activities of the larynx.

Sundberg indicated that a combination of the elastic recoil, muscle-driven rib descent, and diaphragm ascent can generate subglottal pressures in excess of 150 cm of water[12]. This means that the respiratory system is capable of delivering pressures that are five times greater than those needed for most loud singing and almost eight times that required for an average vocal tone.

7.4.2.2 Techniques for the Control of Breathing

Breath control techniques for singing must create a balance between the pressure potential of the forces of exhalation and the desired subglottal pressure. It must be a flexible arrangement that constantly changes with varying pitch and dynamic requirements and with lung volume. There is evidence to suggest that muscles of inspiration are recruited as the natural antagonist to the expiratory forces during phonation. The external intercostals and diaphragm may be most involved in creating the necessary balance of forces.

Watson and Hixon found, during their study of classical singers, that there was a major discrepancy between the way their subjects thought they breathed and their observed patterns[14]. Some singers can easily become tense and awkward if they try to think mechanically, but the process of inhalation for a singer must become more conscious than that for nonsingers so that a full, relaxed breath is taken without extraneous tension.

Breathing in Supine Position. For many singers, the easiest way to gain a sense of the breathing apparatus is to lie flat on the back with a book supporting the head, legs bent with knees pointing upward, jaw relaxed open, and breathing naturally (Figure 7–3). In

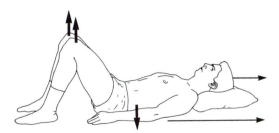

Figure 7–3. Body in the supine position for breathing exercise.

this position, where the alignment of the spine and the position of the thorax is aided by the support of the floor, they will experience expansion at the belt line and in the lower ribs on inhalation. On exhalation, they will feel the initiative taken by the muscles of the epigastric umbilical region of the abdomen to direct the outflow of the air. They will also note that there is little or no rise and fall of the upper chest during the breathing cycle.

Exercise

At a moderate tempo, breathe in for 5 counts, suspend the action for 5 counts, and then exhale for 5 counts. One should feel a complete and unforced expansion of the ribs and upper abdomen during the inhalation phase. The zone of maximum activity will be observed to be between the bottom of the sternum and the navel and to extend all round the body to include the sides and the back. The lips should remain parted during the suspension phase, and there should be no feeling of the breath being held rigidly. The position of the ribs and upper abdomen should be comfortably retained. During exhalation, the position of the sternum and the rib cage should be maintained as long as possible and only allowed to fall if necessary at the very end of the breath supply. The number of counts for each phase of the exercise can be increased steadily with growing efficiency up to a count of 10.

Variations can be made in the count patterns to develop the idea of the shorter inspirations and longer exhalations that musical compositions demand. Quicker inspiration and shorter suspension phases followed by a longer expiratory phase brings the sequence closer to the requirements of normal singing. Additional exercises can be introduced, sustaining for as long as comfortably possible the sibilant /s/ or the fricative /f/.

Breathing in Standing Position. The sensations and movement patterns that were experienced in the supine position should be retained as much as possible when the singer moves into standing position. There obviously will be some physical implications of gravitational down-drag, but the body alignment

should be similar, and most of the feelings learned in the supine position can be transferred to this upright position.

Exercise

Raise the arms above the head, bringing the sternum and ribs into a moderately high position. Allow the arms to fall back to the sides while the rib-sternum position is retained. The sternum should not be too high; this can be checked by seeing if it can be pushed even higher. From this comfortably high position, it should be possible to breathe in and out easily without any rise or fall of the upper chest position. The previous exercises should then be experienced in this new upright position.

Expiratory Phase of the Breath Cycle. The expiratory phase of the breath cycle is best considered in relation to phonation. It is at this point that most of the discord in singing pedagogy occurs because of the need to develop a technique for controlling elastic recoil, airflow, and subglottal pressures. The various schools of pedagogy instruct singers to push out with the stomach muscles, to keep the ribs expanded, to support, to pull the belly in, and even to contract the muscles in their buttocks, all in the cause of achieving the desired control. A great deal of damage is done by this pushing and straining, in fact, more vocal problems are caused by forceful exhalation than by using the voice with no support at all.

7.4.2.3 *Summary of Breathing for Singing*

It is a natural feature of the singing instrument that when a balance between the inspiratory and expiratory forces has been established, the instrument can regulate the airflow rates and pressure values in direct response to the mental demands for pitch and dynamic. It is the singer's responsibility to establish and maintain a physical environment wherein the subtle aerodynamic changes can take place.

Meribeth Bunch aptly summed up the breath action as follows:

> Support of tone is dependent upon maintenance of subglottic pressure. This is done by maintaining the inspiratory position of the rib cage for as long as possible while contracting the abdominal muscles and gradually relaxing the diaphragm. The inspiratory position of the rib cage implies a comfortably high (but not fixed or rigid) chest position so that there is no interference with the vibratory mechanism and no counteraction of expiratory effort. Maintenance of the inspiratory position ensures that at the onset of sound the inspiratory muscles remain in action, checking the elastic recoil of the lungs and rib cage[4].

7.4.2.4 Checklist of General Principles for Good Breath Management

➤ Breathing for singing is dynamic, physical, and muscular, rather than passive and uninvolved. It involves muscular antagonism.

➤ The singer needs an accurate concept of what takes place in the body during the process of breathing in and out. Although many of the same muscles are involved, it is different from weightlifting, vomiting, childbirth, and excretory functions.

➤ Strength and air capacity are of little importance; coordination, skill, and experience are the main requirements. The action of the breathing mechanism should be so flexible that it will allow a new breath to be taken whenever the musical score presents an opportunity.

➤ Singers should not try to inhibit the flow of breath in singing phrases; rather, they should allow the breath to move at all times. Let the voice "call upon" the breath.

➤ Singers should not let the head position be affected by the attack or the release of the note.

➤ Singers should not push or aggressively attempt to support the sound.

7.4.3 Onset and Release of Vocal Tone

7.4.3.1 Onset

The most critical moment in the act of singing is the onset of the vocal tone. The term onset is used in preference to the more frequently used term "attack" because the latter is too suggestive of the clumsy and aggressive action that is at the root of so many singers' vocal problems. At this crucial moment, the total singing instrument must be coordinated, balanced, and finely tuned to the desired pitch, vowel, and tonal quality. In the midst of such a complex operation, the potential for imbalances and problems is great.

Sequence of Events at Tonal Onset. At the end of a full inhalation, the breath pressure in the lungs is equal to that of the surrounding atmosphere. The adductor muscles of the larynx move the vocal folds from their open inspiratory position, to a position where they meet at the midline and close the airway. Also at this time, they are adjusted in length and tension to enable them to vibrate at the desired f_0. Once the airway is closed by the vocal folds, the pressure can be adjusted to meet the pressure requirements of the desired pitch and dynamics. When this is established, vocal fold vibrations can be initiated.

There are three kinds of onset that one observes in singing, which we will label as the **soft** onset, the **hard** onset, and the **balanced** onset. One of these yields good results, another is inefficient, and the third is unhealthy. The type of voice onset used is determined by the timing, positioning, and tension of the vocal fold actions.

Soft Onset. In the soft onset, the sequence of events is slightly rearranged in that there is a flow of breath that precedes the closure of the glottis producing an aspirate /h/ sound. Visual observation often reveals an exaggerated opening in the posterior glottis. The tonal effect is that of a soft, breathy, whispery quality, lacking both vibrancy and dynamic potential. The spectral characteristics of a breathy voice are presented in Chapter 8, Figure 8–16c. This type of onset may represent chronic misuse of the laryngeal mechanism, described in Chapter 2 as the laryngeal isometric.

Hard Onset. This is an action that is deserving of the word "attack." It is produced when the vocal folds are strongly adducted before phonation. The exaggerated adduction and medial compression forces result in high laryngeal resistance, thus demanding higher subglottal breath pressure to initiate phonation. The resulting glottal plosive is an audible, unmusical preface to the sung tone. This kind of onset places considerable stress on the mechanism and carries potential for vocal fold damage. A similar chronic misuse may be noted in the speaking voice as glottal attacks.

Balanced Onset. The desirable, balanced onset occupies a position between these two extremes, and it produces a vibrant, full, resonant tone that has a distinct beginning and is free of any preliminary breathiness or launching bump. W.J. Henderson, the American critic and singing expert who wrote on singing for the *New York Sun* and the *New York Times* from the mid 1880s until 1937 regarded the great soprano Nelli Melba as having the ideal vocal onset. At the time of her death in 1931, he wrote in the *New York Times*:

> The Melba attack was little short of marvelous. The term attack is not a good one. Melba indeed had no attack; she opened her

mouth and a tone was in existence. It began without ictus, when she wished it to, and without betrayal of breathing. It simply was there. When she wished to make a bold attack, as in the trio of the last scene of "Faust," she made it with the clear silvery stroke of a bell[7].

In the balanced onset, the breathing mechanism stays in the expanded suspension position at the moment of onset, and there is no inward movement of the umbilical epigastric region to destroy the balance between the vocal fold tension and the subglottal air pressure that has been established under the mental demand for pitch and dynamic. The result is a clean onset of sound that the singer often achieves by imagining a small aspirate /h/ before the sound but not allowing it to be audible and by eliminating any sense of breath expulsion. In Section 4.4.6 of Chapter 4, the same principles are described to produce the **coordinated voice onset** (CVO) for speech. The relevant research and models of phonatory physiology that are supportive of the concept of **balanced** or **coordinated** voice onset are also discussed in Chapter 4.

It is the manner of onset that determines the vocal sound that must follow, and the quality, intonation, carrying power, ease, and flexibility of the tone in the ensuing vocal phrase is determined at this moment.

7.4.3.2 Release

If the onset is the most critical moment in singing, then the end of the tone—the release—is a close second in terms of importance. The release of a tone should be crisp and clean, with the glottis returning to the fully abducted position of deep inhalation. In other words, the release of the tone triggers a renewal of the breath, which in turn begins a new onset cycle of vocal tone. As was the case with the onset action, there are two undesirable forms of the release in addition to the ideal clean, crisp action. Again, it is possible to have a hard and a soft version of the activity.

A hard gruntlike release causes the muscles to retain tension and prevents the vocal folds from returning to the fully abducted deep breathing position, thus delaying breath recovery and efficient adduction of the vocal folds. In the more common soft release, the muscle action is released slowly and the opening action is delayed, again slowing down the breath renewal action. This is further compounded by the fact that the sloppy, soft, release is usually accompanied by a collapse of the breathing mechanism, and visible changes of posture are necessary during attempts to renew the breath.

Exercises for the onset of tone were a feature of the training manuals of the early singing schools. These consist of vocal-eases using sustained or staccato repeated notes on single or varying pitches, which enable repeated practice of the cycle of onset and release. The ideas that are stressed in these exercises include clean onset, crisp release, and immediate breath renewal at the cessation of sound. These exercise sequences are still used extensively to condition the muscles responsible for vocal fold approximation and glottal flexibility and encourage quick, silent breath renewal.

7.4.4 Resonance

For singing, as for speaking, the sound that the vocal instrument produces is a direct product of the user's tonal imagination exercised within the limits of a naturally endowed physical framework. Speech precedes singing, and with some exceptions, a fine singing voice will be signaled by a fine speaking voice. The size of the voice, its ruggedness, and its resonance potential are basic features of the natural gift, but every singer can maximize the resonance and color of the voice. Beauty of tone is not only a feature of natural gift, it is the result of balanced reso-

nance with unforced, comfortable tone. Unfortunately, many problems arise from the singer's desire to maximize the power and carrying capacity of the voice at the expense of natural free resonance and other, more subtle features.

What must be understood about the singing voice is that it is an instrument that can, for our purposes, be considered to house two vibrating systems: the vocal folds and the air contained in the vocal tract above the larynx (refer to Figures 8–1, 8–9 to 8–14, 8–19, 8–20). Each of these is adjustable, the former by the actions of the intrinsic laryngeal musculature and the latter by adjustments in the size and configuration of the oral and pharyngeal spaces which use the tongue, palate, jaw, and lips to respond to demands for vowel and tonal texture or quality. What is essential for the best quality of sound is that these two systems vibrate in sympathy with each other. Failure to find this sympathetic relationship will be revealed in tones that are lacking in vibrancy, beauty, clarity, and freedom.

To produce a singing tone of acceptable aesthetic quality, the resonance system of the voice selects for enhancement those harmonics from the laryngeal signal that are sympathetic with the overtone series of the desired sung pitch. Only a resonance system that is sympathetically tuned to the frequency of the vibrator can successfully carry out these processes of selection and enhancement. An unsympathetic resonator would be inclined to either enhance the wrong things or to be limited in the extent to which it could enhance the harmonics of the sung pitch. The tonal result would be ugly, weak, or both. For the singer, the feeling would be one of effort, discomfort, and lack of freedom.

7.4.4.1 Tonal Concept as a Control Factor

The major control factor in bringing about this sympathetic relationship between the glottal source vibrator and that of the resonance system is the singer's concept of vocal tone. This tonal model is a mental concept based on imagery and experience and ranks in importance with voice onset and release. It is the device the brain uses to trigger major muscular adjustments in the resonance system, and its model must be appropriate to the natural physical parameters of the instrument and to the aesthetic objectives of the vocal tone.

There are many ways in which this crucial technical requirement can go astray, and in almost every case the cause has its genesis in the singer's desire to create a tonal sound that is not appropriate to his or her natural instrument. A common case is a desire to produce a bigger sound than one can accommodate. Additionally, the tonal model often is distorted by singers who want to make their voices sound like that of their favorite artist, regardless of differences in their age and physical endowment. Among opera singers, the dramatic and tessitura demands of an unsuitable role cause the singer to seek an inappropriate tone. Among pop singers, it is the urge to copy, for obvious monetary reasons, the sound of those who are commercially successful.

The model that the singer creates must contain within it several factors all of which must be appropriate to the natural endowment of the singer in question, including the size, color, emotional quality, and dramatic intent of the tone, plus a precise definition of vowel form and pitch. Any miscalculation in the concept of these elements can have serious implications for the freedom and dynamics of the vocal instrument. For example, attempts to sing too big a tonal sound invariably lead to generation of an excessive respiratory driving pressure and defensive hypervalving in the larynx. This aggressive action of the breath and the consequent laryngeal reaction is highly fatiguing for the larynx and leads to a tonal sound that is shouty and usually faulty in pitch. Attempts to create an inappropriately dramatic sound have some of the problems of the previously described fault pattern plus a tendency to overexaggerate the lower harmonics in the spectrum, making the tonal sound heavy with poor pitch and vowel definition. On the other hand many singers, in their attempts to sing quietly, allow the sound to lose its vibrancy, with weak adduction of the vocal folds and inadequate subglottal pressure that leads to a breathy tone and erratic intonation.

7.4.4.2 An Approach to Vocal Freedom and Tonal Modeling

Perhaps the most constructive approach is to assume that the voice will respond freely to the appropriate mental tonal model if muscle tensions in the throat, jaw, and tongue do not interfere with the natural, effective coordination of the breath and the larynx. The release of these tensions, should they exist, is directed by the singing teacher in a number of ways:

➤ The vowels should be formed with a loose jaw and a forward, relaxed tongue, allowing the resonance of the voice to grow as coordination with the breath increases.

➤ Onsets should be properly coordinated, with no breathiness nor with an exaggerated glottal attack. Staccato exercises have traditionally been used for this, as have long legato phrases for "seating" the vowel in the breath.

➤ Pitch and articulation should be flexible. When the voice is flexible, it is likely that there is good coordination and little unnecessary tension. Exercises in scales, arpeggios, and quick sequential patterns have traditionally helped singers become skillful and relaxed.

➤ Relaxed but refined speech should be practiced, and it should have technical similarities to singing.

Strategies for developing good resonance include the following:

➤ Development of appropriate tonal models: Let singers hear the accomplishments of other singers with similar voices and good techniques.

➤ Use of a variety of environments for singing and alterations of acoustic feedback of the singer's own voice by covering the ears, making a megaphone of the hands, and so forth.

➤ Use of tape recorders to show that the sounds a singer perceives as the most resonant are probably different from those the listener perceives as such.

7.4.5 Imagery in Vocal Pedagogy

In the world of singing pedagogy, extensive use is made of mental imagery to try and gain technical control over the instrument, and some of these images can be considered another aspect of modeling. Terms such as "focus" and "placement," "head voice" and "chest voice" all have the effect of influencing the relationship between the vibratory and the resonance systems of the voice. Although there may be some value to these images, in general they do not provide precise directives and as a result they are the source of much confusion and vocal abuse. Efforts to "place the voice in the mask," in the name of resonance and placement, often are ineffective and usually result in an ugly, pinched tone and a host of other problems.

Although there is potential for problems to develop from the use of ill-defined or vague imagery, it also must be recognized that it is through imagery that we gain access to the control of the voice. The previous discussion on tonal modeling and its influence on pitch, dynamics, and resonance makes that point.

The problem relates to those images that are inspired by the physical sensations that the singer experiences during the act of singing. Focus, placement, forward sound, backward sound, head voice, and chest voice are all products of the real sensory experiences of the singer in action. Unfortunately, many of the sensory impressions that a singer receives convey either vague or inaccurate information about the location or the specific events taking place.

7.4.5.1 Tonal Placement

A good example of this sensory experience is that of the singer who makes a ringing tonal sound having a good, strong **singer's formant** in the 2800–3500 Hz range. He or she often will experience strong sympathetic vibrations in the sinus regions. What the singer is actually experiencing is a strong resonance response from those cavities whose own natural frequencies happen to coincide with those of the singer's formant. To the singer, it feels as though the sound is securely placed "forward" and "in the mask," and it is hard to diminish the conviction that this secure feeling is merely a secondary factor and not the primary cause of such a desired and praised vocal tone. This could be nothing more than a harmless self-deception if it were not for the fact that many schools of vocal pedagogy devote time and effort in placing the vocal tone into particular sinus regions, sometimes, with little regard for what may be going on in the instrument to achieve this result. There are, in fact, several possible ways to achieve this sense of forward placement, some of which can have a negative effect on the singing voice. The sensation of forward placement that comes as a result of a well-produced vocal tone is real to the singer. What must be recognized is that the primary generator of these sensations is located elsewhere in the resonance system, in particular, in the laryngeal cavity.

7.4.5.2 Registers and Range

Similar confusion is created by the sympathetic sensations experienced in the cavities of the skull in the higher pitch range and the chest cavity in the lower pitch range, which gives rise to the images of head and chest voice. These sensory impressions have contributed significantly to widespread confusion in terminology and understanding of vocal registers, and it is hard to convince some singers that these sensations contribute nothing to the tonal quality of the sound product that the audience experiences.

7.4.5.3 Breath Support

The concept of "breath support" also appears to be born out of the singer's sensations of the activity in the lower thoracic and upper abdominal region. In the balanced breath suspension action described earlier, a support-like sensation is associated with the natural antagonistic actions of the diaphragmatic, thoracic, and abdominal musculature, and the intensity of this relationship varies with the rise and fall of pitch and tonal dynamic. Although this feeling of support is a very real sensation to the singer, it is imperative that the singer understand that this range of muscle activities is produced reflexively in response to the mental demands for pitch and dynamic. It must not be construed from these sensations that the way to control pitch or loudness is to deliberately push down on the diaphragm, pull in on the abdomen, or create various deliberate contortions with the thoracic muscles.

7.4.5.4 Open Throat

The concept of an "open throat" is another image that is much sought after by the singer and voice teacher. For the singer whose voice is working well, there is a sensation of freedom, openness, and space in the oropharyngeal cavities. What the singer is responding to is the absence of undesirable, constrictive tension in the system, usually in the posterior part of the tongue, the pharynx, and

within the larynx itself. To the singer the throat feels open, and this is desirable.

Many pedagogic notions are employed to try and remove potential obstructions and recreate this open-throated posture on a regular basis; these include flattening the tongue, raising the soft palate, inflating the pharynx, and lowering the larynx to various levels. Often the yawn reflex is coopted to assist in the cause. It is true that the yawn reflex, in the moment that it begins, causes a sense of release and a comfortable sense of easy increase in the size of the oropharyngeal cavity. If the process stops there, the image of a gentle yawn can have considerable pedagogic value. Because a true yawn reflex is by definition impossible to control, it typically continues to the next stage of its pattern, which is a major distention of the whole oropharyngeal space, tongue retraction, and maximum laryngeal lowering. All this newfound "yawny" space gives singers a feeling of openness of the throat, but all they really have is a retracted tongue, rigidity in the palate, an overly depressed larynx, and a distended pharynx. It may feel open, but in such an environment the essential singing activities of articulation and the constant readjustment of the resonance cavity coupling is rendered virtually impossible. This begs the question, what is the singer's "open throat"? The answer is; there is no such entity in the way we would like to imagine it.

7.4.5.5 Problems of Imagery

The problem with the use of imagery is that it is often inaccurate as a description of events and is usually sufficiently vague as to allow almost infinite interpretation. In 1931, Dr. G.O. Russell published in his book, *Speech and Voice*, some radiographic images of famous singers that were taken during the production of the vowel sounds /i/, /ɑ/, and /u/.[11] These were midsagittal views of the head showing the position of the tongue, palate, epiglottis, and the general configuration of the resonance tract. In 1959, he was able to identify the origin of some of these images: the great tenor Enrico Caruso, who apparently was so dismayed upon seeing them that he refused to allow his name to be associated with them. What concerned him was the fact that they did not bear out his own sensory perceptions: the /ɑ/ and /u/ vowels with their natural constriction between the back of the tongue and the back wall of the throat belied his sensory feeling of an open throat, and the complete closure of his palate did not show the resonance of the nasal passages being properly utilized. As Berton Coffin commented in *Overtones of Bel Canto* "He could not accept the truth of the matter—fancy being stronger than fact."[5]

Coffin also suggested by way of explanation that the so-called huge space of the /ɑ/ vowel in the throat is a fiction, and that, because of the small opening between the epiglottis and the back wall of the throat, a zone of high pressure is felt in this area that is probably what gives the singer a feeling of space.

7.4.5.6 *Images as a Teaching Tool*

The teacher never can be sure that the imagery and terminology used will trigger in the student the same sensations that it does in the teacher. It is important that teachers and singers work together to develop a vocal technique in which the sensations experienced by singers relate to the actual desired physiological and acoustical events. If this can be done, then the sensations that singers feel so strongly can become their confirmation of the correctness of their vocal actions. They can apply whatever imagery they like to these experiences. The images can then become the means that singers use to keep in contact with their instrument in the midst of the complexities and distractions of vocal performance.

If singers and voice teachers could develop a clearer understanding of cause and effect in vocal activity and an exact and direct technical language to communicate that understanding, a great deal could be done to clear away the confusion that bedevils the field of vocal pedagogy.

7.4.6 Registers

Vocal registers and the development of the singer's working range are so bound together that a lack of mechanical understanding and technical knowledge of the former can lead to serious limitations of access and usage of the latter. A review of available literature will quickly show that this is one of the areas of vocal technique about which there is much confusion and disagreement. The modern-day singer is confronted with a set of opinions regarding registers that range from the existence of no registers at all to the possibility of seven, the most popular theory being the idea of 2 registers for male voices and 3 registers for female voices. It is imperative to the development and vocal survival of singers that they make some effort to come to an understanding of this phenomenon and find a practical way to deal with it in their every day vocal activities. Failing to do so can lead to severe limitations in range and tonal quality. Even after singers arrive at some satisfactory concept of the number of registers existing in their voices, they are still confronted with the problem of what to call them.

7.4.6.1 *Register Terminology*

There has developed over time a terminology that, rather than clarifying the issue, has added to the confusion. Maybe the heart of the problem stems from attempts throughout much of the history of singing to explain and label the phenomenon of vocal registers from the point of view of the singer's sensations of physical and resonance phenomena. The understanding and terminology that stems from this process does little to help the singer come to terms with the physiological events that are actually taking place. Let us consider the singers' sensory experiences as they ascend through their vocal ranges. As one progresses from the bottom to the top of the pitch range, one experiences, at certain points in the progression, changes in sensory perception that give one the impression that physical and resonance adjustments are taking place. The lower pitches seem to excite strong vibrations in the chest, whereas on the middle pitches the sensation moves up to the hard palate and into the oropharyngeal cavity. In the higher pitches, it feels as if the vibrations are taking place higher in the head. The series of notes in each of these groups also has a similar tonal timbre (quality), and for each group there is a sense of a specific adjustment of the breathing mechanism.

Because of these powerful subjective experiences, there appeared early in the history of singing an attempt to use the singer's sensations to describe the actual physical events, hence the terms chest voice, head or falsetto voice, and later on, middle voice. This latter was sometimes subdivided into upper middle and lower middle to represent those tones that felt as though they still retained an affinity to the head or the chest voice. There was also a gender difference in this early assessment, with female voices assigned 3 registers (chest, middle, and head) and male voices assigned 2 registers (chest and falsetto).

The term "falsetto" has had a confusing history of its own. On the one hand, it has been used to represent the upper register of the male voice, although some believe the earlier schools of singing employed this term to refer to a more vibrant upper register and not the quasi-feminine sounds that the male voice is capable of making. On the other hand, the great and influential voice teacher Manuel Garcia really muddied the waters when he

used this term to represent the middle register, saying that it constituted a particular register that differed from both the head and the chest register, and was located between them[6]. To the modern-day singer, falsetto has come to represent that quasi-feminine sound that the male voice is capable of producing in the upper part of the vocal range.

What terminology should we use? Voice scientists have suggested that since there is so much confusion and as the old labels do not accurately describe what is occurring mechanically in the larynx, we should adopt the terms applied to speaking voice registers as defined by the vibratory patterns of the vocal folds. Using the speaking register terms, "modal" would incorporate chest voice, and "loft" or "falsetto" might replace head register. This terminology can be used to describe postural and biomechanical aspects of the vocal fold vibratory activity in different pitch ranges. Nonetheless, it is limited in its ability to help singers relate to the precise sensations and timbre differences they feel throughout the pitch range. To be of greatest use to the singer, this type of description may need to be combined with acoustic and sensory aspects of registers, including those sensations associated with vocal tract resonance phenomena.

7.4.6.2 Current Understanding of Registers

One of the best and most comprehensive definitions of singing registers was by Nadoleczeny and Zimmerman[9], and dating back to 1937:

> A register within the human vocal scale is a series of sounds of equal quality. The musical ear distinguishes them from another series of sounds also of equal quality. The limits of each series are marked by "points" of passage sometimes called "lifts". The timbre of each series, or register, is the result of a constant rapport of harmony. To the male singer the

primary register change at the upper part of the scale gives a certain vibrating sensation perceptible to the head. To the female the primary register change at the lower part of the scale gives a certain vibratory sensation in the chest. Each area of identical quality depends upon the adjustment of the resonating cavities. Registers are produced by a mechanism that functions in the production of sound. The principal characteristic of this mechanism is the manner in which a particular vibration is coupled with the supraglottic and the infraglottic resonators.

So where does all this leave would-be singers with their desire to obey both the mechanical and aesthetic rules as they progress up and down the scale? Although the findings of voice scientists have enabled us to understand a great deal about the workings of the laryngeal and resonance mechanisms, unknowns still exist regarding singing registers. Nonetheless, there is sufficient knowledge to plot a strategy and a pedagogical approach to the matter of vocal registers. In a practical approach, there appears to be a need to understand registers as both a resonance and a mechanical phenomenon and to acknowledge that the events coincide and interact.

7.4.6.3 Registers as a Mechanical Phenomenon

To establish a particular fundamental frequency, it is necessary that the vocal folds assume a specific degree of tension and mass per area. Assuming the appropriate driving forces are adjusted to accommodate glottal resistance changes, f_0 rises as length (and thus ligament tension) increases and mass per area decreases, and f_0 falls as the ligament tension relaxes and mass per area increases. The cricothyroid muscles are those principally responsible for adjusting length, but the effective length change depends on antagonistic anchoring forces of the cricoarytenoid

muscles (see Figures 8–9 and 8–14). The thyroarytenoid muscles may contract to adjust tension or mass per area of the folds.

Physiologically, we have on a scalar ascent a gradual increase in vocal fold tension and a diminishing of vocal fold mass per area, which is achieved by the different laryngeal muscle groups taking varying degrees of responsibility as the pitch rises. The ideal, to comply with the aesthetics of most Western music, is that this shifting of responsibility be carried out as smoothly and unobtrusively as possible.

7.4.6.4 Vocal Registers as a Resonance Phenomenon

In Chapter 8, the acoustical characteristics of the harmonic spectrum generated by the vocal folds and the formant structures of the vocal tract transfer function are discussed and demonstrated. We need to review these phenomena because they may account for much of the sensory perception that a singer experiences of the register events. It is by the choice and manipulation of the resonance characteristics that the singer can influence and enhance the pitch progression, and most pedagogical techniques dealing with registration are based on this assumption. This therefore requires an understanding of the interaction of harmonics and vowel formants.

7.4.6.5 Harmonics

The vibratory action of the vocal folds produces a complex signal that delivers into the resonance tract a series of harmonics that are mathematically predictable relative to the f_0 of the sung tone. The first harmonic is always 1 octave above the fundamental ($2 \times f_0$); the second, another octave above ($3 \times f_0$). Figure 7–4 shows the harmonic series assuming for convenience that a bass is singing a low C.

Because of the mathematical designation of harmonics in the voice-source spectrum, the density of harmonics that the vocal tract

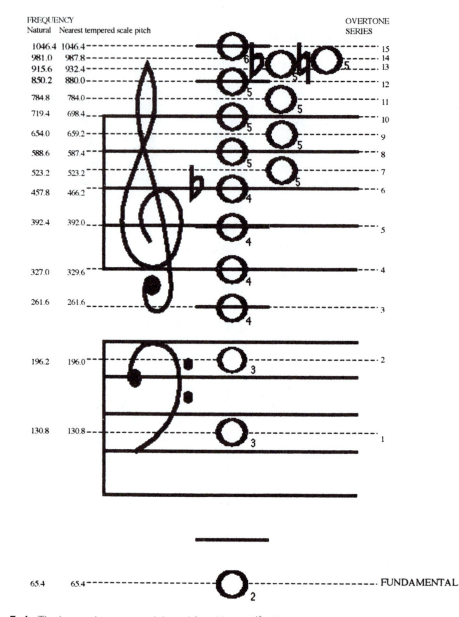

Figure 7–4. The harmonic sequence. Adapted from Vennard[13] with permission.

responds to acoustically depends on the sung fundamental. A bass voice, which operates at relatively low f_0 levels, can generate in the vocal tract a dense spectrum of harmonics because multiplication of the lower f_0 will predict a greater number of harmonics within a given resonator's frequency range. A soprano with her higher f_0 range cannot create so many harmonics for the same frequency range of a resonator. This simple voice source principle accounts for some of the basic differences in the tonal colors of the two voice categories. Luckily, the male and female vocal tracts are designed to enhance different parts of the harmonic frequency range. The larger male tract is particularly suited to resonate lower frequency harmonics, and the resonance capability of the smaller female tract provides potential power to higher frequency harmonics of the voice source spectrum.

7.4.6.6 Interaction of Formants and Harmonics

We see in Chapter 8 that formant frequencies depend on the length and the shape of the vocal tract, and therefore the values will vary for the different voice categories and the size and shape of an individual's vocal tract.

The acoustical effect of the supraglottal cavity shapes is that each subpocket of space tends to be sympathetic to a specific narrow frequency range. Any harmonic whose natural frequency coincides with those favored by the subpockets of a specific resonance tract shape will be reinforced. Other nonsympathetic harmonics are damped. In Chapter 8, we see how the harmonic spectrum is influenced by vocal tract posture to produce various vowels (Figures 8–19 to 8–21).

Appelman has provided us with average frequencies of the first three formant bands for the basic singing vowels in our language (Table 7–1)[2]. It is important to realize that these values mark the center of an allowable range and that some variation in the values will still produce intelligible vowels.

From Table 7–1, we can see that the first formants occur outside the normal working range of most male singing voices, the exception being the very top notes of the bass and baritone and the "head" register of the tenor. In the female voice, we see that the formant values are somewhat higher and that the first formants occur in the pitch range occupied mostly by the middle register of the voice.

To summarize, as the pitch ascends and descends, it is necessary that there be changes in the specific harmonics that the formants choose to boost. These changes of harmonic

Table 7-1. List of Frequencies for the First Three Formants in the Adult Male and Female Voice[2]

	Male				*Female*		
Phoneme	f_1	f_2	f_3	*Phoneme*	f_1	f_2	f_3
/i/	300	1950	2750	/i/	400	2250	3300
/I/	375	1810	2500	/I/	475	2125	3450
/e/	450	1800	2480	/e/	500	1900	3250
/ɛ/	530	1500	2500	/ɛ/	550	1750	3250
/æ/	620	1490	2250	/æ/	600	1650	3000
/a/	650	1200	2500	/a/	675	1555	3300
/ɔ/	610	1000	2600	/ɔ/	625	1240	3250
/o/	450	700	2500	/o/	500	1000	3000
/U/	400	720	2550	/U/	425	900	3375
/u/	350	640	2550	/u/	450	800	3250
/ɑ/	700	1200	2600	/ɑ/	700	1300	3250

selection are influenced not only by pitch variation, but also by changing vowel forms. In plotting the points of change in the harmonic formant relationship throughout all the vowel sounds and ranges of both the female and male voices, it is interesting to note that major changes do tend to take place consistently in certain zones of the voice, and there is a tendency for these formant harmonic changes to shadow the accepted registration change points of traditional pedagogical schools (see Figure 7–5).

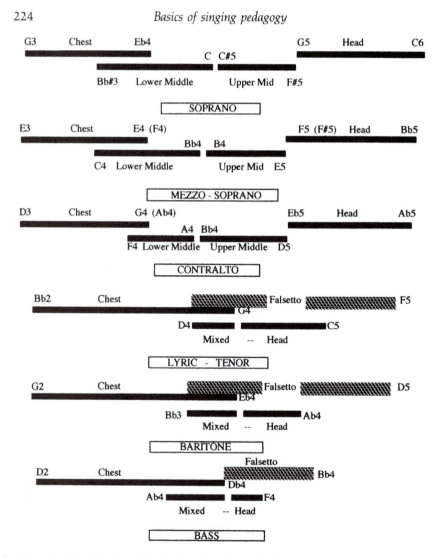

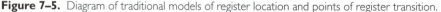

Figure 7–5. Diagram of traditional models of register location and points of register transition.

7.5 Summary

The power of the interdisciplinary approach to voice care extends far-reaching benefits to singers. All aspects of singers' physical and technical processes can be evaluated including an understanding of the impact of the stresses and strains that attend the life and work of the vocal performer. A team approach ensures that all key factors are considered in the development of a rehabilitation program.

It is critical that the singer brings an open-mindedness and a willingness to follow the prescribed strategy to this process. This is not always the case, and there are a number of reasons why singers may be reluctant to consult the medical profession about a voice problem. They may be confronting a strange mixture of fear and hope upon approaching the voice-clinic team. The fear is of the unknown and what terrible tidings may await regarding the state of the vocal apparatus, which for many means the vocal folds. For many singers, nodules are often the worst possible diagnosis that can be pronounced (even cancer pales alongside this). The hope is carried that there will be some simple, quick (sometimes "by tonight") cure. There is always word circulating in the profession of sprays and potions that will provide a quick fix for the problem and get a singer through the coming show. Although the potency of modern drugs can create the occasional minor miracle, many problems need a broader remedy than can be found in the spray or the pill. The problem under consideration is often the product of long-term physical behavior, sometimes under adverse conditions and environments. The proposed rehabilitation strategy may well require a major reevaluation and possible overhaul of vocal techniques, which could mean a recommended change in vocal advisers, voice teachers, or both. A change in performance conditions, frequency, and possibly even in style may be necessary. For many singers, such recommendations could constitute a major upheaval, and the reluctance to cooperate is understandable. Contrary to these fears, the periodic reevaluation of technique and art often can lead to better and maybe greater things.

References

1. Alexander, F. M. (1932). *The Use of the Self.* London: Methuen.
2. Appelman, D. R. (1967). *The Science of Vocal Pedagogy.* Bloomington, IN: Indiana University Press.
3. Barlow, W. (1973). *The Alexander Technique.* Rochester, VT: Healing Arts Press.
4. Bunch, M. (1982). *Dynamics of the Singing Voice.* New York: Springer-Verlag.
5. Coffin, B. (1980). *Overtones of Bel Canto.* Metuchen, NJ: Scarecrow.
6. Garcia, M. (1854;1855). Observations on human voice. *Proceedings of the Royal Society of London, 7,* 399–410.
7. Henderson, W. J. (1968). *The Art of Singing.* Freeport, NY: Book for Libraries.
8. Hixon, T. J. (1987). *Respiratory Function in Speech and Song.* Boston: College-Hill.
9. Nadoleczeny, M., & Zimmerman, R. (1937). Catigories et régistres de la voix. *Revue Francvaise de Phoniatre,* January, 21–31.
10. Proctor, D.F. (1980). *Breathing, Speech and Song.* New York: Springer-Verlag.
11. Russell, G. O. (1931). *Speech and Voice.* New York: MacMillan.
12. Sundberg, J. (1987). *The Science of the Singing Voice.* Dekalb, IL: Northern Illinois University.
13. Vennard, W. (1967). *Singing, the Mechanism and the Technic,* New York: Carl Fischer.
14. Watson, P. J., & Hixon, T. J. (1985). Respiratory kinematics in classical (opera) singers. *Journal of Speech and Hearing Research, 28,* 104–122.
15. Zemlin, W. R. (1998). *Speech and Hearing Science: Anatomy and Physiology* (4th Edition*).* Englewood Cliffs, NY: Prentice-Hall.

CHAPTER

Anatomy and Physiology of Voice Production

8.1 Introduction

Voice production for speech is a psychomotor act that is the result of complex interactions among several anatomical and physiological systems: cognitive-emotional, neuromotor, respiratory, phonatory, resonance, and articulatory (Figure 8–1).

A comprehensive review of the anatomical structures involved in voice production should include all these systems, including those central and peripheral neurological subsystems that initiate and coordinate the voluntary movements of speech. A detailed presentation of the structural aspects of all these system components is beyond the scope of this text. Only aspects of normal structure and function that provide information fundamental to our understanding of voice production and the management of voice disorders will be presented in detail. The reader is encouraged to refer to appropriate texts and anatomical atlases to supplement the material that is offered here. The list of recommended readings at the end of this chapter provides a starting point.

8.2 Function of Phonation in Verbal Communication

Phonation is a term used to refer to the production of sound waves by vibration of structures within the larynx. Under normal circumstances the true vocal folds are the primary vibrators. Phonation with the true vocal folds (or vocal cords) also is referred to as the glottal source of a speech sound, the glottis being the space between the vocal folds on the same horizontal plane. Phonation provides the quasi-regular sound component that gives speech audible or musical tone. The vowel and vowellike phonemes (linguistic sound segments) of English are always characterized by phonation and are the loudest, most intense components of the speech signal. The phonatory system also provides mechanisms for devoicing phonemes that are not associated with vocal tone (and so require that the vocal folds are not vibrating during their production), primarily by contraction of the posterior cricoarytenoid muscles, the intrinsic vocal fold abductors (the muscles that pull the

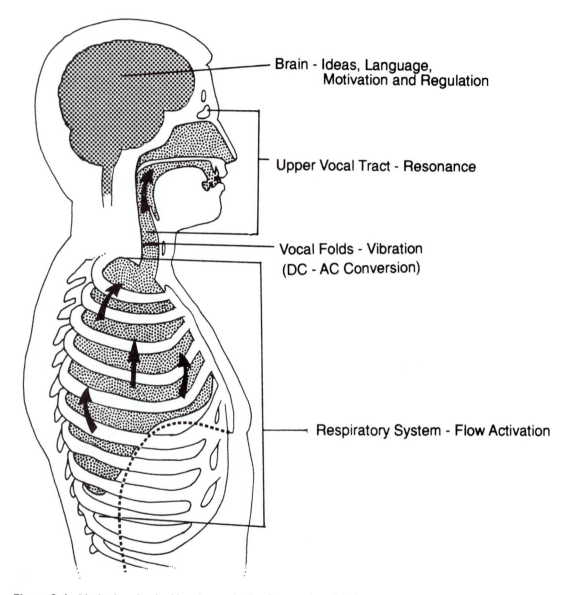

Figure 8–1. Mechanisms involved in voice production for speech and singing.

vocal folds away from each other). The devoicing mechanism is most active during articulation of voiceless phonemes, such as /p/, /f/, /θ/ ("th" as in "think"); /t/, /s/, /tʃ/ ("ch", as in "cheese"); /ʃ/ ("sh" as in "shake"); and /k/.

In addition to providing tone for the voiced speech sounds, phonation for speech includes pitch and loudness mechanisms that create intonation and stress (known as **suprasegmental** features of speech) to help listeners determine the meaning and emotional intent of speech. The suprasegmental function of voice is complex and fascinating. By continuously adjusting laryngeal factors (such as vocal fold length and tension) and other parameters (such as vocal tract length and the rate and amount of airflow from the lungs), we can produce countless combinations of vocal frequencies, intensities, and qualities during speech. We can change the semantics (meaning) and syntax (grammar) of a sentence just by altering the pitch inflections or patterns of vocal emphasis. In addition, we can readily alter the pragmatics (mood and intent) of a particular communicative utterance by varying loudness, pitch, and quality of the voice, without making a single change to the vocabulary. These communication functions are largely dependent on normal phonatory function, and, for the most part, are controlled subconsciously during a typical conversation.

The biological systems for respiration, phonation, resonance, and articulation work together in complex ways during speech. It therefore is difficult to provide accurate and comprehensive descriptions of single component functions of this complex psychomotor act. It is helpful, however, to consider certain aspects of the systems in isolation for the purposes of evaluation and treatment of voice disorders.

8.3 Neuromotor Systems Involved in Speech and Phonation

The true organ of speech and voice is the brain, and to try and describe all the relevant functions would be presumptuous. It may be helpful in understanding voice disorders for us to identify some of the structures that are critical to neuromotor activities during communication and vocal performance. When we study individual neuromotor aspects of communication, several unifying issues must be presumed to overlie and unify the complex system:

First, a thought consists of both intellectual and emotional elements that, when coupled to the underlying personality and style of a speaker, set up the postural and muscle tonus patterns required to deliver the utterance with the needed features. The clinician who evaluates a patient with a voice disorder, and the vocal pedagogue who trains vocal performers must keep this thought-feeling-speech interface in mind because it is here that the source of dysfunction frequently lies. This fact may get lost in the myriad of voice and speech science detail described herein. Chapters 1, 2, and 5 provide more insight into the critical interactions among these functions.

Second, humans use a neuromotor system for voice generation that initially evolved for purposes other than communication, including swallowing, breathing, and airway control. The clinician needs to bear in mind that the larynx, pharynx, and esophagus form an embryologically related neuromuscular tube that is controlled partly voluntarily and partly involuntarily. Sensorimotor reflexes that travel from the pharynx, larynx, and esophagus to the brain and back again are very important, to the extent that voice clinicians tend to form strong reductive biases about the influence of medical factors on voice, such as the effect of chronic gastro-esophageal reflux, which is discussed in Chapters 2 and 3.

Third, the neuromotor activities needed to produce a voice must be delicately coordinated. The vocal athletic gift has been more heavily bestowed on some than others, as has the ability to dance or hit a tennis ball. Training in these skills can enhance voice production of the voice user who has limited natural talent, as well as the gifted person. Much of this book is dedicated to these ends.

Structures of the central and peripheral nervous system are responsible for the act of speech. Within the cerebral cortex, the areas generally recognized as being important to speech and language formulation and processing are the left inferior frontal gyrus of the frontal lobe (Broca's area), the left angular gyrus of the parietal lobe, and the left superior temporal gyrus and temporoparietal region (Wernicke's area). While a person is engaged in conversation, these areas receive input from other cortical and subcortical processing areas as well, including structures of the limbic system, the emotional center of the brain. Within the cerebral cortex, the precentral gyrus or Brodmann's area is also of great importance to vocal communication, because it contains many cell bodies of the motor nerves that operate skeletal muscles during voluntary movements such as speech. The premotor cortex, which includes some of Broca's area, also contains motor cells. The postcentral gyrus is an area for processing various types of sensory input (for example, proprioceptive information regarding the state of muscles and direction and degree of movements), but it also contains cell bodies for motor activity. Within the basal ganglia of the subcortex are important motor and sensory relay and coordination areas such as the thalamus. The cerebellum also plays a role in achieving finely tuned coordinated movements.

The periaqueductal gray matter (PAG) in the midbrain has been identified as a critical mass of neural cells that integrate the precise coordination of respiratory, laryngeal, and oral movements for vocal sounds of an emotional and involuntary nature, and also during speech and singing. Davis and colleagues demonstrated that afferent input to the PAG regarding lung volume contributes to the coordination and control of the various systems involved in vocalization, based on emotional, mechanical, and linguistic influences[12].

Most of the peripheral cranial nerves play a part in speech and voice production. Any disease process that results in cranial nerve dysfunction, in any combination, may have significant effects on speech and voice. The following cranial nerves are particularly important to communication:

➤ The **fifth** or **trigeminal nerve** has a major motor component in its mandibular division that supplies the muscles of mastication and those in the anterior floor of the mouth. The muscles of mastication play an important role in speech production, which optimally involves continuous jaw movements that enhance resonance and articulation. We indicated in Chapter 1 the role of jaw and suprahyoid muscle tension in producing vocal misuse.

➤ The **seventh** or **facial nerve** supplies the muscles of facial expression, which obviously play a role in verbal and nonverbal communication. The lips, served by this nerve, are important speech articulators.

➤ The **eighth** or **auditory nerve** (the "hearing" nerve) plays an important sensory role in monitoring speech and is the afferent (sensory input) component of many sensorimotor reflex arcs.

➤ The **ninth** or **glossopharyngeal nerve** transmits sensory information from much of the posterior oral cavity and pharynx, as well as providing motor supply to some palatal and pharyngeal muscles. Thus, it plays an important role in vocal resonance.

➤ The **tenth** or **vagus nerve** serves both sensory and motor function to the entire pharyngo-laryngo-esophageal tube. The **pharyngeal branch** innervates muscles that effect pharyngeal constriction and elevation of the soft palate during speech and swallowing, including the palatoglossus muscle, which can open the velo-pharyngeal port if the tongue base is anchored. The **superior laryngeal branch** provides sensation to the larynx and pharynx, as well as motor function to the paired cricothyroid muscles, the muscles of vocal pitch. The remaining intrinsic laryngeal muscles receive motor innervation from the **recurrent laryngeal nerve**, also a branch of the vagus nerve. Additionally, the vagus nerve supplies the autonomic function to minor salivary glands, gastric acid secretors, and nerve networks that control peristalsis.

➤ The **eleventh** or **accessory nerve** gives motor supply to the trapezius and sternocleidomastoid muscles. As discussed in Chapter 1, hypertonicity in the trapezius and short rotator muscles are commonly associated with voice misuse.

➤ Finally, the **twelfth** or **hypoglossal nerve** sends motor input to the tongue, the most complex speech articulator. It also combines with some fibers of the cervical plexus to supply the strap muscles of the neck.

The cervical and phrenic nerve plexi of the peripheral spinal nerve system also need to be recognized as important in supporting muscles of respiration and speech-breathing.

Servomechanisms, or feedback devices, within the structures of respiration, phonation, resonance, and articulation are an important part of the neuromotor system for vocal production. These devices may be in the form of cells that are sensitive to air pressure changes within the respiratory system or muscle spindles that detect the state of contraction of the muscles and may also be sensitive to tactile, vibratory, and aerodynamic changes in the vocal tract.

It is imperative that voice clinicians and teachers, regardless of their discipline, maintain a good working understanding of the neuroanatomical connections of the upper aerodigestive tract, particularly of those portions that serve speech and voice. The reader is referred to the many excellent anatomical texts and atlases listed at the end of this chapter for further details.

8.4 Functions of the Respiratory System: Speech-Breathing and Breathing for Vocal Performance

8.4.1 Nature of the Mechanism: An Overview

The process of phonation engages the basic structures of the upper and lower respiratory systems (Figure 8–2). Voice for speech and singing is produced principally during the exhalation phase of respiration. Readers who are unfamiliar with terms related to respiration are referred to the glossary in Section 8.4.4.

In its simplest conceptualization, speech-breathing functions to maintain a relatively constant flow of air to overcome resistance offered by the closed glottis and thus to provide the aerodynamic driving force throughout phonation. In addition, the expiratory flow must provide appropriate aerodynamic forces to allow for the oral, pharyngeal, and laryngeal articulatory effects such as **plosive-aspirate** and **fricative** speech noises. Plosive-aspirate sounds are associated with sudden release of air by a speech articulator, as when the lips are parted (p^h); fricative noise is the hissing sound that is created when air rushes between two articulators that are closely approximated to create air turbulence, for example, the upper teeth and the lower lip: "*ffffffffffff*".

The tissues of the lungs and the rib cage structures have inherent elastic properties that allow them to be stretched and provide recoil forces making them want to return to their respective rest positions after they are stretched. While stretched, they store passive energy that is used in the recoil forces. For example, the lungs have a passive recoil force that makes them want to shrink in volume after they are stretched for inhalation (the in breath). The rib cage structure, on the other hand, has a recoil force that makes it tend to expand back to its neutral rest position after it is pulled in during exhalation (the out breath) or to reduce its dimensions if it is expanded

The Speech Breathing Mechanism

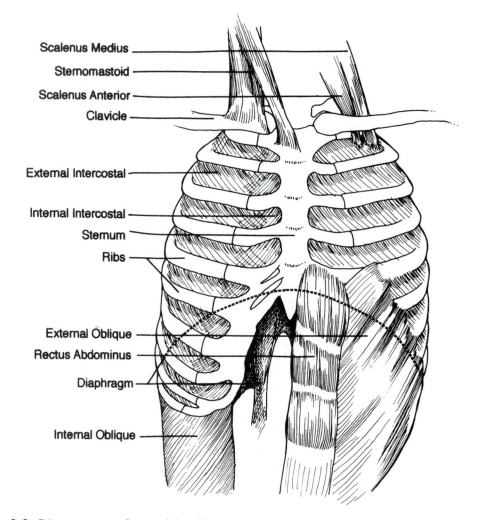

Scalenus Medius

Sternomastoid

Scalenus Anterior

Clavicle

External Intercostal

Internal Intercostal

Sternum

Ribs

External Oblique

Rectus Abdominus

Diaphragm

Internal Oblique

Figure 8–2. Primary structures for speech breathing.

beyond its rest position during inhalation. The respiratory system capitalizes on these recoil forces to a large degree during quiet respiration (non-speech tidal breathing), and the forces vary as a function of lung volume. The respiratory system also engages voluntary muscles to enhance inhalation and exha-

lation activities. Both passive elastic recoil forces and active muscular forces are involved in the maintenance of appropriate expiratory airflow and subglottal pressures required for phonation to occur. Subglottal pressures (pressures below the glottis) are determined by airflow rate and laryngeal or supralaryngeal resistance (resistance in structures above the glottis). During conversational speech at normal loudness, subglottal pressures of from 5 to12 cm H_2O are required to maintain phonation.

Figure 8–3 provides a prototype relaxation curve demonstrating directions and degrees of overall relaxation pressures (P_r), that is, forces, throughout the vital capacity. At resting expiratory level (REL), P_r is 0; above REL, P_r is positive; and below REL, P_r is negative. The relationship of a relaxation curve to force components of the chest wall for various loudness dynamics is shown in Chapter 7 in Figure 7–2.

Figure 8–4 estimates the degree to which passive or relaxation-recoil forces in the respiratory system are available to provide the necessary subglottal pressure for speech over time, within the typical vital capacity range employed for conversation—typically from 60% to 30% of the vital capacity. To meet the

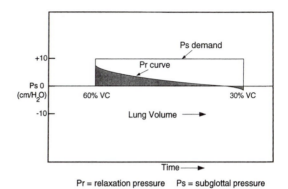

Pr = relaxation pressure   Ps = subglottal pressure

Figure 8–4. Availability of relaxation pressures in the respiratory system to meet subglottal pressure requirements for speech over time and lung volume (see text for detailed description). P_r = relaxation pressure; P_s = subglottal pressure. Adapted with permission from Weismer[122].

average speech requirement, a constant subglottal pressure of 7 cm H_2O could be maintained for only a small part of the vital capacity should one rely only on passive forces of the respiratory system. As seen in the next section, use of the passive expiratory forces during speech-breathing is not simple, nor are interactions between use of passive and active respiratory forces.

Any internal or external situations that require changes in loudness, pitch, or voice quality affect subglottal pressure demands; for example, loud or emotive speech is generally produced with higher subglottal pressure.

In reality, the speech-breathing mechanism must perform a much more complicated task than simply supplying a relatively constant flow of air to maintain steady phonation. Within a spoken phrase, the segmental (single sound unit) and suprasegmental demands of verbal communication result in constantly changing aerodynamic "loading" forces. The segmental characteristics of speech require continual changes in articulatory shapes and vocal tract constrictions, which in turn affect

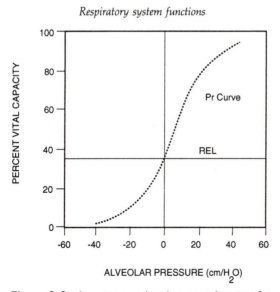

Respiratory system functions

Figure 8–3. A prototype relaxation curve (see text for detailed description). Adapted with permission from Weismer[122].

intraoral pressures and flows and ultimately result in recognizable sound sequences or speech phrases. Articulatory adjustments for speech cause fluctuations in supraglottal loading pressures, which in turn change resistances at the glottis and may even influence vocal fold vibratory patterns. The most dramatic examples of articulatory maneuvers that create rapid resistance changes within the supraglottal vocal tract during speech, are the plosive sounds (such as /p/ or /t/) and fricative sounds (such as /s/ or /f/). Because subglottal pressure should remain relatively constant for phonation to have consistent loudness, pitch, and quality, the aerodynamic driving forces of the respiratory mechanism must have ways of compensating for the changes in vocal tract loading forces, to stabilize phonatory function. Furthermore, suprasegmental effects of intonation (inflections) or stress (emphasis) require that the respiratory system adjust quickly to meet the constantly changing subglottal pressure demands.

Because subglottal pressure during phonation is determined by both respiratory forces and laryngeal resistance, adjustments must be made to the respiratory forces to compensate for or to overcome glottal resistance in cases in which valving at the glottis is compromised or exaggerated. Conversely, if respiratory forces are somehow compromised or exaggerated, the muscles influencing glottal closure may attempt to compensate for or balance the driving forces to maintain phonation.

Our current understanding of mechanics of the respiratory system for speech and vocal performance production embraces the concept of **motor equivalence.** This implies that wide variation in mechanical patterns within the breathing system is observed across individuals when they prepare for, initiate, and sustain phonation[27]. Furthermore, patterns of breathing for singing and theatrical voice use may differ significantly from those associated with speech-breathing[27,28,30,119,120]. Individual variation may be explained by factors such as body

type, training, personality, and vocal performance style. Given the many influences on motor equivalence, we must question the validity of voice training and therapy techniques that use the same speech-breathing or vocal performance breathing instruction model for all students or patients.

8.4.2 Respiratory Kinematics and Dynamics

Traditionally, speech physiologists have differentiated between two functional parts of the respiratory system to study speech-breathing: the rib cage and the diaphragm-abdomen. Together, these functional units comprise the **chest wall**. This delineation continues to be useful in understanding speech-breathing.

Modern concepts of speech-breathing are largely based on findings from the techniques of **kinematics** (movement patterns) and **dynamics** (muscular force functions), as described by Hixon and collaborators[27–29] in the early 1970s for application to speech research. Both techniques use a relaxation curve as a reference for each individual's speech-breathing function. Voluntary closure of the glottis along with relaxation of all respiratory muscles allows for static measures to be made for each individual's reference curves. In the case of kinematic measures, the relaxation curve represents relative positions of displacement for the abdomen and rib cage at various lung volumes. For the dynamic measures, the relaxation curve represents relative pressures within the abdominal and rib cage cavities of the chest wall at various lung volumes.

The relaxation reference charts are assumed to be relatively constant for an individual, although body orientation, such as upright versus supine position, will affect the shape of the curve significantly because of differing gravitational effects on the abdomen and rib cage. In addition, both developmental and aging factors will have an impact on the elasticity and capacity of the involved tissues.

Taken together, the relaxation curves describe the nonmuscular passive chest wall displacement force potentials associated with two recoil reactions over a time-volume history for a specified body orientation. The two relaxation functions include the natural elastic tendency of the lung tissue to compress the air inside the lungs, creating a positive pleural pressure and the opposing tendency of the chest wall structures to expand creating a negative pressure in the lungs. Together with the effects of gravity and abdominal hydraulics, these forces create a passive summation force. To serve as an accurate reference for muscular contributions of speech-breathing, relaxation summation functions must be plotted throughout the relevant ranges of vital capacity for a given posture because the degree of displacement or force varies with lung volume as well as posture.

For the kinematic measures, magnetometers or variable inductance plethysmographs (strain gauges) can be used to measure relative movements of the rib cage and the abdominal wall and thus provide estimates of volume displacement in the lungs (Figure 8–5). Measures, in changes of voltage in chest wall displacements for the rib cage and abdomen during speech can be plotted on an X-Y graph, which uses the position-appropriate relaxation curve for a particular speaker as a reference (Figure 8–6). The tracings that are generated by this procedure during vocal phrases are referred to as "speech limbs." Any deviations from the relaxation curve are considered to be a result of active muscular dynamics, and the direction of the deviation implies which part of the chest wall was moving or providing force (Figure 8–6).

Dynamic measures are generally made with pressure transducers measuring pressures from catheter balloons placed below and above the diaphragm, one in the stomach and one in the esophagus. Because this procedure is invasive, less data is available for study than for the kinematic measures.

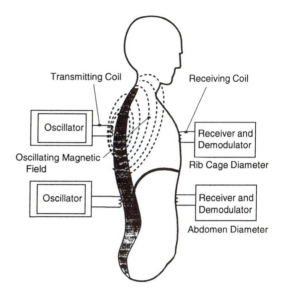

Figure 8–5. Hardware design for measuring kinematics of the chest wall with magnetometers. Adapted with permission from Baken[5].

Results of pressure deviations can be plotted in a manner similar to the motion-motion diagrams for each individual for a variety of speech and phonation tasks. The plots provide information regarding the amount and direction of muscular force. Hixon and colleagues have demonstrated that kinematic measures can be used to estimate active forces of individual chest wall parts during speech-breathing. For detailed descriptions of measurement techniques and interpretations, the reader is directed to texts by Baken[5] and Hixon[27].

Taken together, these sets of speech-breathing measures can provide valuable information about patterns of movement and aerodynamics from which we infer roles of the various structures and muscles of the respiratory system. Figure 8–7 summarizes the relevant pressures, volume displacements, and movements to be considered in describing speech breathing.

In addition to measures of volume dis-

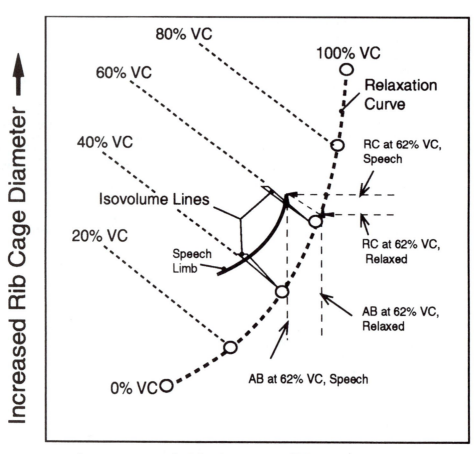

Figure 8–6. Hypothetical expiratory limb for a speech utterance from kinematic measures. VC = vital capacity; RC = rib cage; AB = abdomen. The relaxation reference curve is produced by filling the lungs to a specified volume, then relaxing all voluntary breathing musculature so that only the passive recoil forces are influencing the chest wall shape. The isovolume lines represent the range of potential chest wall shapes at a specific volume when contained air is shifted from the abdomen to the rib cage and vice versa. Vertical shifts indicate rib cage contributions, and horizontal shifts indicated abdominal contributions. By plotting *speech limbs* of relative contributions of the different chest wall parts, we can study the individual characteristics of speech-breathing and compare patterns of speech-breathing across individuals. A sample speech limb is represented by the darkest line, extending from 62% to 30% VC. In this example, muscular abdominal forces are engaged at the outset of the phrase as demonstrated by the limb placement to the left of the relaxation curve; abdominal contributions to the speech phrase are demonstrated by leftward excursion of the limb over time and volume, and rib cage contributions are demonstrated by downward excursion of the speech limb. For this hypothetical speaker, it can be seen that the contribution of the rib cage displacement is large for the first part of the phrase, followed by an increase in abdominal displacement in the latter half. Adapted with permission from Weismer[122].

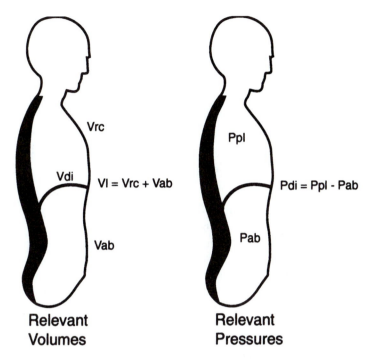

Figure 8–7. Relevant volume displacements and pressures of concern for comprehensive analysis of chest wall function during speech. *V* = volume displacement; *P* = pressure. Subscripts for relevant volumes are: *di* = diaphragm; *rc* = rib cage wall; *l* = lung; *ab* = abdominal wall. Subscripts for relevant pressures are: *pl* = pleural; *ab* = abdominal; *di* = transdiaphragmatic. Adapted with permission from Hixon et al[27] and Hixon, Mead & Goldman[29].

placements and pressures within the chest wall, a limited number of surface electromyographic studies have been undertaken to contribute to our understanding of breathing for speech and performance. These have included studies of activity in the intercostal and abdominal muscles and in the diaphragm[59,62,69,121].

8.4.3 What Do We Know About Speech-Breathing?

The following observations have been confirmed in studies of speech-breathing, and contribute to our current understanding of the mechanisms involved.

8.4.3.1 Inspiration for Speech

Inspiration for speech involves activity in the diaphragm and external intercostal muscles. In cases where a large inspiration is required, often in association with voice disorders, a variety of accessory muscles may be used to facilitate rib cage elevation. The so-called inspiratory muscles (e.g., external intercostals and diaphragm) appear to be engaged during speech as well as during inspiration, probably to offer support in retaining a certain lung volume level or to control flow rates and subglottal pressures. This special use of the inspiratory muscles is even more evident during most vocal performance activities such as singing (see Chapter 7, Section 7.4.2). Vocal performance may also require that the abdominal muscles relax very quickly to allow the diaphragm to lower and a maximum inhalation to occur. Because the abdominal muscles appear to play a dual role, singers may need to distinguish between their inspiratory and expiratory actions[59,60,112].

8.4.3.2 Maintenance of Subglottal Pressure for Speech

Both the rib cage and abdominal mechanisms contribute to maintenance of alveolar pressure (pressure within the lungs) during speech. The internal intercostal muscles are of particular importance in maintaining a fairly steady pressure to ensure constant airflow within the middle range of lung volume during conversational speech. The contributions of rib cage excursion to lung volume change during vocalization are generally larger than those of abdominal movements. This may be explained by the fact that the rib cage covers a relatively larger surface area of the pulmonary system than does the abdomen. When we examine motion-motion graphs for different individuals, their speech-breathing patterns may vary, and the predominant rib cage excursion may not be evident in all vocalizers. During vocal performance, the oblique abdominal muscles may play a role in phasic movements associated with rhythmic singing, and in some cases the diaphragm may contract synchronously with the abdominal muscles[61].

8.4.3.3 Abdominal Muscle Activity

The abdominal muscles are active in all individuals at the outset of phonation for speech and singing[27–32,38,119,120,122,124]. This appears to be the case even when phonation is initiated at lung volumes where relaxation forces alone would be adequate to provide sufficient subglottal pressure. Of particular importance to

voice production is activity in the internal and external oblique abdominal muscles, which pull the rib cage downward and push the abdominal wall inward on contraction and the transverse abdominal muscles, which push the abdominal wall inward on contraction.

Weismer has provided theoretical support for the mechanical advantages of using abdominal muscle forces during speech. He has suggested that the abdominal muscle tone exerts pressure on the diaphragm, which in turn provides a counter force to rib cage compression forces, primarily the internal intercostal muscles, to make them more effective. Without the abdominal pressure, activity of the internal intercostals would result in downward displacement of the diaphragm and no significant respiratory driving force. This counter force role may be particularly important for the rapid pulsatile movements during speech. The upward pressure on the diaphragm may also ensure that it returns to a neutral position following inspiration. Because voluntary muscles contract most efficiently from rest position, this force facilitates rapid diaphragmatic contractions required for quick inspirations during speech and singing[122].

8.4.3.4 Prephonatory Posturing and Speech-Breathing Patterns

An expanded rib cage is often noted at onset, and throughout speech and singing, compared with the position noted for the same lung volume on a relaxation-curve (Figure 8–6). This is represented by a higher position of the speech-limb onset compared with the vertical position for the same lung volume on the relaxation curve. As discussed previously, this position must involve use of the muscle groups generally labeled as inspiratory muscles, in particular the external intercostal muscles, although speech is thought to be an expiratory activity. It appears to contradict previous theory that opposing forces, abdominal-expiratory and rib cage-inspiratory, do not co-occur in speech-breathing[122].

It can be seen that the **typical prephonatory posture** in an upright position is characterized by two apparently oppositional displacements: the abdominal muscles are contracted (an apparent expiratory maneuver), and the rib cage is expanded (an apparent inspiratory maneuver). Several possible combinations of individual chest wall activities have been demonstrated through speech limbs[31,124]. During speech phonation, speech limbs are almost horizontal on the graph for some individuals, suggesting that the predominant activity during the speech phrase is abdominal. Others appear to use predominantly rib cage activity for speech after the initial abdominal and rib cage posturing efforts, and still others appear to shift the activity pattern midphrase. Figure 8–8 demonstrates speech-breathing movement patterns for two individuals across three different loudness or effort levels. For the first individual, the speech limbs for several successive sentences indicate a predominance of abdominal displacement; for the second individual, the speech limbs are principally vertical, indicating predominance of rib cage movement. These movement patterns are consistent for each individual across different phonation loudness tasks.

Most studies of speech breathing in adults note that the speech phrase or "speech limb" is initiated at a lung volume level of about 55% of the vital capacity and that the lung volume level at which individuals finish speech phrases is quite variable, but generally at FRC or below. Hixon has concluded that lung volume levels used for speech in adults are highly dependent on individual rest-breathing levels, suggesting that the equilibrium levels of the respiratory system influence speech-breathing patterns. The speech-breathing system seems to follow an economy of effort principle by operating within the vital capacity range that requires the least overall muscular effort and that takes maximum advantage of the springlike elastic recoil forces available around the REL. Despite the strong mechanical influences on the lung volume levels used in conversational speech, linguistic factors also seem to play a role in determining how speech-breathing is regulated. A linguistic influence also has been observed for more demanding speech tasks, such as reading aloud and loudly. Louder speech, typically studied during a reading task, is associated with use of progressively larger lung volumes, with the speech limb starting at higher lung capacity levels and sometimes finishing at lower levels than is typical during normal speech. In singing, the lung volume ranges used are larger than for spontaneous speech, tending to resemble more those of loud and very loud reading, to meet the higher subglottal pressure requirements of singing (see Figure 7–2).[27,103,126,127]

Sundberg has discussed how lung volume can affect glottal posture and vocal fold vibratory patterns. Of particular interest is the observation that phonation at high lung volumes is associated with a downward tracheal pull, which in turn has an abductory influence on the vocal folds. This tracheal pull also appears to increase the space between the cricoid and thyroid cartilages anteriorly, thus requiring the cricothyroid muscles to contract more to effect pitch increases at high lung volumes[46,101]. If the vocal folds are susceptible to abductory forces at high lung volumes, this may be a factor in the creation of variably breathy voices, which are characteristic of some sociocultural groups. Because vocal fold abduction will contribute to higher flow rates during phonation, larger lung volumes may be required to complete a speech phrase. Individuals using undesirably breathy voices may need to resist the tendency to compensate by using higher lung volumes; a speech-breathing strategy that engages lowered lung volumes may be more likely to rectify the problem.

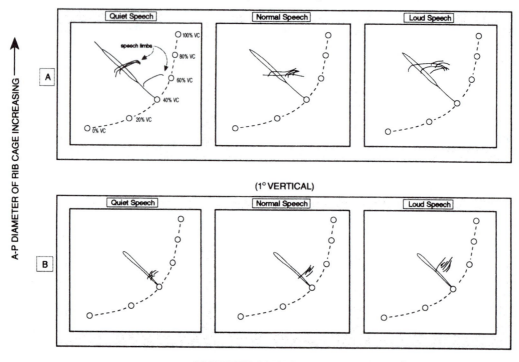

Figure 8–8. Speech limbs for two hypothetical speakers under three different speech effort levels. Speaker A demonstrates predominantly abdominal movement during speech, as represented by horizontal speech limb movement. Speaker B demonstrates predominantly rib cage movements during speech, as represented by vertical speech limb movement. Adapted with permission from Hixon[27].

8.4.3.5 Individual Variation Related to Gender, Body-Type, Developmental,and Aging Factors

Individual variation has been noted in dimensions of the speech-breathing structures, and functional differences have been identified, such as: the lung volume at which individuals start and finish speech phrases, total volume used during speech phrases, predominance of rib cage or abdominal movements during speech-breathing, and aerodynamic measures such as subglottal or tracheal pressure and transglottal flow rates. These individual variations may be explained

in part by gender-based, developmental, aging, and body-type factors.

8.4.3.5.1 Gender-Based Differences

In general, women initiate speech phrases at higher lung volumes and finish at lower lung, rib cage, and abdominal volume levels than do men[97,98]. Women also tend to use higher flow rates[38]. To explain these gender-based differences, it is probably necessary to account for structural and mechanical characteristics at both the respiratory and laryngeal levels. First, when size and shape of the respiratory structures are compared, the chest circumference and lungs are larger in males, most notably after puberty. The rib cage in women has a smaller sternum that rests higher relative to the spine and has greater mobility in the upper ribs. These features may represent an adaptation that allows for greater rib cage expansion required during pregnancy[71]. Differences in average vital capacity for men and women typically are reported as between 1.5 to 2 litres. Differing dimensions of men and women's respiratory structures does not appear to fully explain the variation, however. Lower static recoil pressures in women may account for the need to initiate and end phrases at more extreme lung volumes[97], but one must always keep in mind the gender-based differences in laryngeal structures, postures, and subsequent aerodynamic features, which will be presented in upcoming sections of this chapter. In several cultures and countries, women adopt a glottal posture characterized by an observable posterior glottal chink, which is associated with higher phonatory flow rates[84,95]. If the glottis in women is "leaky," women may compensate by initiating speech at higher lung volumes. We have discussed these potential circular compensatory reactions within the phonatory and respiratory systems in the previous section.

Body type may affect speech-breathing. Hixon and colleagues have suggested that a body type trend exists: lean men, or ectomorphs, tend to use more rib cage activity than abdominal activity, whereas for male endomorphs (more rotund individuals) the opposite is true. In addition, paradoxical rib cage movements have been noted in endomorphs[36]. Gender-based differences in speech breathing patterns paralleling those in men and women have been found in children as young as age 4. This has been explained on the basis of larger lungs and thoraces, creating larger vital capacities in boys and a tendency to use different levels of muscular effort[35,97]. Studies of children under age 4

have not revealed gender-based differences in breathing behavior during vocalization[7,8].

Although current data supports the concept of gender-based differences in speech-breathing, such differences are not apparent during singing in men and women who have undergone extensive classical voice training[119–121]. Perhaps this can be explained by a breathing pattern stereotypy in classical singers that reflects similar training or a common set of physiological strategies that are required to achieve the goals of operatic vocal production.

8.4.3.5.2 Age-Related Differences

Geriatric adults are known to have reduced flexibility and mobility in their respiratory structures due to ossification of ribs and changes in collagen tissue within the lungs. Predictably, geriatric individuals have smaller vital capacities, initiate speech at higher lung and rib cage volumes, use higher lung and rib cage excursions during speech, and some use larger degrees of lung volume per syllable than do younger adults[37,38]. Apart from the known physiological changes in the respiratory system, the speech-breathing changes may be explainable in part on the basis of laryngeal changes. Geriatric individuals, especially men, may experience difficulty approximating their vocal folds completely because of tissue atrophy and thus may need to compensate with larger lung volumes and rib cage excursions to meet voicing and linguistic demands.

Speech-breathing in children is a relatively new area of study. Anatomical details provide some basis for understanding breathing patterns during vocalization. At birth, the thorax rests high, compared with older children and adults. Up to around 2 years of age, the ribs rest in a horizontal position relative to the spine, compared with the more vertical resting position in the adult. Various changes in dimensions reflect adaptation to an upright position in the developing child. The shape of the rib cage and the evolving muscular forces determine that chest volume cannot be greatly increased by rib cage elevation, thus, infants tend to use predominantly abdominal-diaphragmatic movements to support vocal productions. After age 2, a mixed abdominal and rib cage pattern develops to approximately age 8, after which rib cage movements are predominant[48]. Predictably, magnitudes of vital capacity and tidal volume increase with height and age.

The respiratory kinematics of children aged 4 and older have been studied using similar methods to those typically used for adults. Early studies have shown that children, compared to adults, use higher percentages of lung capacity and rib cage excursion and lower lung levels at phrase termination below REL[35,87,99]. Children aged 4 to 10 years may use relatively greater rib cage excursions. Possible explanations for the higher lung volume use and use of FRC in children include lower muscular strength than adults, higher airway compliance, and less efficient laryngeal and articulatory valving[100]. Netsell et al[75] used kinematic measures to interpret subglottal pressure, flow rates, and resistance of children and adults, concluding that sometime after preschool age, children begin to shift speech-breathing patterns from use of primary expiratory muscle force to the more adult pattern of a combined inspiratory-expiratory muscle force. Russell and Stathopoulos noted that children's respiratory patterns were influenced primarily by articulatory demands, and secondarily by vocal loudness, whereas loudness demands appeared to influence the speech breathing patterns of adults to a greater extent[87].

Breathing characteristics during vocalization in children under aged 4 are highly variable across a variety of vocalization types. The variability undoubtedly speaks to the limitations and rapid changes in physiological and cognitive-linguistic skills during this developmental period. Most infants start vocalization at a lung capacity higher than the predicted end-inspiratory level for tidal breathing but avoid initiating vocalization at extreme lung volumes. These behaviors may allow the young child to capitalize on biomechanical properties of the system to realize some economy of effort[7,8].

8.4.3.6 Variability Related to Phonatory Task

Respiratory system activities for singing, chanting, and like vocal activities may be quite different than accounted for above[28,30,59,60,102,119,120]. This may be because of the different temporal, prosody, pitch, and intensity requirements of these vocal activities as well as the different cognitive or emotional goals motivating each activity. The subglottal pressure demands for singing and other vocal performance activities are higher and more varied than for typical conversational speech. Loud singing requires high subglottal pressures, to 30 cm H_2O or higher, for example (Figure 7–2). In general, trained singers use higher lung volumes, exaggerated deformations of the rib cage during prephonatory posturing, specific relationships between abdomen and rib cage volumes, and regionally specific abdominal activity that may contribute to chest wall posturing[119–121]. Classically trained actors also demonstrate speech-breathing patterns during performance that are at variance with their conversational speech patterns. They use relatively wider ranges of volume from the rib cage and abdomen; frequent paradoxical rib cage movements; and chest wall configuration characterized by a relatively larger rib cage and smaller abdominal volume[27].

Training and performance style is likely to have a large influence on the phonatory breathing patterns. In a study of professional country singers, Hoit et al noted that their respiratory patterns during singing activities resembled those of speech, which varies with the distinct performance patterns noted in classically trained operatic singers[33]. Strategies for training breathing for vocal performance are discussed further in Chapter 7.

Hixon and colleagues have described different speech-breathing patterns for sustained phonation or steady speech activities compared with those of conversational speech[27–29]. Activities such as recitation of serial numbers, which are nonemotional, and have limited suprasegmental demands, may use larger ranges of lung volume and take greater advantage of relaxation characteristics or passive expiratory forces, in combination with inspiratory "checking" forces.

A study of the respiratory and laryngeal function of healthy adults during normal and whispered speech demonstrated consistent patterns contrasting these two communicative behaviors. During whispered speech, subjects used lower lung volumes, lower tracheal pressures, higher transglottal flow rates, lower glottal resistance levels, and shorter breath phrase groups than typically used by healthy adults during speech in modal register. Nonetheless, the chest wall configuration (compressed abdomen and expanded rib cage) during whisper resembled that typically used for speech [96].

8.4.3.7 Variability Related to Physical and Emotional Factors

Respiratory function for speech is highly susceptible to differences in physical and emotional states. **Body posture and alignment factors** can greatly influence speech-breathing function. For example, predictable differences in gravitational influence on respiratory function are observed in upright versus supine positions[28,34,105]. Sundberg and colleagues demonstrated that singers used spe-

cific compensatory adjustments to adapt to changes in body position[105]. More subtle differences in body alignment can influence rib cage and abdominal excursion and lung volumes and thus affect speech-breathing patterns. For example, "slouchers" will limit their ability to take advantage of an expanded rib cage and the interplay between the passive and active forces of the two chest wall components.

The respiratory and laryngeal systems work together to produce sufficient subglottal pressure to meet the demands for vocal fold vibration and breath stream resistance produced by supraglottal articulators during speech. Because interaction with the phonatory system is an integral part of speech-breathing, changes to the laryngeal and supralaryngeal structures may cause compensatory changes in use of the respiratory system during speech. Studies of speech-breathing patterns in individuals with voice disorders demonstrate that overvalving or undervalving of the vocal folds during voice production will alter the subglottal pressure requirements for sustained vocal fold vibration, thereby changing the force that various respiratory structures need to contribute to create the expiratory breath stream[27,76,88]. In cases in which laryngeal problems are mild or long-standing, speech-breathing patterns are sometimes remarkably similar to normal patterns, even in the presence of higher laryngeal flow rates[88,89]. This appears to concur with the observations about speech breathing during whispering.

Long-term changes in resistance created by articulatory or resonance structures, such as the tongue or soft palate, also may alter the demand on the respiratory system for speech-breathing. For example, reduced articulatory dynamics or velopharyngeal incompetence will alter demands on the respiratory system during speech because of reduced supraglottal resistance. In some speakers experiencing such supraglottal compromises, compensatory valving may be created within the larynx to help regulate the aerodynamic pressures, which in turn will determine demands on the respiratory system[117,118]. In contrast, if articulatory pressures are increased, as with stuttering, focal dystonia, or muscle misuse voice disorders, the respiratory forces may be increased in an attempt to overcome high levels of glottal and supraglottal resistance.

Emotional states that result in muscular tension and altered motivation for communication can affect function of the respiratory, phonatory, and speech systems because of chronic hypertonicity of muscles normally involved in speech-breathing, phonation, and articulation.

Individuals who are deaf or hard-of-hearing have been studied to determine if any differences exist in their speech-breathing patterns compared with people with normal hearing. In people with congenital deafness or hearing impairment, the pre-phonatory chest wall adjustment patterns were similar to those of individuals with normal hearing. The individuals with hearing impairment, however, demonstrated high levels of lung volume loss before initiating phonation, high lung volume expenditure during speech limbs, initiation of utterances at relatively low lung volumes, termination of utterances below FRC, linguistically inappropriate pauses for inspiration, and wide variability in lung-volume excursions across and within speaking tasks[10,18,123].

Noise is a common environmental factor that may alter speech-breathing patterns. Speech in noisy environments tends to invoke the Lombard effect, a tendency to speak louder, that is generally accompanied by changes in respiratory patterns[27,28]. These speech-breathing changes may reflect both physical demands and emotional reactions to the adverse communication environment[125].

8.4.3.8 Compensatory Mechanisms

Because of a degree of functional redundancy (motor equivalence) in the speech-breathing system, remarkable compensations can be observed in individuals who have experienced anatomical changes in the respiratory system. For example, an individual with diaphragm paresis may compensate with other inspiratory muscle forces to support near-normal speech and voice functions.

8.4.3.9 Servomechanisms In Speech-breathing

The physiological mechanisms that are responsible for pulsatile (rapidly changing) aerodynamic speech events are not fully understood but are likely very complex, probably involving two main types of nerve-muscle systems: extrafusal (large muscle fibers outside the muscle spindle) and intrafusal (fibers inside the muscle spindle). The extrafusal system likely includes alpha motor neuron systems of both the internal and external intercostal muscles. In more emotive or emphatic speech, other muscles (e.g., abdominals) may also be involved. The intrafusal muscle system may act as a servomechanism (feedback device). In this role, a gamma-loop mechanism would operate in response to detection of rapid loading and unloading forces on the respiratory driving mechanism and function to stabilize primary respiratory muscles during these changes, allowing for refinement of compensatory muscular adjustments. Because speech is a motor skill, it is thought that learned patterns of interaction between the different neuromuscular systems are used to regulate the respiratory system during the complex act of verbal communication[27]. We discussed earlier the important role of the periaqueductal gray matter in the brain, which uses afferent input from servomechanisms in the respiratory system to coordinate speech-breathing, phonatory, and articulatory movements during vocalization[12].

8.4.4 Glossary for Respiration

Expiratory reserve volume (ERV): Quantity of air that can be exhaled beyond that of the tidal volume.

Functional residual capacity (FRC): Volume of air in the respiratory system at resting expiratory level (when recoil forces of compression and expansion are balanced). In young, healthy, adult males, a mean FRC of 2.3 liters (2300 mL) is estimated.

Inspiratory capacity: Maximum volume of air that can be inhaled from the resting expiratory level.

Inspiratory reserve volume (IRV): Quantity of air that can be inhaled beyond that in tidal volume.

Residual volume: Quantity of air that remains after a maximum exhalation.

Resting expiratory level (REL): Volume of air in the lungs allowing for a pressure balance between the elastic recoil compression forces of the lungs and the recoil expansion forces of the thorax structure. REL also refers to the typical volume at the end of an exhalation phase of rest breathing.

Tidal volume: Quantity of air inhaled and exhaled during one cycle of respiration, generally in reference to rest breathing. The normal tidal volume represents approximately 10% of the vital capacity, ranges from 0.5 to 0.75 liters (during sedentary activity levels), and occurs from 12 to18 times per minute in adults (up to 70 times per minute in the newborn).[48]

Total lung capacity (TLC): The volume of air in the lungs after a maximum inspiration or at the top of inspiratory capacity.

Vital capacity (VC): Volume of air that can be exhaled following deep inhalation (after inspiratory capacity is reached or from total lung capacity). Normal VC for adults ranges from 3.5 liters for small, young, adult females, to 5 liters for average young adult males.

8.5 Phonation: Conversion of DC to AC Energy

Phonation, or sound-producing vocal fold vibration, is a process by which DC (direct current) aerodynamic energy is converted to AC (alternating current) acoustic energy. This takes place when the vocal folds are adducted sufficiently to offer an adequate resistance to the DC airflow so that they are set into vibration. The vocal fold adducting muscles, principally the lateral cricoarytenoids and interarytenoids, approximate the arytenoid cartilages which effects prephonatory vocal fold closure in the posterior glottis (see Figure 8–9). The degree of resistance offered by the vocal folds determines how much pressure is required from the airflow to initiate and sustain vibratory action. Resistance can be altered at the larynx by varying the tension, the degree of adduction (including that resulting from supraglottal constrictions), or both. This determines in part how hard the respiratory forces must work to sustain phonation. Other influences over laryngeal resistance are intended or required loudness and pitch ranges of a speech or sung phrase and even more subtle linguistic, emotional, and pragmatic requirements. Various combinations of intrinsic muscle contractions serve to adjust the tone, length, shape, and elasticity of the vocal folds according to pitch, loudness, and quality requirements of the phonatory task (See Figure 8–9).

The result of the vocal fold vibration is a series of pressure pulses that disturbs the air molecules in the vocal tract so that they oscillate. Oscillation can be defined as alternate compression and rarefaction of space between the molecules. We refer to the oscillating air column as a sound pressure wave. The shape of the vocal tract resonators determines which components of the glottal source waveform will be enhanced and which will be damped, and thus the nature of sounds we will perceive. The human hearing system is sensitive to the sound pressure changes and

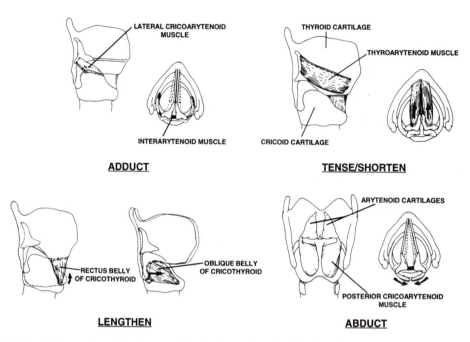

Figure 8–9. Intrinsic muscles of the larynx and their primary functions for phonation.

responds first mechanically, then in turn by sending electrophysiological signals to the brain regarding the nature of the sound.

8.5.1 Histology and Biomechanics of the Vocal Folds

The paired vocal folds consist of several layers of tissues that are quite different in their histological (cellular) structures. Figure 8–10 represents the histology of an adult vocal fold schematically, as studied from a midmembranous frontal section. The most superficial layer comprises stratified squamous epithelium bordered by pseudostratified ciliated epithelium on the superior and inferior edges. The next three layers comprise the **lamina propria.** The superficial layer, also known as **Reinke's space,** consists of pliable areolar tissue, which allows the "cover" to glide easily over the deeper layers of the vocal folds during vibration. The intermediate layer of the lamina propria consists predominantly of elastic tissue, and the

deep layer consists mainly of collagen. The intermediate and deep layers are poorly differentiated at their borders, but deeper tissues are increasingly stiffer compared with the superficial layer. Together they form the **vocal ligament,** a structure that is important during phonation for its elastic biomechanical properties. The deepest layer of the vocal fold consists of striated muscle fibers, the most viscous (stiffest) of the structures. The most medial muscle section often is referred to as the **vocalis** muscle, and the more lateral fibers comprise the **thyroarytenoid** muscle. As is evident in Figure 8–10, the layered structure becomes simpler at the superior and inferior borders. Inferior to and continuous with the vocal ligament, the single-layered conus elasticus provides a sheetlike support for the lower portion of the vocal fold. As will be described later in this chapter, the vocal fold is less developed in infants and children, and neither the vocal ligament nor the conus elasticus are evident in the first few years of life.

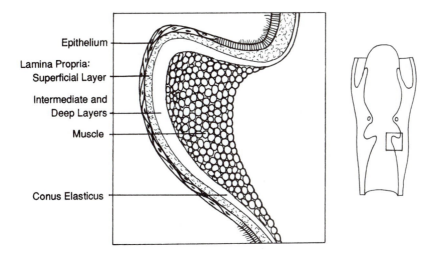

Figure 8–10. Histological structure of the adult vocal fold.

The vocal folds are designed for efficient and effective vibration for phonatory activities. The progressive density and viscosity of the layers contribute to a delicate and complex vibrator system. The tissue fibres in each of the layers run in anterior-to-posterior directions, that is, parallel to the vocal fold margins. Even the laryngeal vascular system provides design features that enhance the complex vibratory behavior. Within the medial portions of the superficial layers of the vocal folds, where phonatory excursion is greatest, the blood vessels are thinnest and run longitudinally, thus providing uniform density and maximum flexibility for vocal fold vibration. The tissues are stiffest in a longitudinal direction and most pliable in a transverse direction. The structure of the true vocal fold determines that the greatest flexibility for vibration is at the medial portion of the vocal folds [22,24,26].

The **"cover-body" theory** helps explain some aspects of vocal fold vibration by relating it to mechanical properties of the different layers and their interactions. At least two distinct layers are described to account for mechanical properties: the cover comprising the epithelium and superficial layer of the lamina propria and the body, which includes the stiffer vocal ligament and muscle layers. It has become evident that we may need to account for more than two layers to thoroughly explain vibratory phenomena. For example, the vocal ligament may serve as a biomechanical transition region because its stiffness is intermediate between the cover and the muscle.

The degree to which the different vocal fold layers function separately during phonation depends on the action of intrinsic and, to some extent, extrinsic muscles of the larynx and the health of vocal fold structures. Muscle groups that serve to lengthen and stiffen the various layers make them function more as if they were one. This is the case during phonation at high frequencies, as in the falsetto or loft register. Disease processes affecting the cover may also unify the function of the layers: edema in Reinke's space increases its viscosity and results in less complex patterns of vibration and surgical scarring may result in tethering of the cover to the body. Muscles that tend to adduct the vocal folds without concurrent increases in muscular tone of the body may result in the two layers functioning more-or-less as if they were one, but in a manner different from the tense state. The acoustic result may include a degree of breathiness because of a lowered resistance to airflow and subsequent longer open phase of the phonatory cycle. Denervation of the vocalis and thyroarytenoid muscle may result in reduced tone and viscosity of the body and mechanical properties more similar to those of the cover. This often is noted in the case of vocal fold paralyses. Contraction of the vocalis and thyroarytenoid muscle group, without a proportional increase in opposing lengthening forces (cricothyroid muscle), will make the body stiffer and the cover looser. This relatively looser cover is the situation in chest or modal register, which is the usual speaking-voice register.

Traditionally, vocal fold vibration for vocalization has been described as a **myoelastic-aerodynamic** activity. Self-sustained vocal fold oscillation is indeed achieved by a number of aerodynamic and mechanical phenomena that essentially transfer energy between a fairly steady airflow and the vocal fold tissues, but the process is much more complex than traditional models would imply.

Titze has used one-mass computer models, multimass models, string models and ribbon models to explain the many interacting biomechanical and aerodynamic features that help explain the self-sustained oscillation that is phonation. He concluded, "asymmetry in the effective restoring force of the system is the essential feature."[112] At least two types of delayed action mechanisms may allow for synchronization of airflow and tissue: 1) a delay in the buildup and collapse of the forward moving air column relative to the opening and closing of the vocal folds in which the resulting asymmetry in aerodynamic pressure relative to tissue velocity allows the vocal folds to move synchronously with their natural movement, and 2) a delay between the movements of the upper and

lower portions of the vocal folds, which creates an asymmetrical driving force[112]. The biomechanical and aerodynamic driving forces are depicted in Figure 8–11

A frontal view of the vocal folds during one phonatory cycle in **modal register** is represented schematically in Figure 8–12. At least four distinct vocal fold shapes may be represented in the phonatory cycle in modal register—convergent, sulcus, rectangular, and divergent[92,112–114]—with the definitions based largely on the nature of vertical phase differences between the upper and lower margins of the vocal folds. Scherer and Titze have demonstrated how each of these shapes must be associated with a different set of aerodynamic and mechanical principles[92]. A three-mass model of phonation has been presented to represent some of these principles (see Figure 8–13). Of particular importance during the vibratory cycle are the **convergent shape** (associated with the onset of the opening phase and a relatively high intraglottal pressure), and the **divergent shape** (associated with the onset of closing phase, and lower intraglottal pressure).

In the past, the aerodynamic aspect of vocal fold self-oscillation focused exclusively on the Bernoulli principle thought to be the primary aerodynamic restoring force for the vocal fold closing phase[116]. The predominant closing influence of this principle depends on an assumption of laminar (smooth, nonturbulent) symmetrical airflow through a rectangular-shaped glottis. It is now clear that the divergent shape of vocal fold closing in modal register must result in other important nonsymmetrical aerodynamic principles contributing to vocal fold closure, principally **flow separation**—separation of the air stream from its boundary at the triangular glottal outlet. Ishizaka and Matsudaira described this aerodynamic principle: Within the divergent glottal channel, the air stream separates from the vocal fold surfaces to create a central jet stream and turbulent flow within the widening glottal margins in the form of

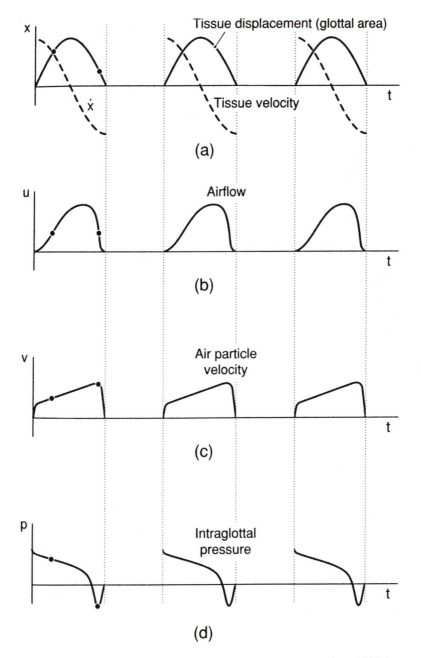

Figure 8–11. Waveforms during sustained oscillation: a) displacement and velocity of vocal fold tissue at the centre of the glottis, b) airflow, c) air particle velocity, and d) mean intraglottal air pressure that drives the vocal folds. Reprinted by permission from *Principles of Voice Production*[112]. Copyright 1994 by Allyn & Bacon.

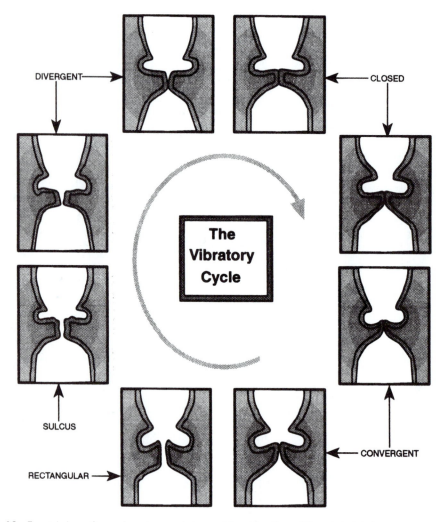

Figure 8–12. Frontal view of one phonatory cycle in modal register. Four different glottal shapes are represented, corresponding to at least four recognized aerodynamic principles that may be in effect during phonation (see text for more details).

eddies[45]. The turbulence can be explained in part by a well-known principle of physics defined by Reynold's number, which demonstrates that maximum turbulent flow is achieved when the glottal outlet is widened, the glottal pressure is high, and the tissue viscosity is low[112]. Further, differential and interacting aerodynamic forces are present at different levels of the glottis throughout the phonatory cycle, and these depend on the shapes the vocal folds assume at any one time, as influenced by the amplitude, frequency, and register of vibration (see Figure 8–13).[44,92,107–109,113] One result of nonlinear characteristics of the flow is a chaotic acoustic pattern[4]. Supraglottal pressures (pressures above the glottis) also contribute to self-sustained oscillation, because of continually

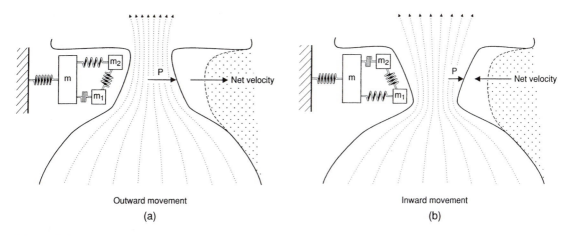

Figure 8–13. A three-mass model of the vocal folds, including airflow and driving pressure in the glottis: a) outward movement with a convergent glottis, b) inward movement with a divergent glottis. Note the direction of net velocity of the tissue in relation to the pressure *P*. Reprinted by permission from *Principles of Voice Production*[112]. Copyright 1994 by Allyn & Bacon.

changing relationships between the upward-moving air column and intraglottal pressures (pressures between the vocal folds). The reader is referred to Chapter 4 of Titze's 1994 text for additional detail regarding the principles of self-sustained vocal fold oscillation[112].

Phonation in other registers, namely **falsetto** or **glottal fry,** is associated with shapes and biomechanical principles that are different from those for modal register. For example, in **falsetto register,** the vocal fold cover is stiffened considerably by anteroposterior lengthening, so the layers act more as one. The vocal fold margins are thinner in the superior-inferior dimension, which affects other aspects of vocal fold vibration to be discussed in the following paragraphs. Finally, reduced contraction of the thyroarytenoid muscles may reduce myoelastic vocal fold adduction properties, so the closed phase of phonation may be incomplete or of short duration. In **glottal fry register,** the cover may be loose and the body stiff, as with modal register, but the closed phase of the vibratory cycle is proportionally longer, and

some syncopated or double-pulsing vibratory action may be observed on acoustic waveforms. Observations of the vocal folds during glottal fry phonation suggest that muscular forces are creating anterior-posterior constriction and high medial compression, which should contribute to a longer closed phase.

An important consequence of the multiple layer structure is the potential for a complex vibratory pattern of the vocal folds. A number of dynamic phenomena may be partially explainable on the basis of the variable layer structure: **longitudinal phase difference, vertical phase difference,** and **mucosal wave.** These three effects are particularly noticeable in modal or chest register phonation, and together determine the potential for a complex sound wave with many harmonic components.

8.5.1.1 Longitudinal Phase Difference

Longitudinal phase difference refers to nonsimultaneous opening and closing of different portions of the vocal folds in the anterior to posterior direction, giving a zipper-type opening and closing effect. The longitudinal phase difference may be a consequence of variable thickness of the different layers from anterior to posterior, variable muscular dynamics from anterior to posterior, different nature of structural attachments of the anterior and posterior portions of the vocal folds, and different mechanical and aerodynamic consequences of all the above factors, from anterior to posterior.

8.5.1.2 Vertical Phase Difference

Vertical phase difference relates to temporal differences in the opening and closing of the bottom and top margins of the vocal folds. This is well represented in Titze's three-mass model of phonation (Figure 8–13).[112] In modal register, the vocal folds open and close from the inferior to superior margins. Because the inferior margins are subjected to subglottal pressures first, the vertical phase difference is easily explainable on the basis of upward-flowing aerodynamic forces and a mechanical linkage dragging the superior edges in the direction of the inferior edges. The inertial elastic forces of the stretched vocal fold tissues, along with any relevant aerodynamic forces, effect the closing phases of the cycle beginning at the lower margins and mechanically drag the upper margins with some phase lag.

8.5.1.3 Mucosal Wave

Mucosal wave is the ripple effect seen along the surface of the vocal folds; this ripple stretches more or less from the anterior to posterior ends and travels from the margin to the peripheral area of each of the vocal folds in the course of each vibratory cycle. It is likely related to several factors including the vertical phase difference and the natural tendency for the cover to move freely when the incompressible vocal folds are subjected to vertical deformation by aerodynamic pres-

sures. Additional factors that may influence the mucosal wave include the impact between the vocal folds when they collide and reflections from the lateral ventricle walls. The velocity of the propagation of mucosal waves influences the phase lag between the upper and lower vocal fold margins.

It should now be evident that self-sustained vibration of the vocal folds during phonation is the result of a complex interaction of aerodynamic and biomechanical forces. Broad has described this relationship succinctly: "Vibrations can be sustained only if the effective aerodynamic coupling between the glottal outlet and inlet is stronger than the mechanical coupling between the corresponding upper and lower parts of the vocal fold"[9, p. 206]. The relative influence of aerodynamic and mechanical forces may be determined by vocal production factors such as vocal effort or tension and pitch. For example, phonation at high pitches is associated with more symmetrical vocal fold margins and a smaller vertical phase difference.

Titze has studied **phonation threshold pressures** (PTP) for different vocal production conditions[110,111]. These studies suggest that phonation at lower fundamental frequencies (f_0) is more responsive to aerodynamic forces than phonation at higher f_0 levels. That is, phonation can be initiated and sustained with lower subglottal pressures when the vocal folds are in their shorter, thicker state, as in the modal speech register. The degree of adduction can also affect PTP, and Titze has speculated on an optimal prephonatory glottal width of only a few millimeters. Because developmental, aging, and gender-based differences predict variability in laryngeal adduction, these factors also may affect PTP profiles. Predicted variability in structure and function because of developmental, aging, and gender characteristics will be discussed at the end of this chapter. The infinite possibilities for different vocal fold vibratory patterns and resultant acoustic products are far from understood at this time. Some recent studies using animal and computer models present the complexity of issues that must be addressed before we can fully understand vocal fold vibratory patterns[1,26,45,79,107,112–115].

8.5.2 Dynamic Control of Pitch, Intensity and Quality

During speech, the intrinsic muscles of the larynx continuously alter the frequency, amplitude, and pattern of vocal fold vibration, causing changes to acoustic and perceptual features of the voice including fundamental frequency (f_0) and pitch, intensity and loudness, and acoustic spectrum and quality. The degree to which biomechanical or elastic properties versus aerodynamic features contribute to changes in f_0 and acoustic intensity depends on the phonation register (mode of vibration), technique, articulatory resistance in the vocal tract, and even motivational and emotional factors. Intrinsic muscles that are involved in various pitch and intensity-changing functions are represented in Figure 8–9.

The **fundamental frequency (f_0)** of vocal fold vibration is the primary determinant of pitch, a perceptual phenomenon. The mean f_0 of an individual's voice is determined anatomically by length of the membranous portion of the vocal folds[24]. A fundamental frequency range of up to 1 octave may be used for speech purposes. In singing, the range used is generally much wider. Mean speaking f_0 values typically cited for North American adults are 200 Hz for women and 100 Hz for men. In the developmental period, the f_0 range tends to decrease with age; preschool children may have mean speaking f_0 levels of around 300 Hz.

Changes in f_0 are undoubtedly as complex as the mechanisms involved. Titze has described the various combinations of passive and active laryngeal tissues that could be involved in altering f_0 to result in perceived pitch changes, as well as effects of respiratory forces, intensity, and biological characteristics of the vocal folds[112]. Our summary of current understanding of these factors is necessarily simplistic, and the reader is encouraged to pursue more detailed descriptions as needed.

Within modal register, changes in fundamental frequency of vibration are related to changes in the stiffness or tension of the vocal folds and may conform best to a body-cover model, which predicts significant contributions by the vocalis-thyroarytenoid muscle body[52,112]. The paired cricothyroid muscles contract to adjust the distance between the two cartilage structures, effecting a visorlike closing and thus lengthening and stiffening the vocal folds. The effectiveness of cricothyroid contraction in achieving this task is dependent on opposing contraction of adducting and abducting muscles that anchor the arytenoid cartilages. Harris has provided a vector model to help explain the delicate balance of intrinsic muscle forces involved in the pitch-changing mechanism (Figure 8–14)[20]. Concurrent contraction of the vocalis-thyroarytenoid complex may increase tension and contribute to pitch increases, particularly in the modal register.

Mechanisms for pitch lowering are primarily related to cessation of activity in the muscles that increase f_0. Both aerodynamic forces and larynx lowering by action of extrinsic muscles have also been implicated in pitch lowering mechanisms[3,11]. Different intonation mechanisms may be used at low versus high pitch, and pitch mechanisms also may vary with syntactic characteristics of speech, such as sentence type[3]. Many questions need to be answered before we fully understand relationships between linguistic and physiological aspects of intonation control. F_0 changes in falsetto register and at low intensities may be explained more simply using a cover model of phonation, which predicts a singularly strong relationship between cricothyroid muscle activity and increases in pitch[112]. Aerodynamic forces may also play a

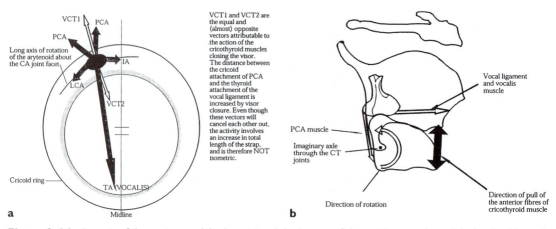

Figure 8–14. Aspects of the vector model relevant to pitch changes. **a**) Isometric muscular activity involved in positioning the right arytenoid cartilage. **b**) The cricothyroid visor mechanism for increasing vocal fold tension. Reprinted with permission from *The Voice Clinic Handbook*[20]. Copyright 1998 by Whurr Publishers Ltd, London.

greater role in effecting f_0 variation because small amplitudes of vibration determine amplitude-dependent f_0 changes[109,110,113,114]. All other factors held constant, f_0 is expected to rise with increases in subglottal pressure and increases in intensity.

Vertical larynx movement has been documented during changes in f_0 due to contraction of extrinsic laryngeal muscles that elevate or lower the larynx[41]. The mechanism by which vertical laryngeal movement contributes to pitch change is not entirely clear, but one explanation suggests that movements of the cricoid cartilage following the spinal lordosis will change vocal fold length[21,41].

Any discussion of vocal pitch ranges inevitably leads to debate regarding vocal registers and their physiological correlates. In speech-science terms, vocal registers may be defined by their characteristic laryngeal postures and subsequent vocal fold vibratory patterns. One of the primary reasons for continued intense interest and debate in this area is the impact that our understanding of vocal registers and pitch changes has on singing and vocal performance pedagogy, particularly as

concerns the modal-falsetto register transition. Based on our current understanding of different biomechanical and aerodynamic principles operating in those two registers, different mechanisms for pitch control would be anticipated and indeed have been documented. Those concerned about vocal performance issues are encouraged to pursue this ongoing study in current journals and texts[47,103,112].

Vocal intensity or power, which contributes to loudness perception, is primarily a function of subglottal pressure and amplitude of vocal fold vibrations; however tuning within the vocal tract and the radiation characteristic of speech also influence the intensity of the final speech product. Acoustic intensity is proportional to subglottal pressure, which is determined by airflow and glottal resistance. Anatomically, lung volume and larynx size are principle determinants of vocal power; all other factors being equal, individuals with larger systems will be capable of generating more intense vocal sounds. Because individuals with larger systems also are capable of producing lower f_0 ranges, which predict a greater number of "audible" harmonic partials within the glottal source spectrum, some dependence on f_0 is recognized (the spectral characteristics of voice will be discussed further in the next section). The efficiency with which an individual converts aerodynamic to acoustic power ultimately determines his or her potential for vocal intensity within the limitations of the anatomical structures involved. This power conversion can be influenced by vocal technique and indeed is often an important goal in vocal rehabilitation and vocal pedagogy. Rapid changes in intensity are required to provide linguistic stress, and production of these linguistic markers involves complex interactions between laryngeal valving forces and aerodynamic driving forces[40].

Because the aerodynamic and biomechanical mechanisms engaged for increases in vocal intensity and f_0 are similar, it is not surprising to discover that these two functions are interdependent to some extent, during vocal productions. When we shout, increases in both intensity and f_0 of the vocal signal can be measured acoustically. This interdependence may also explain why singers comment that it takes more technique to sing a high note quietly than loudly.

Voice quality or timbre is related both to individual structural-mechanical features and to habitual laryngeal and supraglottal postures. Let us look at a graphic representation of the glottal pulse to explore some possible physiological correlates of voice quality at the laryngeal level. In Figure 8–15, one cycle of vocal fold oscillation in modal register is represented by a single glottal pulse, as seen in an inverse-filtered flow glottogram (a product of filtering the upper vocal tract resonance effects from the aerodynamic signal; see Chapter 1 for a description of the instrumental technique). We see that normal phonation in modal register is associated with a skewed waveform. A more gradual slope in the opening phase suggests that the

vocal folds open relatively slowly, and steeper slope in the closing phase suggests they close relatively quickly. This skewed pulse is more noticeable in the average adult male voice than in that of women and children, likely for both structural and physiological reasons. The faster closing phase of phonation has been related to an acoustic signal that is relatively rich in harmonic components of the waveform, especially in those that enhance the important speech and singing formants of the upper vocal tract as seen in Figure 8–16a[103]. If the length of the closing phase is increased (open phase increases) as it tends to be in women and children, then the vocal sound may not be so clear because of relatively lower amplitude of the upper harmonics and formants of the voice, as seen in Figure 8–16b[84,86,93]. The consensus that some North American women have breathier voices than their male counterparts may relate to the slower closing phase in phonation. This voice quality and vibratory feature may also be due to a posterior glottal chink (triangular gap), which has been identified as a frequent characteristic of phonatory posturing in women[6,73,84,85,95]. We already have discussed the role that speech-breathing patterns may have on this phonatory posture. Phonation with a large posterior glottal chink may result in excessive noise in the vocal signal, where harmonics are replaced by air turbulence and a noise peak may be seen in the upper vocal spectrum [84,93]. Earlier we described the conditions defined by Reynold's number that predict an increase in turbulent flow. The glottal chink posture may also be associated with a higher relative intensity of f_0 relative to that of the other areas of the glottal source acoustic spectrum[56,84]. These phenomena are demonstrated in Figure 8–16c. Such an acoustic profile generally results in perceptions of breathiness. The schematic glottal pulse for a clinically breathy voice is seen in Figure 8–15 as the most symmetrical waveform.

The Glottal Pulse

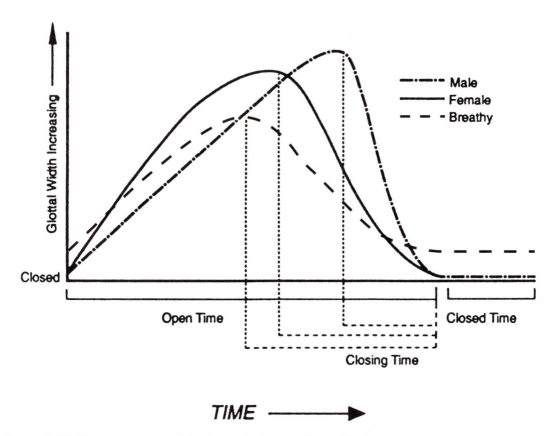

Figure 8–15. Vibratory correlates of the glottal pulse (see text for details).

Harsh or rough voice quality perceptions have been attributed to irregularities or perturbations in consecutive vibratory cycles, resulting in jitter (irregular duration of cycles) and shimmer (irregular amplitude of cycles) in the acoustic waveform[13,72,106]. Figure 8–17 demonstrates schematically these perturbations in the glottal source waveform. Baken has pointed out why physiological and acoustic perturbations are characteristic of the output of the vocal system, even in normally speaking individuals. **Chaos theory** is used to explain the nonlinear function of many major physiological systems, including the respiratory, neuromotor, cochlear, and cerebrocortical systems that form part of the psychomotor act of speech and voice production. Sudden and dramatic changes in physiology and its acoustic product (bifurcations) are present in infant cries and adult speech and represent a particular form of functional integrity of the system, a so-called "unsteady stability"[4].

Extrinsic muscles make many adjustments that may contribute to perceptual changes in the voice (Figure 8–18). For example, unop-

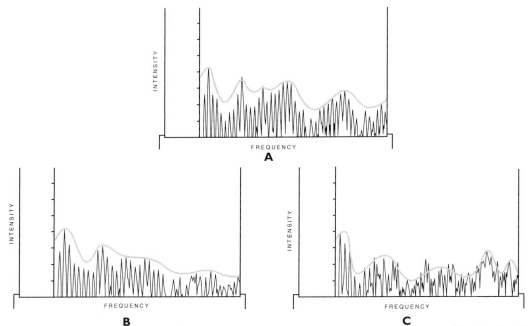

Figure 8–16. Spectra of the glottal source harmonic sequence (vertical spikes) and vocal tract filter function (formants: wavy lines enveloping the harmonic peak pattern). Characteristics of the vibratory pattern of the vocal folds contribute to spectral features. In each spectrum, the abscissa represents frequency and the ordinate intensity. **A**) Intensity-enhanced, high frequency harmonics and speech formants are represented by relative height. Rapid vocal fold closure time, as in men, contributes to high intensity of harmonics in the regions of important speech formants. The density of the spectrum also contributes to acoustic power and is determined by f_0: in men around 100 Hz. **B**) Longer vocal fold closing times contribute to relatively lower intensity in the upper harmonic sequence. This pattern is more typical of women during speech. The higher f_0, 200 Hz, contributes to a spectrum that is less dense. **C**) Phonation with an exaggerated glottal chink often is associated with relatively high intensity in the first harmonic partial (f_0), and noise in the spectrum. The noise may be particularly intense in the region above 5 kHz. These acoustic characteristics may contribute to perceptions of *breathiness* or *whispery voice*.

posed contraction of suprahyoid muscles will cause the larynx to rise in the neck and may change pitch—primarily by affecting vocal fold tension or length, and secondarily by shortening the resonance tube—thus elevating vocal tract resonances or **formants.** Larynx lowering may result in reduced vocal fold tension to lower the f_0 and a longer vocal tract to lower formants and pitch[14,57].

Any long-term postures in muscles of the pharynx, velopharynx, or articulators can influence speech or voice quality. In the next section, we will discuss the opposing effects of rounding or spreading the lips on formant frequencies. We have seen that head and neck posture may alter glottal closure patterns through the extrinsic muscle connections: a jaw-jut posture may be associated with a wider posterior glottal chink and greater breathiness in the voice[95]. The relative degree to which the tongue is held forward or back in the mouth during speech will influence resonance and articulatory qualities. The relative degree to which the jaw is held fixed or is mobile during speech will influence oral-

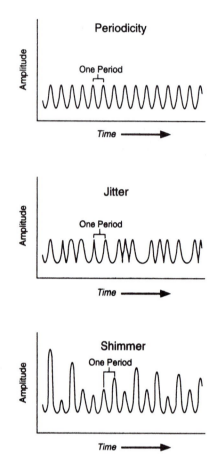

Figure 8–17. Variations or perturbations in the glottal source waveform may contribute to acoustic characteristics such as jitter and shimmer. In reality, absolute periodicity is not a feature of phonatory activity for speech.

nasal resonance balance, and the degree to which the velopharyngeal port is closed or open will determine the perceived nasality [57,58]. Contraction of muscles at the base of the tongue may result in hypernasality, due to a decrease in the size of the oral resonating cavity and a downward pull on the soft palate via the palatoglossus muscle. The complex structural relationships between the larynx and its extralaryngeal attachments are evident in Figure 8–18.

For a detailed and entertaining description of anatomical features and isometric function of the extrinsic and intrinsic laryngeal muscle systems, the reader is directed to *The Voice Clinic Handbook*, Chapter 5[20].

8.6 Acoustic Resonators of Speech

Figure 8–19 shows the structures involved in vocal tract resonance. Figure 8–20 demonstrates the fundamental principles of acoustic waveform transformations during speech. As the glottal pulse propagates along the vocal tract, it is subjected to a variety of resonance effects that are determined by the shape and viscosity of the cavity walls. The principles are based on the acoustic theory of speech production proposed by Fant[14]. The original acoustic theory describes relationships between the glottal source features, vocal tract filter function, and radiation characteristics, and is sometimes referred to as the "source-filter" theory.

The **glottal source** contributes a fairly regular pulselike multifrequency input signal to the vocal tract (Figure 8–20 A and B). In the case of an ideal periodic voice source input signal, the frequencies represented in the glottal pulse are mathematically predictable: the strongest component will correspond to the fundamental frequency and progressively weaker components or harmonic partials will fall at frequencies corresponding to $f_0 \times 2$; $f_0 \times 3$; $f_0 \times 4$, and so forth. An amplitude density spectrum demonstrates that the intensity of progressively higher harmonic partials is reduced by about 12 dB per octave when source characteristics are considered independent of the vocal tract filter function. We have seen that the relatively faster vocal fold closing time during phonation in adult males contributes to enhancement of the upper harmonics (Figure 8–16). Because the f_0 in men is lower (average 100 Hz versus 200 Hz in women), their spectral density is also greater, based on the

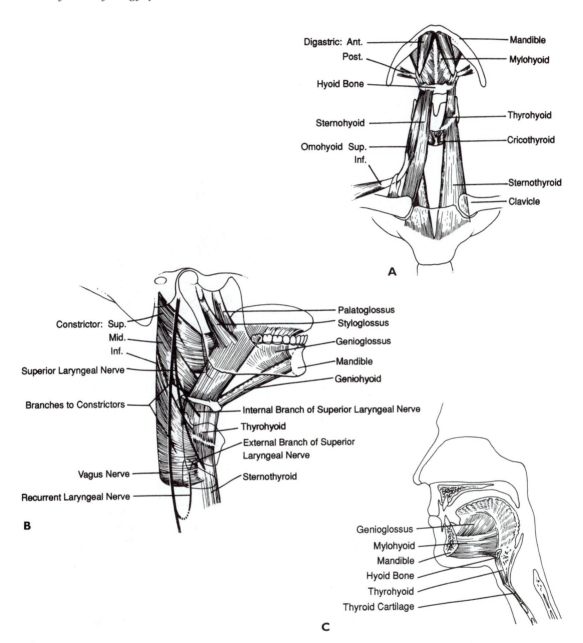

Figure 8–18. Structure and muscles of the larynx and the laryngeal suspension system. The supralaryngeal and infralaryngeal muscles suspend the larynx in the neck and may be active during changes in vocal intensity, frequency, or resonance characteristics. When hypertonic, these muscles in various combinations may contribute to limitations in phonatory function, and to voice disorders. **A)** Frontal view demonstrating extrinsic muscle laryngeal suspension system. **B)** Sagittal view demonstrating relationships of pharyngeal muscles with the larynx and nerve supply. **C)** Sagittal view demonstrating relationships of tongue and mandible with the larynx.

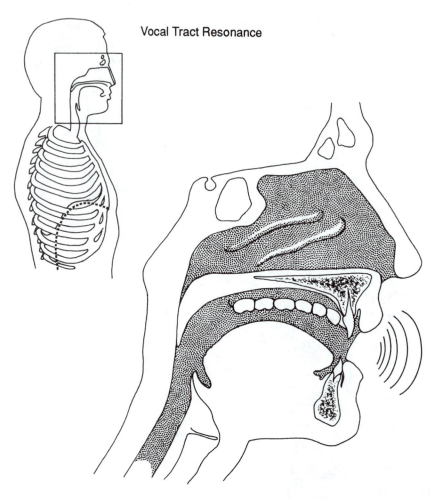

Vocal Tract Resonance

Figure 8–19. Vocal tract resonators for speech are primarily the upper larynx, the pharynx and the oral cavity. The nasal cavities contribute resonance characteristics when the velopharyngeal port is open, most obviously for nasal phonemes: /m/; /n/ /ŋ/. In North America, many individuals have significant nasal resonance contributions to all vocalized sounds in speech.

formula provided above. This is another factor contributing to greater acoustic power in the spectra, greater formant enhancement, and richer quality of adult male voices compared with those of women and children.

As we have discussed, vocal sounds are not perfectly harmonic, and even in normal speech the vocal source waveform may be characterized by minor perturbations and

areas of noise energy. These normal variations from idealized glottal pulses, in addition to the vocal tract filter functions, influence the harmonic energy patterns in speech spectra.

The vocal tract serves as a **filter** to selectively enhance or damp various frequency components or groups of adjacent partials of the glottal pulse waveform (Figure 8–20 C and D).

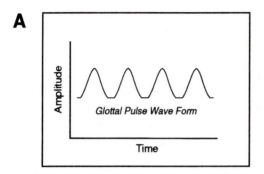

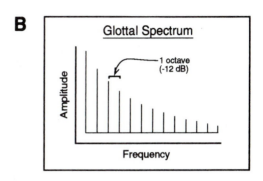

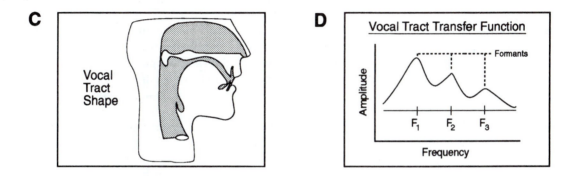

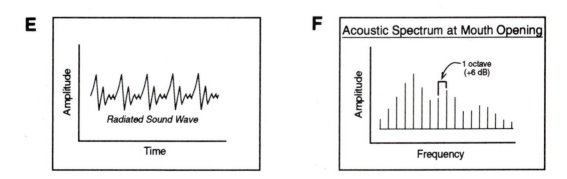

Figure 8–20. Basic components of the acoustic theory of speech production[14,15], the glottal pulse (A and B), vocal tract transfer function (C and D), and radiation characteristics (E and F). (See text for details.)

Positioning of the articulators, including the larynx and cavity walls, results in distinct shapes of the vocal tract corresponding to specific natural resonance characteristics called **formants.** The first two or three formants (and antiformants) can be used to predict and describe articulatory features for continuous sounds of a language, for example, the vowel phonemes. We know that F1 is particularly sensitive to jaw or tongue height, and F2 is sensitive to anterior-posterior place of constriction within the vocal tract (for example whether the tongue is raised in front of the mouth for /i/ ("ee") or in back for /u/ ("oo"). F3 is affected by constrictions at various places throughout the vocal tract. Based on this knowledge, the frequencies of formants can be predicted within a certain range for particular vocal tract lengths: for example, the average formants for North American English /i/ ("ee") are F1 = 270 Hz; F2 = 2300 Hz; F3 = 3000 Hz for an adult male, and F1 = 370 Hz; F2 = 3200 Hz, and F3 = 3700 Hz for a preschool child[54]. As might be predicted, the formant frequencies are lower in longer vocal tracts (such as a man's) than in shorter ones (such as a child's or woman's). An individual can lower his or her vocal tract formants by lowering the larynx or protruding the lips and (assuming other vocal tract postures are kept constant) can raise the formants by elevating the larynx or retracting the lips.

During speech, the formants are in almost constant transition and often do not reach the precise values that predict sound discriminations, owing to continual movement of the articulators and to coarticulatory effects. Even in the brief time that is allotted to a series of speech targets, acoustic filter functions provide the listener with sufficient formant information and other important acoustic cues to recognize speech. Figure 8–21 demonstrates schematically a lateral view of the vocal tract during production of three North American English vowels and their corresponding vocal tract filter spectra.

An understanding of the relationship between vocal tract articulator posturing and formant frequencies is obviously useful for speech clinicians that wish to assist individuals to improve articulation or resonance properties in speech. This knowledge also enhances techniques in singing pedagogy, in which consistency of vocal quality is desired in the presence of a high dependence between the vocal fold oscillator and vocal tract resonance, for example, when singing at high frequencies.

A final important acoustic characteristic encompassed in Fant's theory is that of the **radiation characteristic** of speech (Figure 8–20 E and F). This is the nature of propagation of the speech sounds through the air from the end of the vocal tract, which defines the nature of sound that reaches the listener's ear. The radiation characteristic can be predicted to increase the speech signal by 6 dB per octave. This feature seems to correspond well with the sensitivity of the human acoustic system.

Although the original Acoustic Theory of Speech Production has provided a valuable reference for descriptions of speech function in an idealized fashion, its simplicity limits description of certain aspects of normal and disordered speech function. We have already discussed the inherent "chaotic" nature of the vocal system and its output. A theory that assumes functional linearity is not entirely compatible with the chaotic reality of the human vocal system. The source-filter theory also assumes relative independence between the vocal fold oscillators and the articulatory function, and indeed such independence is desirable and to some extent achievable during speech. Nonetheless, there are known interactions between the glottal source function and vocal tract adjustments that may influence the nature of the final radiated acoustic signal due to mechanical-aerodynamic loading forces and acoustic interactions. This may be particularly important in influencing fine-tuning during singing or other vocal performance. Further, the supra-

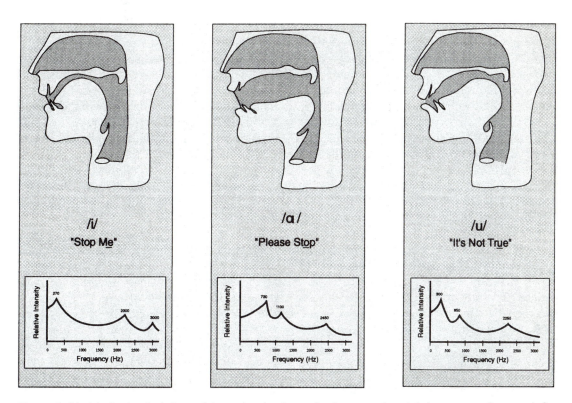

Figure 8–21. Idealized sagittal views of the oral cavity shapes for three vowels and their corresponding speech formants.

glottal and subglottal spaces may be coupled to varying degrees during speech and phonation, depending on the length of open phases in the phonatory cycle and the degree of approximation of the vocal folds[15–17,54,86,104].

8.7 Normal Variability in Structure and Function

8.7.1 Normal Development and Aging

A comprehensive treatment of issues related to voice development and aging should include consideration of not just the larynx, but the developmental and aging patterns and schedules for all structures and systems involved in speech and vocal production. Presentation of such details is beyond the scope of this text. Developmental and aging patterns in speech breathing have been highlighted in a previous section. The reader is referred to the excellent reviews by Kahane[48–50], Kent and Vorperian[53], and Mackenzie Beck[71] for detailed descriptions of developmental aspects of head and neck structure and function and their effects on communication.

Kent and Vorperian have presented a hierarchy of development for the head and neck structures: the head (particularly the cranium and brain) reach their full size by about 6 years of age, followed by the face-jaw, the larynx, and then the tongue, which continue their development into the adolescent years[53].

Neurological development plays a major role in communication maturation and continues into the adult years. Beyond the different laryngeal structures in infants, children, and adults, one must consider the significant developmental differences in the lower face, including the lips, tongue, hard and soft palate, and jaw to account for all variations in speech and singing characteristics at different ages. Schematic midsagittal sections of the lower face and vocal tract of an infant, child, and adult are represented in Figure 8–22.

In the infant, the larynx is positioned differently than in the adult, and structural development is incomplete. The larynx is high in the neck at birth and apparently continues to descend during the life cycle (studies report variable locations from second to fourth cervical vertebrae in infants and between C5 and C7 in adults). During respiration, the epiglottis may touch the uvula. With the larynx positioned thus, tucked close to the tongue and soft palate, the infant is able to alternate rapidly between suckling and breathing without aspirating, but this position limits its phonetic repertoire[53]. Articulatory structures are also not fully developed at birth. Muscle coordination and strength of the tongue is inferior to that of adults. Nevertheless, the infant is capable of producing a wide enough repertoire of vocal sounds for communication of basic needs to take place. Mothers quickly learn to distinguish among the various cries in order to oblige the appropriate requests.

In infancy, the opening to the larynx is narrow, due in part to the shape of the laryngeal cartilages. The hyoid bone and thyroid cartilage function as one and the cartilage structure is more flexible. The infant's vocal folds are 4 to 8 mm long, compared to a typical adult male length of approximately 29 mm and adult female length of approximately 21mm, and the posterior 50% is composed of cartilage (the vocal processes of the arytenoid cartilages)[49,53]. The vocal fold layer structure is much simpler than in the adult:

Newborns have very thick mucosal layers, and there is no vocal ligament apparent, but a uniform lamina propria structure more like that of the superficial layer (Reinke's space) in adults[25]. Histological studies have suggested that infant laryngeal muscles have fewer type 1 muscles (those known to have slow and prolonged contraction). One possible function served by a large proportion of type 2 muscles in infants is effective and rapid opening and closing of the glottis to allow for rapid inspiration without aspiration during feeding[55].

In older children and adults, a larger proportion of type 1 muscle fibers in laryngeal muscles may assist in prolonged vocal fold adduction for the purposes of verbal communication. The formation of a poorly differentiated vocal ligament begins in the preschool years, and two layers become more apparent before puberty. Some developmental features of the vocal folds, as identified during laryngoscopy and histological studies, are represented in Figure 8–23.

Gender differentiation at puberty is accompanied by many aspects of vocal development. By the end of puberty, the larynx has assumed a lower position in the neck, where it rests between C5 and C7 of the cervical vertebrae (Figure 8–22). In concert with other growth spurts, under the influence of increasing testosterone levels, the male larynx virtually doubles in size, usually in a short period of a few months. Increases in neck and vocal tract sizes usually occur before or concurrent with the laryngeal growth spurt. The male larynx has reached its full adult size before age 20. The vocalis-thyroarytenoid muscle bulk increases, creating a more rectangular (than convergent wedge-shaped) glottis, so that a greater proportion of the vocal fold is involved in the vibratory cycle[112]. The overall acoustic effect of the growth spurt is a dramatic drop in the natural fundamental frequency range of vocal fold vibration, usually at least a 1-octave change, and a richer timbre.

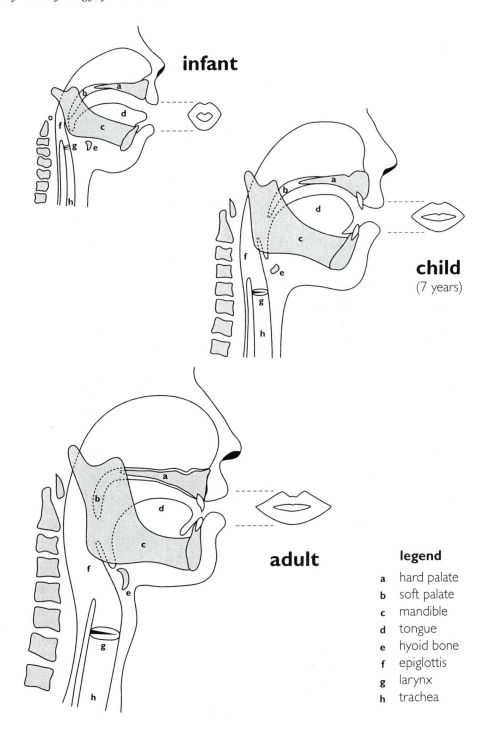

Figure 8–22. Sagittal views of the vocal tracts and lower face structures in a newborn infant, 7-year old child, and adult male (see text for details).

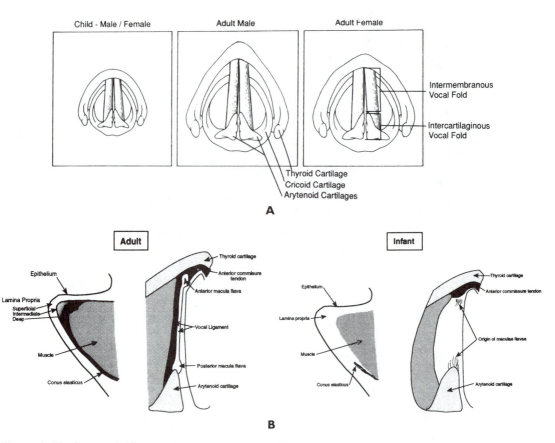

Figure 8–23. Structural differences in the larynx and vocal folds for adults and children. **A**) The proportion of cartilaginous glottal area decreases after puberty, most notably in the adult male. **B**) Histological development in the vocal fold. The newborn has poorly differentiated layer structure, with no obvious vocal ligament. The origins of the anterior and posterior macula flava may represent the developing ligament. The full layer structure is not evident until age 12 or later. (Adapted with permission from Hirano and Kurita[25].)

In addition, because the resonance chamber increases in length and width, the formant frequencies drop to contribute further to a deep masculine voice. The angle of the thyroid cartilage decreases from 120° to 90° in the mature male larynx. The epiglottis may change shape, becoming less omega shaped. An increase in the anterior portion of the cricothyroid muscle contributes to the ability to produce a falsetto register in men. A continuous lowering of f_0 has been noted in males up to age 50, which is difficult to explain based on the schedule for larynx maturation, and may be due to subclinical trauma associated with daily voice use[39].

The growth of the female larynx during puberty is directed by increasing levels of estrogens and progesterone, which become particularly influential on the subglottal and supraglottal mucosa during the menstrual cycle and may cause premenstrual voice changes of lowered pitch and f_0 range. Laryngeal growth is slower and less dramatic than in the pubertal male and may continue into the early 20s. The size and angle of the thyroid cartilage do not change dramatically during puberty, and although both larynx and vocal tract increase in size, the overall pitch and resonance changes are less dramatic than in the male counterpart. In addition to a difference in overall size, gender-based differences in the shape of the vocal tract have been reported in the adolescent larynx. In men, the pharynx grows proportionally larger than the oral cavity[49,54].

Hirano has suggested that male and female adolescents have developed full vocal ligaments by age 15[25], but the morphology suggests subsequent gender-based differences. Histological study has suggested some basic gender-based cellular and chemical differences. Of particular interest is the observation that mature males have thicker vocal ligaments and higher levels of hyaluronic acid within the vocal ligament layer of the lamina propria. Hyaluronic acid is known to provide the vocal folds with a greater impact resistance and may aid in growth of the lamina propria[19]. This information has been used to help interpret the apparent resilience of men's voices to vocal abuse and the relatively lower prevalence of voice problems in men engaged in certain vocally active occupations[94]. The absence of the vocal ligament in young children may contribute to a more delicate system that is susceptible to vocal fold lesions due to vocal overuse or abuse.

Growth of the larynx and vocal tract has some predictable effects on acoustic properties of voice and speech. With vocal tract growth, formant frequencies lower, and a general lowering of formant frequencies can be expected through the entire life span because the vocal tract continues to grow[53]. In the developing larynx, the vocal f_0 is inversely related to vocal fold length, but other factors may play a role in the f_0 decrease in men into middle age and later on in women, as will be discussed in the next section. Figure 8–24 demonstrates the relationship of f_0 changes to vocal fold length, with age as a factor.

Several changes in laryngeal and vocal tract structure and histology may contribute to the sounds of aged voices. Researchers

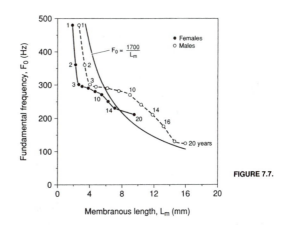

FIGURE 7.7.

Figure 8–24. Fundamental frequency as a function of membranous length of the vocal fold, with age as a parameter. Reprinted with permission from *Principles of Voice Production*[112]. Copyright 1994 by Allyn & Bacon.

have investigated acoustic aspects of aging, and changes in f_0 and pitch with age. F_0 appears to be a particularly salient cue in perception of age, but elevated jitter and shimmer, high standard deviation of f_0, and reduced articulatory dynamics and speaking rates are also cues to aging[63,64,90].

Studies of the laryngeal cartilage, muscle, connective tissue and mucosa have yielded a strong consensus about expected effects of aging. These include the following:

➤ ossification of laryngeal cartilages
➤ atrophic changes in the lamina propria and muscle layers of the vocal folds, more pronounced in men, and often of concern to them because of increased pitch and a thin, reedy voice
➤ edema and polypoid change in the superficial lamina propria, more pronounced in women, which may bother them if vocal pitch drops into the typical "male" range
➤ vocal instability, including wobbling and tremolo

These effects may be less evident in the presence of good physical conditioning. Some of the changes and schedules contributing to aging voice perceptions are different for men and women. In the male larynx, histological changes may be noted in the fourth decade of life, whereas female aging signs do not generally appear until the fifth decade.

Ossification of laryngeal cartilage continues until age 65[80]. Islands of cartilage remain in the thyroid cartilage in the male larynx, and preservation of cartilage exists in the upper portion of the female larynx. The cricoid may ossify almost completely[50]. The arytenoids undergo ossification of the body and muscular process, with the apex remaining cartilaginous. In general, the onset of ossification is later and less extensive in women, and the entire process is variable between individuals. There is nothing to suggest that this ossification process is related to laryngeal dysfunction except where changes occur in the cricoarytenoid joints. Kahn and Kahane have shown that older articular surfaces undergo fibrillation and other changes in collagen fiber arrangement, as well as ossification that may limit the range of arytenoid excursion[51]. When this leads to an inadequate posterior glottal closure, there may be a degree of air leakage that alters voice quality and intensity.

Connective tissue changes also show a gender difference. In the elderly man, the elastin fibers are fewer, fragmented, and clumped into groups. The number of collagen fibers is decreased with the remaining fibers being thinner, separate from each other, and more wavy. In women, the dense packing and linear relationship is preserved. The muscles of the larynx show general thinning and decreased fiber density, as well as fragmentation of the intermuscular septae[50,80]. Sato and Tauchi have shown a significant decrease in the number of both red and white muscle fibers with some increase in fiber volume after 50 years of age. After age 80, the changes are even more significant, but while increased fiber volume compensates to some degree for the loss of red fibers, the white fibers simply are reduced in number[91]. Finally, there is a

decrease in the number of fibroblasts seen in the conus elasticus. These changes are more prevalent in male than in female larynges[50,80].

The mucous membrane becomes thinned and atrophic with age. Mucous glands become atrophic and reduced in number, which probably has a drying effect. Metaplasia of the epithelium is seen. The underlying tissue may be subject to fatty infiltration, and the number of lymphatic channels is reduced[50,68].

Laryngeal findings on physical examination are familiar to most practicing voice clinicians. Honjo and Isshiki found 39% of male and 47% of female larynges examined to have significant abnormalities[41]. They also noted that 67% of the men had a glottal gap, a similar portion had atrophy, and 56% had edema. Women had significant edema in 74%, a glottal gap in 58%, and only 26% had atrophy. About 1 in 10 of each gender had vocal fold sulci.

A number of studies have looked at changes in speaking fundamental frequency with age. Mysak compared middle-aged sons to their elderly fathers and discovered an increased f_0 in the older group[74]. Hollien and Shipp studied males aged 20 to 80 and found increased f_0 with age, with a saucer-shaped curve describing the relationship when younger subjects were included. They theorized that the vocal folds were thickest in the 40s and 50s and that the increasing f_0 was secondary to thinning and stiffening of the vocal folds with declining levels of testosterone[39]. In a longitudinal study of three aging males, increases in f_0 were noted for all three over a span of 30 years. In two of the subjects, an increase was noted in the tilt of the acoustic spectrum of the glottal source, that is, reduced intensity of high-frequency components relative to lower frequency partials[43]. The suspected cause of this acoustic change is reduced glottal closure. Elderly men may subconsciously resist the age-related elevation in vocal f_0 by adopting postures to lower the larynx or making other compensatory adjustments to lower their vocal pitch to one their ears recognize as theirs.

In the woman, atrophic changes may be less significant, but increased edema in the superficial layer of the lamina propria accounts for greater bulk of the vocal folds after menopause (most notably in smokers). Reduced estrogen levels may contribute to the mucosal thickening. The overall effect on phonation is to produce a lower fundamental frequency of vibration and subsequent lower speaking pitch[63]. Linville and Fisher, however, have shown that the first formant frequency is also lowered for both phonated and whispered voice, thus suggesting that both phonatory and resonance features play a role in defining age characteristics of women's voices[64,65]. Women may resist the change to a more masculine pitch by tensing muscles, raising the larynx, or engaging other mechanisms to elevate the voice to a level their ears can accept.

There is less agreement in findings regarding pitch range. McGlone and Hollien[70] determined that pitch range was largely preserved in elderly women, whereas Ptacek et al[81] found a loss of the high-tone production in both men and women, and Luchsinger's study supported this[68]. Aronson's data supported the preservation of pitch range in both sexes[2]. Peppard found that elderly trained singers maintained a wider pitch range than elderly nonsingers[78]. Methodology differences in each series may be responsible for the apparently conflicting results.

Other age-related voice changes include a wobbling of the voice, attributed to irregular respiration, and the tremulous voice or senile tremolo. Some of these changes can be demonstrated as increased f_0 standard deviations and altered jitter levels[66].

In addition to gender-specific changes, characteristics of the aging voice can be influenced by systemic diseases such as arthritis, respiratory ailments, and neuromuscular disease such as the various dysarthrias (see Chapter 2).

When considering effects of age on the vocal system, it is important to keep in mind that physiological age is a more accurate predictor of state of function than is chronological age[82,83]. Lowery noted that older women who engaged in regular aerobic exercise had lower stroboscopic ratings of vocal fold aperiodicity, asymmetry, and supraglottal constriction patterns and were rated as having relatively younger voices for their ages than were women who were not aerobic exercisers[67]. Physical conditioning specifically targeting vocal functioning may also minimize aging effects. According to Peppard, voice training may have an effect of maintaining lower perturbation, noise levels, and aberrant acoustic-perceptual features in voices of older women due to greater flexibility, regularity, and symmetry of vocal fold movements; greater glottal efficiency; and lower degrees of supraglottal activity in senescent trained singers[78]. Voice changes are part of the overall physical dynamic that accompanies human development and aging. A particularly graphic representation of the changes in stature in the aging human is reprinted in Figure 8–25.

8.7.2 Other Variability Factors in the Human Vocal System

We have discussed the potential impact of aging on voice, but we have not addressed the issue of vocal differences in populations across time. A recent study demonstrated that a group of young Australian women had significantly lower speaking fundamental frequencies than an age-matched group recorded 50 years previously. The apparent explanation for this difference is primarily psychosocial: society condones lower-pitched voices in men and women and reinforces it through modern media resources that were less available to us 50 years ago[77].

Studies of voice differences among people of different countries and cultures have been sparse. A few studies have focused on speak-

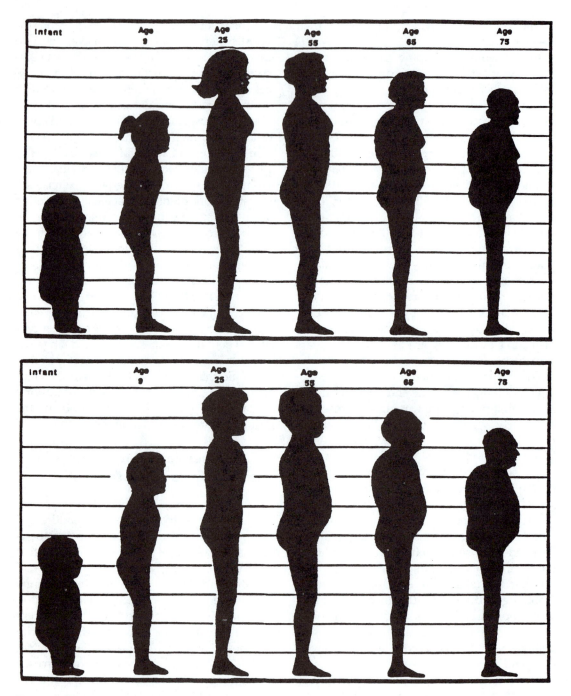

Figure 8–25. Postural changes related to the normal aging process. Reprinted with permission from *Videostroboscopic Examination of the Larynx*[23]. Copyright 1993, Singular Publishing Group, Inc.

ing voice f_0 in different countries, but much is yet to be learned about physiological and cultural influences on voice features and behaviors. Little is known about racially based differences in structure and histology of the human vocal system. Given the differences observed in physical stature, skull and facial shapes, and disease susceptibility among people of different races, it is worth speculating that there are differences in structure and function that influence vocal production and speech. This is a topic of great relevance to vocalists, clinicians, and pedagogues, and it is hoped that more knowledge in this area will be provided in the future.

8.8 Summary

Voice production for speech is a psychomotor act that is the result of complex and dynamic interactions among several anatomical and physiological systems: cognitive-emotional, neuromotor, respiratory, phonatory, resonance, and articulatory. Professional members of the voice care team must be knowledgeable about structural and functional aspects of the complex voice production system and its normal variability to formulate accurate diagnoses and develop appropriate preventive, treatment, and pedagogical programs. This foundation of knowledge has been presented to help voice care professionals best use the information provided in the remainder of this textbook.

References

1. Alipour-Haghighi, F., & Titze, I. R. (1991). Elastic models of vocal fold tissues. *NCVS Status and Progress Report-I*, 39–48.
2. Aronson, A. E. (1985). *Clinical Voice Disorders: An Interdisciplinary Approach*. New York: Thieme-Stratton.
3. Atkinson, J. E. (1978). Correlation analysis of the physiological factors controlling fundamental voice frequency. *Journal of the Acoustic Society of America, 63*, 211–222.
4. Baken, R. J. (1995). Between organization and chaos: A different view of the voice. In F. Bell-Berti, & L. J. Raphael (Eds.), *Producing Speech: Contemporary Issues—for Katherine Safford Harris* (pp. 233–246). New York: AIP.
5. Baken, R. J. (1987). *Clinical Measurement of Speech and Voice*. Boston: College-Hill.
6. Bless, D. M., Biever-Lowery, D. M., Campos, G., Glaze, L. E., & Peppard, R. C. (1989, July). Videostroboscopic, acoustic and aerodynamic analysis of voice production in normal adults. Proceedings of the Vocal Fold Physiology Conference, Stockholm, Sweden.
7. Boliek, C. A., Hixon, T. M., Watson, P. J., & Morgan, W. J. (1996). Vocalization and breathing during the first year of life. *Journal of Voice, 10*(1), 1–22.
8. Boliek, C. A., Hixon, T. M., Watson, P. J., & Morgan, W. J. (1997). Vocalization and breathing during the second and third years of life. *Journal of Voice, 11*(4), 373–390.
9. Broad, D. J. (1979). The new theories of vocal fold vibration. In N. J. Lass (Ed.), *Speech and Language: Advances in Basic Research and Practice, Vol.2* (pp. 203–255), New York: Academic Press.
10. Cavallo, S. A., Baken, R. J., Metz, D. E., & Whitehead, R. L. (1991). Chest wall preparation for phonation in congenitally profoundly hearing-impaired persons. *Volta Review, 93*, 287–300.
11. Collier, R. (1975). Physiological correlates of intonation patterns. *Journal of the Acoustical Society of America, 58*, 249–255.
12. Davis, P. J., Zhang, S. P., Winkworth, A. & Bandler, R. (1996). Neural control of vocalization: Respiratory and emotional influences. *Journal of Voice, 10*(1), 23–38.
13. Davis, S. B. (1979). Acoustic characteristics of normal and pathological voices. In *Speech and Language: Advances in Basic Research and Practice* (Vol I). New York: Academic Press.
14. Fant, G. (1960). *Acoustic Theory of Speech Production*. The Hague, Netherlands: Mouton.
15. Fant, G. (1983). The voice source-theory and acoustic modeling. In I. R. Titze, & R. C. Scherer (Eds.), *Vocal Fold Physiology: Biomechanics,*

Acoustics and Phonatory Control (pp 453–464). Denver: Denver Center for the Performing Arts.

16. Fant, G. (1986). Glottal flow: Models and interaction. *Journal of Phonetics, 14*, 393–399.

17. Fant, G., & Lin, Q. (1991). Comments on glottal flow modeling and analysis. In J. Gauffin, & B. Hammarberg (Eds.), *Vocal Fold Physiology: Acoustic, Perceptual and Physiological Aspects of Voice Mechanisms* (pp. 47–56). San Diego: Singular Publishing Group, Inc.

18. Forner, L. L., & Hixon, T. J. (1977). Respiratory kinematics in profoundly hearing-impaired speakers. *Journal of Speech and Hearing Research, 20*, 373–408.

19. Hammond, T. H., Zhou, R., Hammond, E. H., Pawlak, A., & Gray, S. D. (1997). The intermediate layer: A morphologic study of the elastin and hyaluronic acid constituents of normal, human vocal folds. *Journal of Voice, 11*(1), 59–66.

20. Harris, T., Harris, S., Rubin, J. S., & Howard, D. M. (1998). *The Voice Clinic Handbook.* London: Whurr Publishers Ltd.

21. Hirai, H., Honda, K., Fujimoto, I., & Shimada, Y. (1994). Analysis of magnetic resonance images on the physiological mechanisms of fundamental frequency. *Journal of Acoustic Society of Japan, 50*, 296–304.

22. Hirano, M. (1977). Structure and vibratory behavior of the vocal folds. In M. Sawashima, & F. S. Cooper (Eds.), *Dynamic Aspects of Speech* (pp. 13–27). Tokyo: University of Tokyo Press.

23. Hirano, M., & Bless, D. M. (1993). *Videostroboscopic Examination of the Larynx.* San Diego: Singular Publishing Group, Inc.

24. Hirano, M. (1983). Structure of the vocal fold in normal and disease states. Anatomical and physical studies. In *Proceedings of the Conference on the Assessment of Vocal Pathology, ASHA Reports 11* (pp. 11–26). Rockville, MD: American Speech-Language-Hearing Association.

25. Hirano, M., & Kurita, S. (1986). Histological structure of the vocal fold and its normal and pathological variations. In J. A. Kirschner (Ed.), *Vocal Fold Histopatholog,* (pp. 17–20). Boston: College-Hill.

26. Hirano, M., Kakita, Y., Ohmaru, K., & Kurita, S. (1982). Structure and mechanical properties of the vocal fold. In N. J. Lass (Ed.), *Speech and Language: Advances in Basic Research and Practice* (Vol. 7, pp. 271–297). New York: Academic Press.

27. Hixon, T. J. et al (1987). *Respiratory Function in Speech and* Song. Baltimore: Williams & Wilkins.

28. Hixon, T. J., Goldman, M. D., & Mead, J. (1973). Kinematics of the chest wall during speech production: Volume displacements of the rib cage, abdomen, and lung. *Journal of Speech and Hearing Research, 16*(1), 78–115.

29. Hixon, T. J., Mead, J., & Goldman, M. D. (1976). Dynamics of the chest wall during speech production: Function of the thorax, rib cage, diaphragm, and abdomen. *Journal of Speech and Hearing Research, 19*(2), 297–356.

30. Hixon, T. J., Watson, P. J., & Maher, M. Z. (1987). Respiratory kinematics in classical (Shakespearean) actors. In T. J. Hixon et al (Eds.), *Respiratory Function in Speech and Song* (pp. 375–400). Boston: College-Hill.

31. Hixon, T. J., Watson, P. J., Harris, F. P., & Perlman, N. B. (1988). Relative volume changes of the rib cage and abdomen during prephonatory chest wall posturing. *Journal of Voice, 2*(1), 13–19.

32. Hodge, M. M., & Putnam Rochet, A. (1989). Characteristics of speech-breathing in young women. *Journal of Speech and Hearing Research, 32*(3), 466–480.

33. Hoit, J. D., Jenks, C. L., Watson, P. J., & Cleveland, T. F. (1996). Respiratory function during speaking and singing in professional country singers. *Journal of Voice, 10*(1), 39–49.

34. Hoit, J. (1995). Influence of body position on breathing and its implications for the evaluation and treatment of speech and voice disorders. *Journal of Voice, 9*(4), 341–347.

35. Hoit, J., Hixon, T., Watson, P., & Morgan, W. (1990). Speech breathing in children and adolescents. *Journal of Speech and Hearing Research, 33*, 51–69.

36. Hoit, J. D. & Hixon, T. J. (1986). Body type and speech-breathing. *Journal of Speech and Hearing* Research, 29(3), 313–324.

37. Hoit, J. D., & Hixon, T. J. (1987). Age and speech-breathing. *Journal of Speech and Hearing Research, 30*(3), 351–366.

38. Hoit, J. D., Hixon, T. J., Altman, M. E., & Morgan, W. J. (1989). Speech-breathing in women. *Journal of Speech and Hearing Research, 32*(2), 353–365.

39. Hollien, H., & Shipp, T. (1972). Speaking fundamental frequency and chronological age in males. *Journal of Speech and Hearing Research, 15*, 155–159.

40. Holmberg, E. B., Hillman, R. B., & Perkell, J. (1988). Glottal airflow and transglottal air pressure measurements for male and female speakers in soft, normal, and loud voice. *Journal of the Acoustical Society of America, 84*, 511–529.

41. Honda, K. (1995). Laryngeal and extra-laryngeal mechanisms of f_o control. In F. Bell-Berti, & L. J. Raphael (Eds.), *Producing Speech: Contemporary Issues* (pp. 215–232). New York: AIP Press.

42. Honjo, I., & Isshiki, N. (1979). *Laryngoscopic and Vocal Characteristics of Aged Persons.* Osaka, Japan: Kansai Medical University.

43. House, A. S., & Stevens, K. N. (1999). A longitudinal study of speech production, I: General findings. Princeton, NJ: IDA Center for Communications Research.

44. Ishizala, K., & Flanagan, J. L. (1977). Acoustic properties of longitudinal displacement in vocal fold vibration. *Bell System Technical Journal, 56*, 889–918.

45. Ishizaka, K., & Matsudaira, M. (1972). Fluid mechanical considerations of vocal fold vibration. *SCRL Monograph, 8.*

46. Iwarsson, J., Thomasson, M., & Sundberg, J. (1998). Effects of lung volume on the glottal voice source. *Journal of Voice, 12*(4), 424–433.

47. *Journal of Voice* (1987-) San Diego: Singular Publishing Group, Inc.

48. Kahane, J. C. (1988). Anatomy and physiology of the organs of the peripheral speech mechanism. In N. J. Lass, L. V. McReynolds, J. L. Northern, & D. E. Yoder (Eds.), *Handbook of Speech-Language Pathology and Audiology.* Philadelphia: B.C. Decker Inc.

49. Kahane, J. C. (1983). Postnatal development and aging of the human larynx. *Seminars in Speech and Language, 4(3),* 189–203.

50. Kahane, J. C. (1983). A survey of age-related changes in the connective tissues of the human adult larynx. In D. M. Bless, & J. H. Abbs (Eds.), *Vocal Fold Physiology* (pp. 44–49). San Diego: College-Hill Press.

51. Kahn, A. R., & Kahane, J. C. (1986). India ink pinprick assessment of age-related changes in the crico-arytenoid joint (CAJ) articular surfaces. *Journal of Speech and Hearing Research, 4,* 536–543.

52. Kakita, Y., & Hiki, S. (1974). A study of laryngeal control for voice pitch based on anatomical model. Proceedings of Speech Communication Seminar, Stockholm, SCS-74, 45–54.

53. Kent, R. D. & Vorperian, H. K. (1995). Development of the Craniofacial-Oral-Laryngeal Anatomy: A Review. *Journal of Medical Speech-Language Pathology, 3,* 145–190.

54. Kent, R. D. & Read, C. (1992). The *Acoustic Analysis of Speech.* San Diego: Singular Publishing Group, Inc.

55. Kersing, W. (1986). Vocal musculature, aging and developmental aspects In J. A. Kirchner (Ed.), *Vocal Fold Histopathology,* 11–16. Boston: College-Hill.

56. Klatt, D. H., & Klatt, L. C. (1990). Analysis, synthesis, and perception of voice quality variations among female and male talkers. *Journal of the Acoustical Society of America, 87*(2), 820–857.

57. Laver, J. (1980). *The Phonetic Description of Voice Quality.* Cambridge: Cambridge University Press.

58. Laver, J., & Mackenzie Beck, J. (1991). *Vocal Profile Analysis.* Edinburgh: University of Edinburgh.

59. Leanderson, R., Sundberg, J., & von Euler, C. (1984). Effects of diaphragm activity on phonation during singing. *Transcripts of the Thirteenth Symposium on Care of the Professional Voice* (pp. 165–169). New York: Voice Foundation.

60. Leanderson, R., Sundberg, J., von Euler, C., & Lagercantz, H. (1983). Diaphragmatic control of the subglottic pressure during singing. *Transcripts of the Twelfth Symposium on Care of the Professional Voice* (pp. 216–220). New York: Voice Foundation.

61. Leanderson, R., Sundberg, J. & van Euler, C. (1987). Breathing muscle activity and subglottal pressure dynamics in singing and speech. *Journal of Voice, 1*(3), 258–261.

62. Leinonen, L., & Laakso, M. L. (1990). Control of static pressure by expiratory muscles during expiratory effort and phonation. *Journal of Voice, 4*(3), 256–263.

63. Linville, S. E. (1996). The sound of senescence. *Journal of Voice, 10*(2), 190–200.

64. Linville, S. E. & Fisher, H. B. (1985a). Acoustic characteristics of perceived versus actual vocal age in controlled phonation by adult females. *Journal of the Acoustical Society of America, 78,* 40–48.

65. Linville, S. E., & Fisher, H. B. (1985b). Acoustic characteristics of women's voices with advancing age. *Journal of Gerontology, 3,* 324–330.

66. Linville, S. E., & Korabic, E. W. (1987). Fundamental frequency stability characteristics of elderly women's voices. *Journal of the Acoustical Society of America, 4,* 1196–1199.

67. Lowery, D. B. (1993). Aerobic exercise effects on the post-menopausal voice. Doctoral dissertation, University of Wisconsin-Madison.

68. Luschinger, R., & Arnold, G. (1965). Vocal involution or senescence of the voice. In *Voice-Speech-Language.* Belmont, CA: Wadsworth.

69. McFarland, D. H., & Smith, A. (1989). Surface recordings of respiratory muscle activity during speech: Some preliminary findings. *Journal of Speech and Hearing Research, 32*(3), 657–667.

70. McGlone, R., & Hollien, H. (1963). Vocal pitch characteristics of aged women. *Journal of Speech and Hearing Research, 6,* 164–170.

71. Mackenzie Beck, J. (1997). Organic variation of the vocal apparatus. In W. J. Hardcastle, & J. Laver (Eds.), *The Handbook of Phonetic Sciences* (pp. 256–297). London: Blackwell Publishers.

72. Moore, G. P. (1971). *Organic Voice Disorders.* Englewood Cliffs: Prentice-Hall.

73. Morrison, M. D., Rammage, L. A., Belisle, G., Nichol, H., & Pullan, B. (1983). Muscular tension dysphonia. *Journal of Otolaryngology, 12*(5), 302–306.

74. Mysak, E. D. (1959). Pitch and duration characteristics of older males. *Journal of Speech and Hearing Research, 2,* 46–54.

75. Netsell, R., Lotz, W. K., Peters, J. E., & Schulte, L. (1994). Developmental patterns of laryngeal and respiratory function for speech production. *Journal of Voice, 8*(2), 123–131.

76. Netsell, R., Lotz, W., & Shaughnessy, A. (1984). Laryngeal aerodynamics associated with selected voice disorders. *American Journal of Otolaryngology, 5,* 397–403.

77. Pemberton, C., McCormack, P., & Russell, A. (1998). Have women's voices lowered across time? A cross-sectional study of Australian women's voices. *Journal of Voice, 12*(2), 208–213.

78. Peppard, R. C. (1990). Effects of aging on selected vocal characteristics of female singers and non-singers. Doctoral dissertation, University of Wisconsin-Madison.

79. Perlman, A. L., & Durham, P. L. (1987). In vitro studies of vocal fold mucosa during isometric conditions. In T. Baer, C. Sasaki, & K. Harris (Eds.), *Laryngeal Function in Phonation and Respiration* (pp. 291–303). Boston: College-Hill.

80. Pressman, J. J., & Keleman, G. (1955). Physiology of the larynx. *Physiology Reviews, 35,* 513–515.

81. Ptacek, P., Sande, E. K., Malone, W., & Jackson, C. C. R. (1966). Phonatory and related changes with advanced age. *Journal of Speech and Hearing Research, 9,* 353–360.

82. Ramig, L. (1983). Effect of physiological aging on speakers and reading rates. *Journal of Communicative Disorders, 16,* 217–226.

83. Ramig, L., & Ringel, R. (1983). Effects of physiological aging on selected acoustic characteristics of voice. *Journal of Speech and Hearing Research, 26,* 22–30.

84. Rammage, L. A. (1992). Acoustic, aerodynamic and stroboscopic characteristics of phonation with variable posterior glottis postures. Doctoral dissertation. University of Wisconsin-Madison.

85. Rammage, L. A., Peppard, R. C., & Bless, D. M. (1989). Aerodynamic, laryngoscopic and perceptual-acoustic characteristics in dysphonic females with posterior glottal chinks: a retrospective study. *Journal of Voice, 6,* 64–78.

86. Rothenberg, M. (1983). Source-tract interaction in breathy voice. In I. R. Titze, & R. C. Scherer (Eds.), *Vocal Fold Physiology Biomechanics, Acoustics and Phonatory Control* (pp. 465–481). Denver Center for the Performing Arts. Denver, CO.

87. Russell, N. K., & Stathopoulos, E. T. (1988). Lung volume changes in children and adults during speech production. *Journal of Speech and Hearing Research, 31,* 146–155.

88. Sapienza, C. M., & Stathopoulos, E. T. (1994). Respiratory and laryngeal measures of children and women with bilateral vocal nodules. *Journal of Speech and Hearing Research, 37,* 1229–1243.

89. Sapienza, C. M., Stathopoulos, E. T., & Brown Jr., W. S. (1997). Speech breathing during reading in women with vocal nodules. *Journal of Voice, 11*(2), 195–201.

90. Sataloff, R. T., Rosen, D. C., Hawkshaw, M., & Spiegel, J. R. (1997). The three ages of voice: The aging adult voice. *Journal of Voice, 11*(2), 156–160.

91. Sato, T., & Tauchi, H. (1982). Age changes in human vocal muscle. *Mechanisms of Aging Development, 18,* 67–74.

92. Scherer, R. C., & Titze, I. R. (1981). A new look at van den Berg's glottal aerodynamics. *Transcripts of the Tenth Symposium on Care of the Professional Voice* (pp. 74–81). New York: Voice Foundation.

93. Shoji, K., Regenbogen, E., Yu, J. D., & Blaugrund, S. M. (1992). High-frequency power ratio of breathy voice. *Laryngoscope, 102,* 267–271.

94. Smith, E., Kirchner, H. L., Taylor, M., Hoffman, H., & Lemke, J. H. (1998). Voice problems among teachers: Differences by gender and teaching circumstances. *Journal of Voice, 12*(3), 328–334.

95. Sodersten, M. (1994). *Vocal Fold Closure During Phonation: Physiological, perceptual and acoustic studies.* Stockholm: Huddinge University Hospital, Department of Logopedics and Phoniatrics.

96. Stathopoulos, E. T., Hoit, J. D., Hixon, T. J., Watson, P. J., & Pearl-Solomon, N. (1991). Respiratory and laryngeal function during whispering. *Journal of Speech and Hearing Research, 34,* 761–767.

97. Stathopoulos, E. T., & Sapienza, C. M. (1997). Developmental changes in laryngeal and respiratory function. *Journal of Speech, Language, and Hearing Research, 40,* 595–614.

98. Stathopoulos, E. T., & Sapienza, C. M. (1993a). Respiratory and laryngeal function of women and men during vocal intensity variation. *Journal of Speech and Hearing Research, 36,* 64–75.

99. Stathopoulos, E. T., & Sapienza, C. M. (1993b). Respiratory and laryngeal measures of children during vocal intensity variation. *Journal of the Acoustical Society of America, 94,* 2531–2543.

100. Stathopoulos, E. T., & Weismer, G. (1986). Oral airflow and air pressure during speech production. A comparative study of children, youths, and adults. *Folia Phoniatrica, 37,* 152–159.

101. Sundberg, J. (1999, May). Breathing and phonation. Presentation at the 4th International Care of the Professional and Occupational Voice Symposium. Canadian Voice Care Foundation, Banff, Alberta.

102. Sundberg, J. (1990). What's so special about singers? *Journal of Voice, 4*(2), 107–119.

103. Sundberg, J. (1987). *The Science of the Singing Voice,* Delkalb: Northern Illinois University.

104. Sundberg, J., & Askenfelt, A. (1983). Larynx height and voice source: A relationship? In D. M. Bless, & J. H. Abbs (Eds.), *Vocal Fold Physiology: Contemporary Research and Clinical Issues* (pp. 307–316). San Diego: College-Hill.

105. Sundberg, J., Leanderson, R., von Euler, C., & Knutsson, E. (1991). Influence of body posture and lung volume on subglottal pressure control during singing. *Journal of Voice, 5*(4), 283–291.

106. Takahashi, H., & Koike, Y. (1975). Some perceptual dimensions and acoustic correlates of pathologic voices. *Acta Otolaryngologica 338,* 1–24.

107. Titze, I. R. (1973). The human vocal cords: A mathematical model. Part I, *Phonetica, 28,* 129–170.

108. Titze, I. R. (1974). The human vocal cords: A mathematical model. Part II. *Phonetica, 29,* 1–21.

109. Titze, I. R. (1980). Comments on the myoelastic-aerodynamic theory of phonation. *Journal of Speech and Hearing Research, 23,* 495–510.

110. Titze, I. R. (1988). The physics of small-amplitude oscillation of the vocal folds. *Journal of the Acoustic Society of America, 83*(4), 152–153.

111. Titze, I. R. (1992). Phonation threshold pressure: A missing link in glottal aerodynamics. *Journal of the Acoustical Society of America, 91*(5), 2926–2935.

112. Titze, I. R. (1994). *Principles of Voice Production.* Prentice-Hall, Englewood Cliffs, NJ.

113. Titze, I. R., & Strong, W. J. (1975). Normal

modes in vocal cord tissues. *Journal of the Acoustical Society of America, 57*, 736–744.

114. Titze, I. R., & Talkin, D. T. (1979). A theoretical study of the effects of various laryngeal configurations on the acoustics of phonation. *Journal of the Acoustical Society of America, 66*(1), 60–74.

115. Titze, I. R., Jiang, J., & Druker, D. G. (1987). Preliminaries to the body-cover theory of pitch control. *Journal of Voice, 1*(4), 314–319.

116. van den Berg, J. W., Zantema, J. T., & Doorenball Jr., P. (1957). On the air resistance and the Bernoulli effect of the human larynx. *Journal of the Acoustical Society of America, 29*, 626–631.

117. Warren, D. W., Dalston, R. M., Morr, E. K., Hairfield, W. M., & Smith, L. R. (1989). The speech regulating system: Temporal and aerodynamic responses to velopharyngeal inadequacy. *Journal of Speech and Hearing Research, 32*, 566–575.

118. Warren, D. W., Rochet, A. P., Dalston, R. M., & Mayo, R. (1992). Controlling changes in vocal tract resistance. *Journal of the Acoustical Society of America, 91*, 2947–2953.

119. Watson, P. J. & Hixon, T. J. (1985). Respiratory kinematics in classical (opera) singers. *Journal of Speech and Hearing Research, 28*(1), 104–122.

120. Watson, P. J., Nixon, T. J., Stathopoulos, E. T., & Sullivan, D. R. (1990). Respiratory kinematics in female classical singers. *Journal of Voice, 4*(2), 120–128.

121. Watson, P. J., Hoit, J. D., Lansing, R. W., & Nixon, T. J. (1989). Abdominal muscle activity during classical singing. *Journal of Voice, 3*(1), 24–31.

122. Weismer, G. (1988). Speech production. In N. Lass, L. McReynolds, J. Northern, & D. Yoder (Eds.), *Handbook of Speech, Language and Hearing Pathology* (pp. 215–252). St. Louis: Mosby Year Book.

123. Whitehead, R. L. (1983). Some respiratory and aerodynamic patterns in the speech of the hearing impaired. In I. Hochberg, H. Levitt, & M. Osberger (Eds.), *Speech of the Hearing Impaired: Research, Training and Personnel Preparation* (pp. 97–116). Baltimore: University Park Press.

124. Wilder, C. N. (1983). Chest wall preparation for phonation in female speakers. In D. M. Bless, & J. H. Abbs (Eds.), *Vocal Fold Physiology* (pp.109–123). San Diego: College-Hill.

125. Winkworth, A. L., & Davis, P. J. (1997). Speech breathing and the Lombard effect. *Journal of Speech, Language, and Hearing Research, 40*, 159–169.

126. Winkworth, A. L., Davis, P. J, Adams, R., & Ellis, E. (1994). Variability and consistency in speech breathing during reading: Lung volumes, speech intensity, and linguistic factors. *Journal of Speech and Hearing Research, 37*, 535–556.

127. Winkworth, A. L., Davis, P. J,, Adams, R., & Ellis, E. (1995). Lung volumes and breath placement during spontaneous speech. *Journal of Speech and Hearing Research, 38*, 124–144.

Recommended Reading

Baken, R.J. (1987). *Clinical Measurement of Speech and Voice,* San Diego: Singular Publishing Group, Inc.

Davis, P. J., Zhang, S. P., Winkworth, A., & Bandler, R. (1996). Neural control of vocalization: Respiratory and emotional influences. *Journal of Voice, 10*(1), 23–38.

Harris, T., Harris, S., Rubin, J. S., & Howard, D. M. (1998). *The Voice Clinic Handbook.* London: Whurr Publishers Ltd.

Hirano, M., Kirchner, J. A., & Bless, D. M. (1987). *Neurolaryngology: Recent Advances.* Boston: College-Hill.

Hixon, T. et al. (1987). *Respiratory Function in Speech and Song.* Boston: College-Hill.

Journal of Voice (1987–) San Diego: Singular Publishing Group.

Kahane, J. C. (1988). Anatomy and physiology of the organs of the peripheral speech mechanism. In N. J. Lass, L. V. McReynolds, J. L. Northern, & D. E. Yoder (Eds.), *Handbook of Speech-Language Pathology and Audiology.* Philadelphia: B.C. Decker Inc.

Kahane, J. C., & Folkins, J. W. (1984). *Atlas of Speech and Hearing Anatomy.* Columbus: Charles E. Merrill.

Kent, R. D. (1997). *The Speech Sciences.* San Diego: Singular Publishing Group, Inc.

Kent, R. D., & Vorperian, H. K. (1995). Development of the Craniofacial-Oral-Laryngeal Anatomy: A Review. *Journal of Medical Speech-Language Pathology, 3,* 145–190.

Kirchner, J. A. (1986). *Vocal Fold Histopathology.* Boston: College Hill.

Linville, S. E. (1996). The sound of senescence. *Journal of Voice, 10*(2) 190–200.

Sundberg, J. (1987). *The Science of the Singing Voice,* Dekalb, IL: Northern Illinois University.

Titze, I. R. (1994). *Principles of Voice Production.* Englewood Cliffs, NJ: Prentice-Hall.

van den Berg, W. (1960). The *Vibrating Larynx* (videotape).

Weismer, G. (1988). Speech production. In N. Lass, L. McReynolds, J. Northern, & D. Yoder (Eds.), *Handbook of Speech, Language and Hearing Pathology* (pp. 215–252). St. Louis: Mosby Year Book.

Subject Index

A

Abdominal muscle activity, 262
Abduction and adduction movements, rate, range
    and symmetry of, 41, 43
Abductor spasmodic dysphonia, 92, 123
Abuse of voice, 82
  lesions due to, 111–113
  mucosal changes caused by, 82
Abuse-related vocal fold hemorrhaging, 113
Accessory or eleventh nerve, 255
Acoustic and perceptual acoustic assessment
  acoustic analysis of speech, 22–23
  form for, 14
  instrumentation, application, protocols and
    interpretation, 13–22
  rationale, environment and basic recording
    hardware, 12–13
Acoustic recordings, high quality, 13
Acoustic resonators of speech, 282–287
Acquired motor speech disorders, 85–86
Adduction, as facilitation technique, 56
Adductor breathing disorders, therapy for, 182
Adductor laryngeal breathing disorders, 123–124
Adductor spasmodic dysphonia, 122
Adenoviruses, 81
Adolescent transitional voice disorders, 215
  falsetto register in, 79–80
Adults, differences in voice disorders from
    children, 207–209
Aerodynamic evaluation of voice, 23–27
  flow glottograms, 27
  flow volume, 25

mean phonatory flow rate, 23–25
pressure and resistance, 25–26
Aging factors
  and normal development, 287–293
  normal, changes due to, 125
  voice variation related to, 264
Alignment-posture training, 141–142
Allergic laryngitis, 111
Allergies and voice disorders, 82
Amplitude of vibrations, 45
Amyloidosis, 111
Anatomy and physiology of voice production
  acoustic resonators of speech, 282–287
  function of phonation in verbal communication,
    251–253
  functions of respiratory system, speech-
    breathing and breathing for vocal
    performance, 255–269
    glossary for respiration, 269
    knowledge of speech-breathing, 261–269
    respiratory kinematics and dynamics, 258–261
  neuromotor systems involved in, 253–254
  normal variability in structure and function,
    287–295
    and aging, 287–293
    other variability factors in human vocal
      system, 293–295
  phonation, conversion of DC to AC energy,
    269–282
    dynamic control of pitch, intensity and
      quality, 277–282